T0184820

APPLIED EPIGENOMIC EPIDEMIOLOGY ESSENTIALS

This applied clinical medicine and public health text introduces the fundamental concepts in epidemiological investigation and demonstrates how to integrate emerging research on epigenomics into practice.

Epidemiology has a vital strategic role in facilitating and leading evidence discovery in all aspects of human health, with the intent of improving patient and public health through disease control and health promotion practices. It emphasizes what we now know about the transformation the human body and the ecosystem undergo as a result of social structure, environment, daily challenges and mutation. The first part of this text explores the origin of epidemiology, its relationship with medicine and public health, and its role in assessing disease distribution as occurrence or frequency, risk factors, treatment and management. The main direction of this text is to explore the assessment of how gene and environment interactions, termed epigenomic modulations, aberrantly predispose to morbidity, prognosis, survival and mortality at the individual as well as the specific population level.

This text presents a novel approach based mainly on epigenomic modulations in the application of epidemiologic investigation in disease incidence, morbidity and mortality at a specific population level for graduate education in public health and clinical sciences as well as medical education.

Laurens Holmes, Jr. is a specialist in Immunology and Infectious Disease as well as an expert in cancer epidemiology and biostatistical modeling. He is a major proponent of aberrant epigenomic modulations in disease incidence, morbidity, prognosis, mortality and survival; and a former Head of the Epidemiology Laboratory at the Nemours Center for Childhood Cancer Research, Wilmington; former clinical and translational science education and training director, Medical College of Wisconsin, Milwaukee; as well as a former Professor of Molecular Epidemiology and Clinical Trials at the University of Delaware, USA. Professor Holmes is currently the Director of the Graduate Public Health Program at Delaware State University, Dover, USA.

APPLIED EPIGENOMIC EPIDEMIOLOGY ESSENTIALS

A Guide to Study Design and Conduct

Laurens Holmes, Jr.

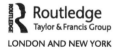
Routledge
Taylor & Francis Group

LONDON AND NEW YORK

Designed cover image: © Getty Images

First published 2024
by Routledge
4 Park Square, Milton Park, Abingdon, Oxon OX14 4RN

and by Routledge
605 Third Avenue, New York, NY 10158

Routledge is an imprint of the Taylor & Francis Group, an informa business

British Library Cataloguing-in-Publication Data
A catalogue record for this book is available from the British Library

Library of Congress Cataloging-in-Publication Data
Names: Holmes, Larry, Jr., 1960– author.
Title: Applied epigenomic epidemiology essentials : a guide to study design and conduct / Laurens Holmes, Jr.
Description: Abingdon, Oxon ; New York, NY : Routledge, 2024. | Includes bibliographical references and index. | Summary: "This applied clinical medicine and public health text introduces the fundamental concepts in epidemiological investigation and demonstrates how to integrate emerging research on epigenomics into practice. This text presents a novel approach mainly epigenomic modulations in the application epidemiologic investigation in disease incidence, morbidity, and mortality at specific population level for graduate education in public health and clinical sciences as well as medical education"— Provided by publisher.
Identifiers: LCCN 2023034170 | ISBN 9780367556426 (hardback) | ISBN 9780367556273 (paperback) | ISBN 9781003094487 (ebook)
Subjects: MESH: Epidemiologic Research Design | Epigenomics—methods | Epigenome | Epidemiology
Classification: LCC RA651 | NLM WA 950 | DDC 614.4—dc23/eng/20231006
LC record available at https://lccn.loc.gov/2023034170

ISBN: 978-0-367-55642-6 (hbk)
ISBN: 978-0-367-55627-3 (pbk)
ISBN: 978-1-003-09448-7 (ebk)

DOI: 10.4324/9781003094487

Typeset in Galliard
by codeMantra

Access the Support Material: https://www.routledge.com/Applied-Epigenomic-Epidemiology-Essentials-A-Guide-to-Study-Design-and/Jr/p/book/9780367556273

Mom, KMIA (in memoriam), Grandma, NUA (in memoriam), Dad, Morrison Holmes (in memoriam) and Granddad, Duke Holmes (in memoriam), who dedicated their lives to ensuring that children and families in need (food insecurity and shelter environment) were provided with basic needs (health, food and shelter) in normal epigenomic modulation, thus improving health outcomes and transforming health equity.

CONTENTS

An appendix discussing Epigenomic Determinants of Health (EDH) is also available to download via https://www.routledge.com/ Applied-Epigenomic-Epidemiology-Essentials-A-Guide-to-Study-Design-and/Jr/p/book/9780367556273

FORWARD

"Novel Epidemiology—Epigenomic Epidemiology"

Epidemiology, which reflects the core function of public health assessment and the preventive aspect of clinical medicine, remains applied and translational in the process of improving individual patient care and public or societal health. Since epidemiology involves the distribution and determinants of disease, and health-related events at a specific population level, the understanding of the environment in these predispositions and risks remains a unique and reliable pathway in clinical care and public health improvement via specific intervention mapping based on epidemiologic findings.

Epigenomic epidemiology is the study of gene and environment interactions in disease causation/risk, prognosis, mortality and survival in specific human and non-human animal populations. This course requires the understanding of several environments, such as chemical, physical, psychological, isolation, stress, exogenous, endogenous, toxic waste, pollutants, air quality, discrimination, social economic statutes and social gradients, and interactions with specific genes in gene expression, transcriptomes, protein synthesis and cellular functionality. Since aberrant epigenomic processes result in inverse gene expression, adversely impacting cellular functionality, the understanding of DNA methylation as the most utilized mechanistic process in epigenomic modulations and gene downregulation at specific population levels allows for intervention mapping in achieving an optimal environment for normal epigenomic modulations. This initiative remains to transform public health as well as health equity across subpopulations such as race, ethnicity, age, sex, disability, socio-economic status and urbanicity. Since epigenomic modulation is transgenerational but reversible, transforming the human environment based on epigenomic data will result in the improvement of health nationally and globally.

Specifically, epigenomic epidemiology is the study of the distribution and determinants of disease and health-related events at a specific population level with a unique focus on gene and environment interactions and the utilization of these findings in intervention mapping, implying specific risk characterization and induction therapy prior to the standard of care. This course initiative remains translational, transdisciplinary and team science (3Ts). Epigenomic modulation reflects the gene and environment interaction but not genomics (DNA sequencing), implying the genetic activities within the genome. Specifically, epigenomic modulations involve the binding of a methyl group (CH_3) to the prompter/enhancer region of the gene, termed the shores or islands as the CpG region, reflecting the non-coding region of the gene. This binding results in methyl-cytosine that adversely impacts the transcriptomes, resulting in impaired protein synthesis and cellular functionality due to inverse gene expression. With this approach, epidemiology as the core function of public health assessment will allow for the understating of subpopulation variances in CVDs, cerebrovascular accidents, malignant neoplasms, diabetes and other endocrinologic disorders, depression, anxiety, obesity, suicide, PTSD, pre-eclampsia, preterm birth, infant mortality and maternal mortality, thus applying a reliable and functional perspective to intervention mapping.

The specifics of this novel epidemiology will enhance the knowledge and understanding of how environmental conditions predispose to adverse health outcomes, including but not limited to incidence, risk determinants, association, causality, prognosis, mortality and survival, by addressing the following dimensions, namely:

a **Epigenetics/Epigenomics**: Epigenetics is the study of specific gene and environment interactions while epigenomics involves the assessment of multiple genes as a genome and their implications for a specific disease process, prognosis, and mortality and survival outcomes.

b **Epigenomic Study Design**: Experimental design as human subject experiment and non-experimental designs are very briefly and accurately explained in this text with examples.

c **Aberrant Epigenomic Modulations and Disease Effect and Causal Inference:** The disease frequency and occurrences are explained, as well as the measure of association, causal inference and quantitative evidence synthesis (QES) as applied Meta-Analysis.

d **Molecular Sequencing and Subgroups/Types**: Cytogenetics allows for the understanding of molecular sequencing in a disease process that facilitates disease subtypes. The understanding of subtype of a given disease, such as a brain/CNS tumor termed ependymoma, facilitates specific treatment, improving prognosis and survival.

e **Epigenomic Laboratory Techniques, Methods/Mechanistic Process and Design**: Epidemiology remains the study of diseases in a specific population with respect to distribution/determinants and the utilization of these findings in intervention mapping in disease incidence and mortality associated with aberrant epigenomic mechanistic processes as modulations. The mechanistic processes in the epidemiologic designs will focus on DNA methylation, histone modification in the acetylation process, phosphorylation, etc.

With the ongoing climate changes that adversely impact individual and population health, there is a need to transition clinical medicine and public health to epigenomic clinical medicine and epigenomic public health. This initiative requires the understanding of how gene and environment interaction, as epigenomic modulations alters the biologic system, and the application of a reliable and accurate epidemiologic design and bioinformatics in this direction. Very substantial and pragmatic to health outcomes improvement is the application of these findings from epigenomic investigations in induction therapy, therapeutics, intervention and disease prevention and control.

Laurens Holmes, Jr.
Major Epigenomic Epidemiology Proponent, Clinical Medicine and Public
Health Translational Research, therapeutics, intervention and prevention

PREFACE

Applied Epigenomic Epidemiology Essentials

Currently, disease determinants or predisposing factors are not driven by aberrant genomic factors such as DNA sequencing, genetic damage or injury but by aberrant epigenomic modulation, indicative of the gene and environment interaction in morbidity, treatment, prognosis, survival and mortality. Epidemiologic training and education should emphasize what we can contribute to the clinical, biomedical and public health fields and not what we can profit from these fields, with such a perspective enhancing unequivocal commitment to knowledge acquisition and skills development by future translationists and epidemiologists as well as clinicians.

Over the past five decades, we have experienced a dramatic transformation in epidemiologic thoughts and reflections, requiring a current approach to evidence discovery in the advancement of medicine and public health to meet the current challenges of increasing individual treatment effect heterogeneity and sampling variability in finding generalizability. Since genes or DNA have no destiny with respect to disease incidence, mortality and survival, gene and environment interactions—implying aberrant epigenomic modulation—remain a human destiny in disease development, causation, prognosis and survival.

With the rapid social and environmental changes having a fundamental exposure effect on human health, epidemiology deserves a re-invention as a profession and not a discipline, implying its strategic role in facilitating and leading evidence discovery in all aspects of human health with the unique intent of improving patient and community/public health through disease control and health promotion practices. As the human society changes structurally and socio-politically, given daily challenges and "mutations" accumulation, the biologic and ecosystem undergoes transformation that requires a reliable and valid understanding of such alterations and their roles in the human biologic organ-system and its adaptation to health and disease. Therefore, a reliable and valid epidemiologic approach to research and evidence discovery provides this profession with such an opportunity in a translational context.

Epidemiology is conceived as translational in this text, given its strategic position in facilitating meaningful, valid, reliable and generalizable study design and conduct for improving human health. With this challenge, this text extends the notion of epidemiology to embrace human and non-human animals, given the increasing involvement of non-human animals in the daily interactions of human animals. Therefore, epidemiology reflects the study of disease, disabilities, injuries, natural disasters, and health-related events distribution and determinants at specific human and animal population levels. Additionally, with the consequentialist direction of epidemiology, epidemiology in this current context involves the application of reliable findings in policy development and intervention mapping to improve individual patient and public health.

The origin of epidemiology is presented as the study of the underlying causes of a disease at a population level and implies that when such diseases occur out of proportion, it is indicative of an outbreak of food poisoning following an ingestion of contaminated food and beverages. We currently perceive epidemiology as a scientific discipline with investigative strategies for understanding how diseases, injuries, disabilities, natural disasters and health-related events are distributed and the factors that determine this distribution among subpopulations, implying etiologies and risks as well as predisposing factors. Currently, epidemiology remains a profession charged with the assessment (design and conduct), interpretation and application of such findings in addressing disease, health, health-related issues and other environmental and exogenous conditions related to human health, including but not limited to social and health inequities.

Epidemiologic investigation is neither simple nor complex as conceived by most researchers in the health and healthcare fields, but requires a basic understanding of the biologic, behavioral, genetic, epigenomic, social, neurobehavioral and environmental factors that collectively alter the adaptation required in the human organ-system due to the inability to rapidly respond to cellular injury due to the adverse interaction of these factors. With such an approach, a basic knowledge of epidemiologic principles involves an understanding of the population at risk and what characterizes such a population in terms of descriptive epidemiologic notions such as person, place and time of health and health-related event occurrence. Further, potential scholars or students of epidemiology require the basic integrative determinants of cellular and biobehavioral alterations that predispose to disease processes, namely agent, host and environment as the epidemiologic triangle. Basically, while the agent refers to the pathogen, such as microbes in infectious diseases, the host is the individual's immunologic surveillance and the environment is the condition, such as nutrients, hormones and endogenous temperature, that may alter the host factor. The environment, as currently conceived, involves in utero, postnatal hormones, diet and physical settings such as housing arrangements and settings.

Whereas the traditional notion of epidemiology focuses on disease effect or association, clinical medicine and public health require the understanding of the causal pathway in the development of disease for an effective treatment and preventive intervention, since modern epidemiology is concerned with disease causation given the complex etiologic process today as a result of the changing pathologic environment (highly processed food, genetically engineered produce, sedentary lifestyle, increasing air pollution, climate modification— global warming, digital/electronicity). Furthermore, for proven effectiveness of treatment or intervention modalities, knowledge and skills in evidence-based approaches to treatment and intervention mapping, systematic review and applied Meta-Analysis, such as quantitative evidence synthesis (QES), are required. This approach remains one of the perspectives available for epidemiologic causal inference.

Given epidemiologic investigation, genetic heterogeneity is complex and requires the knowledge and application of confounding, effect measure modifiers and bias as systematic errors such as measurement or observation errors. Scholars of epidemiology require an understanding of bias identification and minimization in study conduct, confounding assessment and adjustment, as well as effect measure modification identification and data interpretation based on such heterogeneity. Systematic error refers to bias which could result from information misclassification regarding exposure or outcome/disease, with such misclassification leading to selection bias. A confounding, which is not a bias, is the mixing effect of the third variable termed extraneous in the association between exposure and disease and may result in a biased estimate of the effect or association. An effect measure modification, also termed heterogeneity of effect, is a third external variable on the pathway of the association between exposure and outcome.

With the ongoing recognition of the impact of social inequity implying the unfair and unjust distribution of social, economic and environmental conditions related to health as social determinants of health and the biologic consequence therein, epidemiology requires an understanding of how racial differences in health outcomes relate to the biologic consequence of racial discrimination, employment-related stress, excess incarceration and a lack of appropriate and reliable access to and utilization of the healthcare system. Social determinants of health and racial discrimination as well as incarceration are defined by social stressors that have adverse implications for disease causation, poor prognosis and excess mortality or survival disadvantage. With the complex disease etiology implying an integrative etiologic model, epidemiology deserves an opportunity to assess the conjoint effect of disadvantaged neighborhood environment factors with exogenous physical environment in disease causation and prognosis. Scholars of epidemiology are expected to understand and apply multivariable design and analytic models in assessing the contributions of these multiple factors or multi-factoriality as causal webs in disease development, prognosis and outcomes.

While epidemiology is fundamentally concerned with design, its public health perspective requires epidemiologists to apply the knowledge of health and health-related issues in research conceptualization, hypothesis testing and study interpretation. In effect, design transcends analysis, and regardless of the statistical or probability model used in data analysis, sampling and design errors remain. Scholars of epidemiology are required to acquire the knowledge and understanding of design strategies for appropriately addressing the research question/s by reflecting on the sampling techniques that allow for an unbiased sample for the external validity of the study as well as the statistical power of the study that reflects an appropriate sample size.

However, in the era of "big" data where data size and not sample size is the application, caution is required in the interpretation of the findings to avoid the rejection of a true null hypothesis based on the data size and not a clinically meaningful difference as reflected in the marginalized effect size. Specifically, if the point estimate with respect to inverse gene expression correlation variance is <0.1 on a scale of 0.10–1.00, comparing DNA methylation of a specific gene such as ACE II in essential hypertension, and the "big data" is implicated, with a random error quantification of <0.001, this finding remains clinically and biologically non-meaningful in clinical and public health decision-making in therapeutics and intervention mapping.

This material is conceived to provide the basics of epigenomic epidemiology to students pursing master's degrees (MS, MPH, MSPH) and doctorate degrees in clinical sciences and medical education, namely MD, MD/PhD, MD/MS, PhD, DrPH and ScD. In providing the knowledge and skills in applied epidemiology, an effort is made to present this material in a practical manner by clarifying concepts and their applications in evidence discovery, hence enhancing therapeutics and intervention. There are three parts in this book, namely: (a) epidemiology and epigenomic epidemiology contribution in public health and clinical medicine, (b) traditional and modern epidemiologic designs and (c) laboratory techniques and epigenomic mechanistic process in epidemiologic principles, concept and application.

Part I. Epidemiology and Epigenomic Epidemiology Contribution in Public Health and Clinical Medicine

This text explores the origin of epidemiology and its relationship with medicine and public health. As the basic science of public health and medicine, the role of epidemiology is to assess disease distribution as occurrence or frequency, risk factors, treatment, management and intervention (behavioral and medical). As an integral part of this section, disease screening and diagnosis are explained with examples that illustrate the sensitivity and specificity of a diagnostic test and their applications in disease control and prevention. While the goal of clinical medicine remains to diagnose and treat disease at the individual patient level, public health is charged with disease control and prevention as well as health promotion at the specific population level. The core function of public health includes the assessment of health and health-related issues which is a shared responsibility and function of clinical medicine as well. These aspects are covered in a simplified and practical manner in this text to allow for the extended role of epidemiology which is the application of the findings from epidemiologic investigation in intervention mapping to improve the health of the public, especially the populations at risk. Surveillance and monitoring are essential components of disease control and prevention, and are covered in this text in order to provide entry-level public health professionals and students of epidemiology with an overview of the overall and extended role of epidemiology in improving public health.

Part II: Traditional and Modern Epidemiologic Designs

The main and most relevant aspect of this book is this part, which reflects the concepts, principles and methods of epidemiology. Basically, all quantitative research or investigation employs one form or another of design in its conduct, which is all epidemiologic in nature except for qualitative methods. Epidemiologic designs are employed in basic sciences, biomedical research, clinical studies and population-based research, and remain the foundation of evidence discovery. While probabilistic models are utilized in these designs, inappropriate designs yield erroneous inferences or conclusions regardless of the statistical sophistication utilized, since no statistical model can rectify the error of sampling or design. The type of design deemed appropriate should be based on the nature of the research, namely the research question, as "PE-ICO," and specific aims and hypotheses as applicable in inferential studies. For example, if a study is proposed to examine the DNA methylation signature in pediatric acute lymphoblastic leukemia (ALL) causation, such a design cannot be cross-sectional or case-control but prospective cohort that will involve the collection of blood samples from the exposed and unexposed to certain nutrients observed to be high in the methyl (CH_3) group, DNA methylation analysis and follow-up for the development of ALL (ALL incidence data). In contrast, samples collected from children with ALL will result in reverse causation since feasible designs such as cross-sectional or case-control are clearly limited with respect to causal inference. This text covers the conceptualization, design, conduct and interpretation of experimental (clinical trials) and non-experimental designs (prospective and retrospective cohort, case-control, cross-sectional, etc.), which are inaccurately characterized as observational since all studies, regardless of the design utilized, are observational in the sense that the outcome of any study requires the observation of the occurrence of the outcome. Specifically, designs include traditional (case report, case series, ecologic, cross-sectional, cohort and clinical trials) and modern (ambi-directional cohort, case-cohort, nested case-control, case-crossover, atypical case-noncase, prospective case-control).

An overview of epidemiology is presented with the types of epidemiology, mainly genomic, epigenomic, epigenetics, genetics, cancer, reproductive, pediatric, chronic disease, aging, neurology, health disparities science, cardiovascular, neonatal, clinical, health outcomes, health services, medical care, molecular, occupational, environmental, social, maternal and child, psychiatric, orthopedic, etc. The current attention on precision medicine in addressing individual treatment effect heterogeneity, pharmaco-genetics and unequal outcomes of health signals the need for specific risk characterization on cellular level changes that are driven by gene-environment interaction, namely epigenomics. Epidemiology is placed in a leadership position in a team science environment, given its responsibilities in monitoring reverse causation in causal inference on the pathway of disease development as observed in aberrant epigenomic modulations, namely DNA methylation, histone modification and non-coding RNA.

The traditional designs, typically ecologic, cross-sectional, case-control, prospective or longitudinal, and retrospective cohort and clinical trials, are characterized based on the timing of the study and the exposure or outcome status at the time of the design. This text explains in practical terms the principles and methods of these designs, mainly (a) description, (b) exposure and outcome characterization, (c) design and conduct, (d) measures of effect or association, and (e) strengths and limitations as perspectives and challenges. For example, if a study is proposed to examine the epigenomic modulations in hypertension involving angiotensin converting enzyme (ACE) inhibitors in predisposition to elevated systolic and diastolic blood pressure, and the design involves blood samples from hypertensive (case) and non-hypertensive (non-case) subjects, a feasible design remains case-control or case-comparison. A case-control study is therefore based on the availability of well-characterized and defined cases (preexisting outcomes) to determine the exposure and establish an effect or association that is not necessarily causal. Alternately, a longitudinal or prospective study will involve blood samples from healthy individuals exposed to a certain exposure, such as a high-methylated diet, that may result in increased methylation at the enhancer or promoter region of the gene, thus inhibiting the transcription factor, resulting in impaired gene expression and abnormal protein synthesis as well as abnormal cellular proliferation (neoplasia). Such designs partly explain the causal effect of exposure (DNA hypermethylation of ACE) on the outcome (hypertension). This text characterizes the measures of effects in these designs and applies these measures to the interpretation of the findings. Since no design is without limitations, this text delves into the design's benefits and limitations by observing the approximation of causality based on the measures of effect and conduct.

Since all studies, regardless of the design, portray some uncertainties in terms of inference, reliable and applicable findings must examine the potential for uncertainties and the communication of such uncertainties in clinical medicine and public health decision-making to improve patient and public health. Specifically, epidemiologic or all research findings, irrespective of the field, are subjected to bias, confounding and effect measure modification. This book explains in detail the challenges of epidemiologic studies since inconsistent findings are driven by sample variability, despite unbiased samples from a probability sampling technique which is often ignored in public health and clinical medicine investigations. Future epidemiologists are provided with the knowledge and skills to assess effect measure modifiers and confounding in this text, a concept not clearly covered by most basic epidemiologic literature.

Causal inference is covered in this text, which renders this presentation very unique, given that the overall purpose of epidemiologic studies is causal association , not causal inference, as commonly claimed by most epidemiologic literature. Since effective intervention or therapeutics requires the knowledge of the underlying cause of the condition, causal inference is necessary for the success of public health in controlling and preventing disease, and the same applies to clinical medicine. This text explores the concept of effect and cause and describes the causal criteria as well as evidence-based approaches, including applied Meta-Analysis and QES.

Part III. Laboratory Techniques and Epigenomic Mechanistic Process in Epidemiologic Principles, Concept and Application

This part describes epigenomic epidemiology which emerges as a result of the pressing need to examine injuries at the cellular or molecular level that are not responsive to rapid repair and hence disease development. These molecular changes, though reversible, do not directly result from changes in the DNA sequence but from gene and environment interactions, which may ultimately affect gene expression and hence disease development, causation and impaired prognosis. For example, stress, social stressors, racial discrimination, oppression and abuse as social signal transduction may result in excess elaboration of catecholamines from the sympathetic nervous system and glucocorticoids from the hypothalamus-pituitary-adrenal axis which may affect genes by binding to receptors involved in social signal transduction, thereby inhibiting the transcription factor on the promoter region of the gene (5′C---). Epigenomic epidemiology is concerned with the assessment of individual differences in the promoter region of the gene, as seen in the effect of mDNA and transcription factor inhibition, resulting in restricted or impaired gene expression, and the related disease development and impaired prognosis. A chapter in this section examines the aberrant epigenomic mechanistic process that results in malignant neoplasms, with a specific focus on ALL, prostate cancer, major depressive disorder and essential hypertension.

Aberrant Epigenomic Modulations and Disease Causation

Environment either social, psychosocial or physical interaction with gene if adverse as aberrant epigenomic modulation reflects impaired gene expression, predispose to biological system alterations, implying disease development and causation. While DNA sequence as genomics does not remain a static blueprint to human health, but epigenomic modulations, understanding of these implications in human health remains a reliable pathway in individual patient and subpopulations health improvement and care optimization.

The materials covered in this novel epigenomic epidemiology text allow for the understanding of the types of genes implicated in epigenomic modulations in disease causation, such as ACE-II, NR3C1 and CTRA. Specifically, social isolation, discrimination, rejection and social disconnection as socio-environmental alterations adversely affect self-regeneration, implying the inability of the human biologic system to replace dead or impaired cells as well as decayed proteins. Since human proteins have an estimated half-life of 80 days, implying an estimated 1–2% of the entire molecular makeup replacement daily, this process involves normal gene expression. Simply, all cells have status of limitation, and failure to achieve this normal cellular functionality results in abnormal cellular proliferation, implying malignant neoplasm. Specifically, with an estimated 21,000 genes as DNA, the biological system regeneration gene expression implies DNA transcription into RNA regulated by intracellular proteins as transcription factors. Typically, transcription factors alter gene expression as observed in response to extracellular signals, namely hormones such as androgen, testosterone, estrogen and progesterone, and neurotransmitters (dopamine, norepinephrine, serotonin). With respect to social and psychosocial factors, stress or anxiety, glucocorticoid (NR3C1) receptors or catecholamine (dopamine, norepinephrine) receptors are observed on the cell surface, resulting in the activation of transcription factors, namely cyclic AMP response element-binding protein and/or glucocorticoid receptor elaboration.

Simply, a stressful environment implicates exogenous control or regulation of human gene expression. For example, cell surface receptors experience extracellular signals from either endocrine and/or sympathetic nervous system in response to social isolation, discrimination, stressful environment, racism, low SES, etc. With this observation, intracellular transcription factors such as cyclic

AMP response element-binding protein (CREB) relay signals to the cell nucleus, hence the binding of transcription factors such as glucocorticoid receptor (GR) or CREB to gene enhancer or promoter region (CpG), implication in DNA replication and transcription to tRNA, mRNA and translational RNA, and hence amino acid elaboration and protein synthesis. With this perspective or direction, variabilities at individual or subpopulation levels within social, psychological or psychosocial contexts may adversely affect the transcription factor binding to the CpG enhancer region of the gene (DNA) through DNA methylation, histone modification or non-coding RNA epigenomic mechanistic processes, implying impaired gene transcription, inverse correlation gene expression and cellular dysfunctionality. Therefore, given aberrant epigenomic modulation in this context, there is a predisposition to disease development, impaired prognosis and survival disadvantage (Figure 0.1).

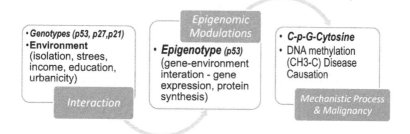

Notes and Abbreviations: Epigenomic Modulation via Methyl group (CH3) – Methylcytosine and Transcriptome Inhibition & inverse gene expression that implicates impaired protein synthesis, Cellular dysfunctionality and abnormal cellular proiiferation as malignant neoplasm. The p53, p21 and p27 are tummor suporessor genes, involved in programmed cell death, given all cells within the biologic system with "apoptosis" as programmed cell death" and cellular replication.

With the observed social determinants of health (SDH) such as educational level, low SES, race/ethnicity, age, social inequity and health inequity, as well as isolation, subordination, rejection and discrimination that adversely impact gene expression, the mechanistic process in this direction remains social signal transduction (SST). This approach or trajectory involves the critical role of the central nervous system (CNS) in adversity data transduction such as discrimination, isolation and rejection experiences into hormonal (estrogen) and neurotransmitter (5-HT) alteration, hence inverse gene expression, cellular dysfunctionality and disease causation such as malignant neoplasm. Specifically, the sympathetic nervous system (SNS) and the hypothalamic-pituitary-adrenal (HPA) axis, based on the SST, tend to suppress antiviral genes such as IFN-α, IFN-β and pro-inflammatory cytokines, namely IL-6 and IL-8.

With these gene expression alterations, disease causation remains, implying aberrant epigenomic modulation in this circumstance, requiring social, physical and chemical environment normalization and improvement in optimized health and health outcomes at a specific population level as well as individual patient care.

ACKNOWLEDGMENTS

Evidence discovery and application depends on team science, transdisciplinary and translational (3Ts) initiative, requiring scientific collegiality, as well as mutualistic, symbiotic and dynamic direction in epigenomic understanding in disease process, therapeutics, prognosis, survival and mortality.

Laurens Holmes, Jr. Medical College of Wisconsin,
Population Health Seminar, Podcast, 2017

Scientific knowledge remains dynamic rather than static in clinical and public health decision-making, while the gene and environment interaction as epigenomic modulation is our destiny, not DNA sequencing or genomic modulation. This approach requires time and dedication to assess aberrant epigenomic modulations via reliable study design, conduct, analysis and interpretation.

The initiation of this book reflects the interest and dedication of the fellows from a Translational Health Disparities Research Program, who remain passionate and committed to the application of aberrant epigenomic modulations in the understanding of subpopulations such as race, ethnicity, sex, age, poverty, SES, imbalanced nutrients, physical inactivity, discrimination, air pollutants and toxic waste differentials in disease outcomes. With this direction, subpopulation differentials, variabilities or disparities in health outcomes driven by social injustice, health inequity and environmental injustice remain to be transformed, implying the utilization of findings from epigenomic epidemiology studies in health equity transformation as well as transitioning clinical medicine and public health to epigenomic clinical medicine public health.

One is extremely grateful to all those who facilitated some of the changes and modifications in enhancing the readability of the information in this book, namely Dr. D. Ogungbade, Dr. Prachi Carvan, Dr. Valecia John, Dr. Tatina Picolli, Dr. Doriel Ward, Dr. Monica Garrison, Dr. Justin Williams, Dr. Aidina Williams, Dr. Maura Poleon, Jannaile Williams, MPH, PhD(c), Dr. Pascal Ngalim, Dr. Fancis Kate, Benjamin Ogundele, MPH, PhD(c), Dr. Michael Enwere, Kume Nsongka, MHA, Dr. Cailin Nelson, Dr. Gilberta St. Rose, etc.

Professor (Dr.) Holmes wishes to thank his entire family—Maddy Holmes, Kenzie Holmes, Landon Holmes, Devin Holmes, Aiden Holmes, Larry Holmes, III, Anne, Victor, Nkoyo, Ima, Julie, Brian, Paul, Dr. Ene Abi, Thomas, Charles, Victor II, Fidelis, Elizabeth, Paula, Faith St. Rose, Quan St. Rose, Dr. Glen Philipcien, Chenna Philipcien (in memoriam), etc.—for the time away from them during the preparation of this book. Immense thanks to all those who encouraged and motivated me during the preparation of this book, including Ms. Grace McInnes and Ms. Amy Thomson from Taylor & Francis Publisher.

Laurens Holmes, Jr.

Scientific Uncertainties

Epidemiology, as an applied science in public health and clinical medicine with a primary focus on disease and health-related event distribution and determinants at a specific population level, remains an ever-changing discipline and profession. The author has consulted with various scientific information sources that have been ascertained to be reliable in the presentation of these materials on Epigenomic Epidemiology, namely epigenomic modulation concepts and applications, laboratory techniques, bioinformatics, design, conduct, analysis, interpretation, limitations and recommendations for improving clinical medicine and public health outcomes. The author or publisher is not responsible for any error arising from the use of these materials in the future advancement and improvement of this novel science in epidemiology. Therefore, readers are advised to consult related scientific texts, should such texts exist, in the design and conduct of epigenomic epidemiology studies.

Laurens Holmes, Jr.

PART 1

Epidemiology and Epigenomic Epidemiology Contribution in Public Health and Clinical Medicine

1

INTRODUCTORY EPIGENOMIC EPIDEMIOLOGY

Basic Concepts and Application

1.1 Introduction

Epigenomic epidemiology presents the opportunity to understand the mechanistic process of disease and remains instrumental in the precision medicine initiative that depends on specific risk characterization for risk-adapted treatment protocols. However, this initiative is challenged by design, analytic and interpretation issues in the appropriate transformation of such findings to therapeutics in enhancing precision medicine initiatives, thus addressing treatment effect heterogeneity, especially in malignancies, given the complex and several pathways of cellular proliferation, prognostic biomarkers and anti-apoptotic dynamics.

The precision medicine initiative in clinical care improvement is based on patient outcomes differences due to individual treatment effect heterogeneity, rendering therapeutics ineffective and non-beneficial in some settings despite comparable side effects. Epigenomic alterations or modulations reflect heritable, although reversible, changes in the gene and environment, not DNA sequence, but influence gene transcription and expression, nuclear organization, genomic instability and imprinting. Whereas attempts at understanding treatment effect heterogeneity have been made through sub-subpopulation analysis of treatment outcomes, there remains a feasible approach through epigenomic investigations for specific risk characterization and risk-adapted intervention mapping.

Specifically, epigenomics reflects the molecular modulation of DNA with respect to gene activity regulation which is independent of DNA sequencing and mitotic stability [1]. Over the past few years, there have been some studies on epigenetics and epigenomics. Epigenomic epidemiology remains a

DOI: 10.4324/9781003094487-2

meaningful pathway in the understanding of the distribution of aberrant epigenomic modulations and their determinants at a specific population level as well as the application of these data in related diseases such as asthma, cancer and hypertension and prevention at subpopulation levels. Specifically, the most utilized epigenomic mechanistic process involves DNA methylation (mDNA), histone modifications and non-coding RNAs (ncRNAs) [1, 2]. These methods, as well as many others presented in this specific issue, provide comprehensive guidelines and advanced technologies in the area of epigenetics that facilitate further developments in this promising and rapidly developing field.

The unique purpose of this introductory chapter is to provide a basic understanding to researchers in epidemiology, health disparities epidemiology, biomedical sciences, translational sciences and clinical sciences with respect to the epigenomic mechanistic process, laboratory techniques and reliable study designs concerning the association and causal inference on the implication of aberrant epigenomic modulation or mechanistic processes in disease causation and outcome modifications. The inherent approach is relatively basic and explains the challenges in epigenomic studies as the process of specific risk characterization and risk-adapted treatment narrows subpopulation prognostic and survival variances. Stress is placed on the ongoing emphasis in precision medicine today that reflects the challenges with current therapeutics in terms of individual response, mainly treatment effect heterogeneity or subpopulation variability in therapeutics, driven in part by pharmaco-genetics and within-individual differences in gene expression or epigenomic alteration as a function of gene-environment interactions.

Epigenomic studies contribute to the mechanistic understanding of disease etiology and biomarkers of disease severity or prognosis, enabling specific risk characterization in defining the causal pathway and hence specificity in therapeutics and preselection treatment induction. Since disease processes are complex and multifactorial, neither genetic nor epigenomic studies per se are capable of providing data on meaningful disease etiology, requiring the need for epigenomic studies, especially epigenomic interaction with social determinants of health, namely socio-epigenomics, in reliable causal correlation investigations. Epigenomic alterations or modulations, study designs, analysis and challenges in translating the data from epigenomic studies to precision medicine initiatives in addressing the persistent and reoccurrence treatment effect heterogeneity management are addressed.

Specifically, epigenomics reflect the modulation of the gene and environment by gene-environment interactions, with such modulation or modulation not affecting the DNA sequence but messenger RNA (mRNA) transcription and translation, implying gene expression downregulation if the modulation remains aberrant [2]. The interaction between the environment and genes results in epigenomic modulation or changes that influence the pathway of the disease, thus resulting in disease manifestation through processes such as mDNA process and histone protein modulation as post-translational events, which could depend on diet, lifestyle, alcohol, pollutants, drugs, hormone (endogenous environment), physical activities, in utero environment, etc. Epigenomic modulations or modulations reflect dynamic changes commencing in utero and continuing till the "oldest old" life course [1], with such alterations remaining causal in disease development or prognostic as biomarkers of survival but reversible.

Whereas epigenomic modulation via "gene" and environment interaction does not involve the DNA sequence, but results in gene transcription impairment via methylation—CH_3- (mDNA) as well as altered transcriptional activator proteins activities (histone methylation and acetylation) [3]. The observed alteration has a direct impact on specific genes involved in cellular functionality, disease progression, prognosis and mortality.

The design of studies in epigenomic research depends on the biomarkers and the measurement scale, implying consideration of the biosample in terms of timing and storage [4]. Additionally, the design varies depending on the hypothesis proposed to be tested or the epigenomic approach for assessment of epigenomic alterations or aberrant epigenomic modulation as in a morbidity pathway or as a biomarker of disease severity or prognosis. Such designs could be prospective or longitudinal as well as cross-sectional, case-control or hybrids of case-control and cohort designs. However, the use of these designs requires a specific outcome for the epigenomic alterations to avoid reverse causation that may occur from "diseased samples" while attempting to assess the causal mechanism of a disease. Further, studies on epigenomic modulations must consider sample size and power estimations since small samples are more likely to result in statistically insignificant gene expression findings despite the obvious correlation between hypo- or hyper-methylation (CH_3) and disease causation or prognosis. Further, for the internal validity of epigenomic studies in providing valuable data for precision medicine, epigenomic design and interpretation should minimize systematic error and examine false error rates. Furrthermore, random error quantfication as probaility value (p vlaue), althpough not a maesure of precision, but confidence interval (CI) ,confounding and effect maesure modifier assessement should be applied in accurate and reliable understanding of aberrant epigenomic modulations in disease causation, prognosis, survival and mortality.

1.2 Genomic and Epigenomic Epidemiology

Traditional epidemiology aimed at assessing the correlation or association between exposure and outcome, implying the risk factor that resulted in disease development or a health-related event [5]. However, despite the traditional epidemiologic investigation notion of non-causal association, this correlation has a causal trajectory in terms of intervention mapping and therapeutics. Such traditional attempts focused less on the cellular or molecular-level events or exposures without penetrating the "black box" of epidemiology. With molecular epidemiology, the interest shifted to molecular events such as disease and prognostic biomarkers—causal association through black box penetration. Additionally, the genetic predisposition to disease is traditionally assessed as single and polygene associations with disease process, as observed in conditions such as trisomy 21 (Down syndrome), XYY (Klinefelter syndrome) and phenylketonuria—an inborn error of metabolism associated with tyrosine hydroxylase enzyme deficiency and mental retardation. With the challenges related to treatment effect heterogeneity, multiple causal pathways in disease development and pharmaco-genetics, gene expression presents an added opportunity to explore disease processes, prognosis and survival. Specifically, early childhood trauma, social disadvantage and a disadvantaged neighborhood environment characterized by living conditions, socio-economic status and health inequity as systemic and unfair allocation of economic, social and environmental conditions related to health have been observed to influence biologic processes resulting in disease development, progression and subpopulation survival differences (3-NR3C1). In effect, such influence has been implicated in gene-environment interactions resulting in epigenomic modulation of gene expression and disease propagation as well as severity, prognosis and survival. Consequently, disease propagation is driven by biologic, genetic, epigenomic, epigenomic, socio-epigenomic, behavioral, social, environmental and psychological predispositions. These predispositions including culturally and linguistically competent care also influence response to treatment, prognosis and survival.

Simply, epigenomics refers to any process that alters gene activity without changing the DNA sequence, and leads to modulations that can be transmitted to daughter cells, but not without reversibility. Epigenomics controls genes, implying the switching on and off mechanism of the gene, and genes are specific sequences of bases that provide instructions for proteins synthesis (transcription to translation). Whereas the same or comparable DNA is expected to predispose to the same functions and alterations in function, that is not the case given distinct gene expression due to different cell types for differential functional activities. Specifically, the changes in epigenome reflect the influence of environment, such as indicated earlier, namely stress, diet, drugs, exogenous environment and pharmacologic agents (treatment effect) on a defective or diseased gene that do not affect the DNA sequence but mRNA and gene expression.

1.3   DNA Molecule and Structure

Simply, DNA comprises four nucleotides, namely adenine (A), thymine (T), guanine (G) and cytosine (C), along with sugar and phosphate molecules. These compositions, termed the backbone or core of DNA molecule, allow for the understanding of epigenomic alterations induced by mDNA. The basics of molecular genetics illustrate the organization of nuclear DNA into 46 chromosomes, implying 22 autosomes and one sex chromosome derived from each human animal parent. The synthesis of protein, either structural or regulatory, follows the central dogma of molecular biology, implying an information pathway or flow from DNA to mRNA and then the synthesis of proteins. Therefore, since genes consist of the base sequences or nucleotides that map the direction of the complimentary mRNA, the specific protein produced depends on this translation. The functionality of the synthesized protein in effect depends on the accuracy of such translation in the formation or development of a specific amino acid (AA-building block of protein), which supports the role of mDNA in the gene expression and the subsequent protein production, whether regulatory or structural.

1.4 Human Gene, DNA, mRNA and Protein Synthesis

The appraisal of terms used in epigenomic modulation is essential for mDNA processes such as promoter, enhancer, transcription factors and transcriptional control. Genes, as indicated earlier, are components of DNA, and the bases or nucleotides that code the AA are organized as exons and group into blocks. The introns comprise bases that are not specific to AA and hence protein synthesis but may contain the control regions located between the exons. In a typical gene, DNA strands have one side referred to as the 5′ end while the other side is termed the 3′ end. The promoter or enhancer region of the DNA strand is associated with the 5′ end, and is enriched with cytosine (C) and guanine (G) bases. The transcription process in the central dogma theorem involves the binding of this region, the 5′ end, with the transcription factors, resulting in the synthesis of complementary mRNA thanks to RNA polymerase [3]. Protein synthesis involves the new primary copy of the gene, the removal of introns, and binding or stitching together of exons. As the process evolves, the ribosomes then utilize the mRNA as a template in the synthesis of the polypeptide chain as the basic structure for proteins, whether structural or regulatory [6].

1.5 DNA Methylation (mDNA)—Covalent Binding of Methyl Group to Gene Promoter Region (CpG)

mDNA is a process by which cells create epigenomic markers. As observed above, the promoter regions of genes contain sequences, namely cytosine (C), alternating with guanine (G), expressed as 5′-CG-3′ (CpG). However, CpG is located in other areas besides the promoter region of the gene. The C of the CpG is predisposed to modulation by the DNA methyltransferase; thus, a covalent reaction involving the addition of the methyl (CH_3) to this portion (C) results in the formation of 5´-methylcytosine. *What is the cellular or physiologic consequence of this formation, 5´-methylcytosine?* Since the promoter region of the gene is involved in the transcription process, methylation of C (cytosine), which is an enduring process, may result in the inability of this region to bind relevant transcription factors as observed above, thus inhibiting and stopping transcription (Figure 1.1).

1.6   Epigenome and Epigenomic Concepts in Epidemiology

Traditionally, modern epidemiology emerged from clinical medicine in an attempt to quantify the risk and predisposing factors in disease, implying the role of exposure in the causal pathway of disease despite the stress on association as the core of epidemiologic investigation. While exposure was traditionally and initially conceived at a non-cellular level, such as cigarette smoking in bronchial carcinoma risk, epidemiologic evidence indicated a factual association as well as a causal inference based on the magnitude of effect and dose-response explanation as implied in causal inference. Epidemiologic investigation continues to evolve with the examination of cellular level exposure, namely biomarkers of disease, thus the penetration of the "black box" to the emergence of molecular epidemiology. With the worldwide genomic project that opened the window for the total gene study, the role of epigenomics in epidemiology has emerged. Basically, this initiative is the assessment of hereditable changes in gene expression that occur in the absence of underlying DNA sequence as observed in epigenomic regulators, namely mDNA (addition or removal of a methyl group (CH_3), predominantly where cytosine bases occur consecutively), histone modulations, prions, microRNA and DNA microarray. Besides

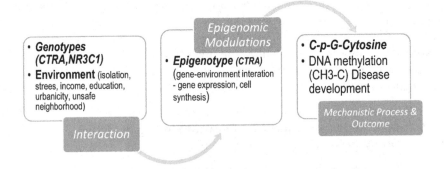

Epigenomic modulation via Methyl group (CH3) – Methyl-cytosine and Transcriptome Inhibition & inverse gene expression ⟶ Impaired protein synthesis ⟶ Cellular dysfunctionality and abnormal proliferation

FIGURE 1.1   Epigenomic mechanistic process.

methylation, other processes could alter gene activities without affecting DNA sequence, such as acetylation, phosphorylation and ubiquitylation. However, mDNA remains the most common mechanism for epigenomic epidemiologic investigation due to its relative stability with storage and several processes and technologies for analysis [6]. The mDNA study or assessment measures the percentage of methylated cytosine residues within CpG dinucleotides.

1.7 Epigenomic Role in Epidemiologic Investigation of Disease Causation

In a broad sense, epigenomics is the study of heritable changes in gene expression, implying the examination of active versus inactive genes that do not involve changes to the underlying DNA sequence. Simply, it implies a change in phenotype without a change in genotype, but it affects how cells read the genes. While epigenomic change is a regular (ongoing cellular process) and a natural occurrence, these changes are also influenced by multiple factors such as age, environment, lifestyle, in utero environment and disease status (epigenomic prognostic biomarkers). Epigenomic modulations can manifest as mild and physiologic or normal, involving cell differentiation in skin, liver and brain cells. Additionally, epigenomic change can have more damaging effects, resulting in disease development as well as severity. Currently, these systems include, though not limited to, mDNA, histone modulation and ncRNA that are associated with gene silencing and are involved in initiating and sustaining epigenomic change.

Genetic epidemiology emerged as an attempt to associate disease predisposition with genetic inheritance and heritability and the environment. *The application of environment in environmental epidemiology is very broad and involves in utero exposure, social determinants of health, physical and social exposures (exogenous), and endogenous exposure (hormones—testosterone and prostate cancer, estrogen and breast cancer).* The process by which disease is claimed to run in families opened the window for traditional epidemiologic studies on the familial origin of disease. For example, phenylketonuria, an inborn error of metabolism that involves a deficiency in the enzyme phenylalanine hydroxylase, influences the metabolism of an essential AA, phenylalanine, which is associated with mental retardation. This inborn error of metabolism requires an environmental factor prior to the development of mental retardation, the related phenotype. Environmental factors thus interact with genes to predispose to disease manifestation, such as in gene-environment interactions. In effect, the current epidemiologic approach to epigenomic modulations reflects a departure from the traditional model of investigation, namely: (a) family aggregation studies, (b) twin/adoption/half-sibling/migrant studies, (c) segregation analysis, (d) linkage analysis and (e) association studies.

Epigenomic changes underlie developmental and age-related biology. Genetic epidemiology implicates epigenomics in disease risk and progression, and suggests that epigenomic status depends on environmental risks as well as genetic predisposition. Epigenomic epidemiology represents a mechanistic link between environmental exposures, or genetics, and disease development and prognosis, and attempts to provide a quantitative biomarker for exposure or disease in areas of epidemiology currently lacking such measures.

Specifically, epigenetic or epigenomic epidemiology provides an additional understanding of the biologic mechanism involved in disease causation and severity or survival. Therefore, epigenomic modulations allow for the examination of disease causality through: (a) a direct link or effect on disease risk characterization, (b) risk modulation implying impact on exploring disease association via epigenomic alterations, (c) disease and environment biomarkers, and (d) mechanisms for transgenerational effects or impacts. In terms of the direct link with disease, epigenomic studies have demonstrated that Rett syndrome is due to genetic mutations (genotype) caused by an epigenomic mechanism as a result of spontaneous mutations in the methyl-CpG-binding protein 2 (MECP2) gene on the X chromosome [7]. Specifically, MECP2 is relevant for identifying epigenomic modulations that control gene expression. Additionally, mutated MECP2 has been observed to alter the expression of other genes that are usually regulated by epigenomic alterations. Another example has been illustrated by a single nucleotide polymorphism (SNP) in the COMT gene, which is associated with a new CpG site and correlates with lifetime stress level and memory and the methylation level of the variant allele [8]. Epigenomic alterations may serve as biomarkers of disease, implying no role in the mechanistic process of the disease. Such biomarkers could serve as prognostic factors that drive severity and survival, implying their role in patients' responses to a given therapeutic agent. For example, epigenomic epidemiologic data have observed tumor hypermethylation of the DNA repair enzyme O^6-methylguannine-DNA methyltransferase (MGMT) to be associated with increased favorable response, increasing survival [9].

1.8 Challenges in the Design, Conduct and Interpretation of Epigenomic Studies

The challenge in epigenomic epidemiology lies in the clarity and feasibility of study design, measurement tools, statistical methods, and biological, physiological and clinical interpretation. These aspects are required in this attempt to provide a causal inference on the pathway of epigenomic alteration as an exposure function of disease, severity, prognosis and survival.

Genome-wide association studies (GWAS) of conditions have identified hundreds of genomic regions containing variants robustly associated with disease. These variants have been shown to reside in large regions of strong linkage disequilibrium and most do not index coding variants involving or affecting protein structure. In effect, there are substantial uncertainty regarding the causal genes involved in disease and the way in which they are functionally regulated by associated risk variants. Therefore, in an attempt to localize the functional consequences of disease-associated variants, there is a need to characterize mDNA quantitative trait loci (mQTLs) in organ-system and relate these to genetic findings from clinical conditions and disorders.

While there is optimism in the field of epigenomic epidemiology for informing precision medicine, the challenges are obvious given the differences between genetic epidemiology and epigenomic epidemiology. Primarily, the approach to epigenomic studies requires an understanding of the level of epigenome of interest, namely mDNA, histones and microRNA, which depends on the stability of the epigenomic marker as well as the sensitivity to changes in the external and internal environment. Additionally, the location of the marker is important, given millions of epigenomic markers in a cell. For instance, the mDNA process places emphasis on CpG islands and CpG island shores, stressing inter-individual variability in epigenome. Since epidemiology is concerned with determining the differences, epigenomic investigation must examine between and within variance to gain a better understanding of epigenomic alterations that result in a disease or serve as a biomarker of disease severity or prognosis. For example, mDNA studies for epigenomic variation require cross-tissue (intra-individual and within subject) and cross-population (between subjects, inter-individual) assessment in determining the variability in methylation as a function of disease as well as the topography or location (spatial relationship). Very importantly, and a departure from genetic epidemiology, epigenomic epidemiology requires an understanding of the temporal variation or changes in the epigenome, implying dynamic changes and the timing of the sample collection and processing.

1.8.1 Epigenomic Study Design

The *study design* requires uniqueness relative to traditional epidemiologic or genetic epidemiology design, as mentioned earlier, implying differences in study timing, samples (frozen or fresh) and the type of epigenome. Samples must be collected in a manner that preserves the epigenomic mark of interest to the investigators, since these are dynamic exposures that can undergo changes or vary over a short period. In traditional epidemiology, if exposure and disease variables are collected simultaneously, it is difficult to establish causality, and the same applies to epigenomic markers or alterations. Similarly, the assumption that epigenomic markers are causal in the disease pathway requires attention to the timing of sample collection, namely at the disease state or pre-disease state, as well as the type of non-experimental or experimental epidemiologic design. Because of the stress on epigenomic investigation in addressing mechanistic processes in disease, genomic epidemiologic studies require prospective or longitudinal designs. Such designs that implicate repeated prospective epigenomic measures are highly likely to establish causal inference in epigenomic alterations and disease causation. Like in traditional epidemiologic risk studies, epigenomic epidemiologic studies can be used to characterize risk if samples are collected at the pre-disease or subclinical stage of disease manifestation. In addition, because epigenomic alterations may be influenced by aging, stratification by age remains an important approach in the design of epigenomic epidemiologic studies. While cross-sectional and case-control traditional epidemiologic designs are applicable in epigenomic studies, caution is required in the causal interpretation, thus avoiding reverse causation. Design, in this context, should be planned a priori in terms of disease causation or a biomarker of disease, given epigenomic alterations as the function of these outcomes (epigenomic as causal or biomarker of disease severity/prognosis).

1.8.2 Bio-Specimen and Analysis

An estimated 28 million CpG sites with mDNA targets had been observed in human genome. This process of mDNA on a genome-wide scale involves the application of next-generation sequencing (NGS) as well as the hybridization of microarrays. The microarray system allows for robust quantification of the mDNA levels based on the targeted CpG sites or islands. Specifically, the mDNA detection within the enhancer or promotion region of the gene involves (a) digestion with methylation-sensitive restriction enzymes, (b) methylated genomic position enrichment and (c) sodium bisulfite treatment, implying the conversion of the unmethylated cytosine residues into thymine, while the methylated cytosine is not converted but protected. This simple approach, although with variability, involves DNA input, genomic resolution degree and coverage, as well as quantification capability. In the process of comparing mDNA levels with several studies in QES as an applied Meta-Analysis, the specific methods used should be very carefully considered.

Over the past years, the genome-wide methods involved the enrichment of the methylated DNA fragments by the application of methylation-specific restrictive enzyme digestion and polymerase chain reaction (PCR), as well as immunoprecipitation of methylated DNA fragments and thereafter, reading out the results by utilizing hybridization microarrays. Despite the effectiveness and strength of this enrichment method, this process does not provide single-base resolution of mDNA at individual or specific CpG sites or shores. Currently, the methods used are the Infinum BeadChip assays (Illumina) with the ability to achieve single-base resolution of a bisulfite-converted DNA with high-throughput analysis of many CpG sites. The BeadChip assays require the interrogation of the methylation status of the cytosine residues by genotyping cytosine or thymine, implying contrast between methylated and unmethylated cytosine residues based on a predetermined set of probes in microarray format, while the Infinum assay provides the quantitative measure of mDNA.

Very relevant to the current epigenomic mechanistic process is the application of the sodium bisulfite procedure in the measurement or assessment of the methylation status of individual cytosine residues at a single-base resolution. While the BeadChip assays remain reliable in mDNA analysis with respect to a large patient cohort, an estimated 3% of the 28 million CpG sites remain their target.

Of interest in epigenomic studies is the *availability of biosample*. With specific reference to the method of examination of the epigenomic alterations, the sample storage method may not be appropriate. For example, histone modulation and microRNA samples are considered unstable in frozen form while mDNA is not, implying the use of frozen samples for mDNA studies [10]. The *statistical approach* to the analysis of epigenomic studies requires both a traditional inferential approach and reliable modeling of complex data. The cell type distribution with disease may serve as confounding, requiring stratification or a multivariable regression model once the cell types are identified and isolated. A reliable analytic approach to causal inference in epigenomic studies should conform to reality in the modeling of biomedical and epidemiologic research data by addressing issues arising from batch, normalization and confounding by cell type distribution. Currently, a statistical approach involves single-CpG statistical tests and region-based tests, also termed bump hunting. This technique derives information from neighboring sites and examines the correlation of methylation signals [11]. While *sample size and power estimations* require a clinically meaningful effect size, which is difficult to estimate with epigenomic alteration studies, power and sample size estimations are needed in these studies. Additionally, since the absence of evidence does not imply evidence of absence and small studies are likely to yield a statistically insignificant finding, the probability value (p) is a function of sample or study size and not a measure of evidence which is provided by the parameter values or estimates.

However, since many epigenomic marks are easily influenced by several factors, including external and internal milieu, epigenomic epidemiology remains an attempt to provide a mechanism for the interaction of the genome with environmental exposures, an essential pathway to disease etio-pathogenesis and prognosis. Therefore, epigenomic epidemiology explores how disease-associated nutritional or dietary chemical, physical and psychosocial factors mediate changes to the epigenome, specifically at the level of mDNA, implying the mediation of cellular responses to several environmental agents such as drugs, physical environmental chemical exposure such as pollutants, dietary exposure and lifestyle by epigenomic processes. In addition, socio-epigenomic epidemiology attempts to specifically examine the interaction between social determinants of health and health inequity factors and epigenomic process in disease predisposition, causality, prognosis and mortality outcomes. As previously observed, the mDNA induced by diet, for example, results in the formation of 5′-methylcytosine that may halt the transcription process, affecting gene expression.

1.8.3   Challenges: Design, Conduct, Analysis and Interpretation

A feasible approach in epigenomic epidemiology is the use of prospective cohort studies that allow for the assessment of epigenomic changes over time and the ability to assess these patterns in relation to temporal changes in exposure and disease prevalence. The longitudinal analysis of epigenomic changes in a population cohort of monozygotic (MZ) twins is a strategy that can be particularly informative for understanding epigenomic variation and its causal association with disease. MZ twins share their DNA sequence, parents, birth date and sex, and are likely to have experienced a very similar prenatal environment. Therefore, epigenomic epidemiologic investigations involving twin cohorts serve to provide a direct understanding of the causal pathway from gene and environmental exposure to disease development.

While the epigenomic epidemiology endeavor remains to benefit clinical medicine and public health, this approach is translational in understanding the mechanistic basis of disease in humans or non-human animals. These challenges are obvious, including but not limited to collaboration, consortia, data sharing and dataset development and maintenance. Additionally, the sample and the context of the design are challenging since epigenomics may reflect biological decline with aging and not necessarily be a disease biomarker. A further challenge in this epidemiologic attempt at disease causal mechanisms with epigenomics is not only the location of the changes or differences but also the timing of the epigenomic changes during gametogenesis/embryogenesis and disease. With an epigenomic epidemiologic approach to the timing of epigenomic changes, intervention mapping is feasible if a time point sensitive to the epigenomic changes is identified, enhancing public health and clinical medicine intervention mapping initiatives. Furthermore, epigenomic epidemiologic studies are challenged with the inherent interpretation regarding gene-epigene nexus, the impact of inherited genes relative to environment, aging as a decline in biologic function, random errors and false discovery rate (FDR) on epigenomic landscape.

Despite these limitations, epigenomic modulations have been shown to be beneficial in assessing causal mechanisms in certain malignant neoplasms [12], neurodegenerative diseases such as Alzheimer's disease and twin studies. With respect to twin studies, there is a greater epigenomic difference across lifespan due in larger part to accumulated environmental stress (physiologic) and disease causation [13–15]. The basis of precision or personalized medicine today lies in the ability of collaborative and team science efforts in epidemiologic investigation of the role of epigenomics in disease causation, prognosis, survival and mortality [16]. Genomic and epigenomic epidemiology remain a challenge in this context, requiring a meaningful and objective team science initiative, an assessment of reliable, factual and non-confounded data (minimized confounding), and implying a causal association between epigenomics and disease development or prognosis. The data from these initiatives and epigenomic epidemiology remain a reliable source for clinical trials and translational clinical trials in testing therapeutics in precision, individualized and personalized medicine.

1.9 Summary

Epigenomic epidemiology presents the opportunity to understand the mechanistic process of disease via "extra-gene," gene and environment interaction, and remains instrumental in precision medicine initiative that depends on specific risk characterization for risk-adapted treatment protocols. However, this initiative is challenged by design, analytic and interpretation issues in the appropriate transformation of such findings to therapeutics in enhancing precision medicine, thus addressing treatment effect heterogeneity, especially in malignancies, given the complex and several pathways of cellular proliferation, prognostic biomarkers and anti-apoptotic dynamics.

The complexities of disease etiology and therapeutics remain challenging, requiring some novel approaches, including but not limited to epigenomic modulations. Currently, there are reliable and accurate mechanistic processes or procedures required for understanding epigenetic functions or roles, transcriptomes and proteomics. There are several methodologies, as observed in this chapter, that provide a better understanding of the information derived from epigenomic mapping and the associated morbidity, prognosis and survival. Furthermore, the application of relevant and accurate bioinformatics as well as computational science as translational tools in epigenomic epidemiology with respect to epigenomic function based on multi-omics data facilitates clinical medicine and public health understanding of the disease process based on aberrant epigenomic modulations.

1.10 Questions for Review

1 Differentiate between genomics and epigenomics.
2 Describe the DNA structure and identify DNA replication and RNA transcription and translation.
3 Explain epigenomic epidemiology and the application of this discipline in morbidity risk determinant.
4 Discuss the benefit of this discipline in precision medicine initiative.
5 Mention a brief challenge in the application of a frozen bio-specimen in histone acetylation compared with DNA methylation.

Abbreviations—Genomic/Epigenomic

ChIP	Chromatin immunoprecipitation
DNMTs	DNA methyltransferases
HATs	Histone acetyltransferases
HDACs	Histone deacetylases
HMTs	Histone methyltransferases
5mC	5-methylcytosine
5hmC	5-hydroxymethylcytosine
MSP	Methylation-specific PCR
NSG	Next-generation sequencing
WGBS	Whole-genome bisulfite sequencing
RRBS	Reduced representation bisulfite sequencing
MRE-seq	Methylation-sensitive restriction enzymes-sequencing
MeDIP	Methylated DNA immunoprecipitation
PBAT	Post-bisulfite adaptor tagging
ChIP-seq	ChIP-sequencing
ChIP-BMS	ChIP-bisulfite methylation sequencing
BisChIP-seq	Bisulfite-treated ChIP DNA-sequencing
ncRNAs	Non-coding RNAs
miRNA	MicroRNA
siRNA	Short interfering RNA
lncRNA	Long non-coding RNA
RISCs	RNA-induced silencing complexes

References

1 Holmes L Jr et al. DNA methylation of candidate genes (ACE II, IFN-γ, AGTR 1, CKG, ADD1, SCNN1B and TLR2) in essential hypertension: a systematic review and quantitative evidence synthesis. *Int. J. Environ. Res. Public Health.* 2019;16(23):4829. doi: 10.3390/ijerph16234829.

2 Brueckner B, Garcia Boy R, Siedlecki P, Musch T, Kliem HC, Zielenkiewicz P et al. Epigenetic reactivation of tumor suppressor genes by a novel small-molecule inhibitor of human DNA methyltransferases. *Cancer Res.* 2005;65:6305–6311.

3 Chen RZ, Pettersson U et al. DNA hypomethylation leads to elevated mutation rates. *Nature.* 1998;395:89–93.

4 Cervoni N, Szyf M. Demethylase activity is directed by histone acetylation. *J. Biol. Chem.* 2001;276:40778–40787.

5 Holmes L Jr. *Applied Epidemiologic Principles and Concepts.* (Boca Raton, FL: Taylor & Francis Publisher, 2018).

6 Bakulski KM, Fallin MD. Epigenomic epidemiology: promises for public health research. *Environ. Mol. Mutagen.* 2014;55(3):171–183.

7 Amir RE, Van den Veyver IB et al. Rett syndrome is caused by mutations in x-linked mecp2, encoding methyl-cpg binding protein 2. *Nat. Genet.* 1999,23;185–196.

8 Ursini G, Bollati V, Fazio L et al. Stress-related methylation of the cathecol-o-methyltransferese al 158 allelle predicts human prefrontal cognition and activity. *J. Neurosci.* 2011;107(31):6692–6698.

9 Esteller M, Garcia-Foncillas J, Andion E et al. Inactivation of the DNA-repair enzyme mgmt. and the clinical response of gliomas to alkylating agents. *N. Engl. J. Med.* 2000;343:1350–1354.

10 Deng J, Davies DR, Wisedchaisri G et al. An improved protocol for rapid freezing of protein samples for long-term storage. *Acta Crystallogr. D Biol. Crystallgr.* 2004;60:203–204.

11 Jaffe AE, Murakami P, Lee H. Bump hunting to identify differentially methylated regions in epigenomic epidemiology studies. *Int. J. Epidemiol.* 2012;41: 200–209.

12 Feinberg AP, Tyoko B. *The history of cancer epigenomics. Nat. Rev. Cancer.* 2004;4:143–153.

13 Javierre BM, Fernandez AF et al. Changes in DNA methylation associate with twin discordance in systemic lupus erythematosus. *Genome Res.* 2010;20:170–179.

14 Ribel-Madsen, R, Fraga ML et al. Genome-wide analysis of DNA methylation differences in muscle and fat from monozygotic twin discordant for type 2 diabetes. *PLoS One.* 2012;7:e51302.

15 Bob Weinhold. Epigenomics: The science of change. *Environ. Health Perspect.* 2006;114(3):A160–A167.

16 Feber A, Guilhamon P et al. Using high-density DNA methylation arrays to profile copy number alterations. *Genome Biol.* 2014;15:R30.

2

PUBLIC HEALTH, EPIDEMIOLOGY AND TRANSLATIONAL EPIGENOMIC EPIDEMIOLOGY PERSPECTIVE

2.1   Introduction

Public health reflects what we as a society aim to achieve in order for all individuals to remain healthy, implying all aspects of life, survival and existence. With the notion of health as not a mere absence of a physical disease process but a complete and total state of physical, psychological, social, economic and mental well-being [1], public health involves the objective evaluation of these conditions in ensuring that society remains healthy. In this process of achieving these outcomes, a reliable and objective assessment of these elements of human health—namely essential health services, optimal preventative care, value care, disease control and health promotion practices—is necessary.

While epidemiology remains the basic and applied science of clinical medicine and public health, disease at the individual and specific population level requires the understanding of the genetic and environmental predisposition and etiology prior to an effective intervention, implying treatment and prevention. With the evolution of molecular sequencing in disease classification prior to reliable and appropriate therapeutics, the understanding of the gene and environment interaction in disease causation, prognosis and survival, implying epigenomic modulations, allows for specific risk characterization and induction therapy prior to the standard of care. Such initiatives with respect to chemotherapeutics in cancer treatment result in marginalized dose escalation, chemotoxicity and enhanced malignant neoplasm survival.

Care provisions for patients require the healthcare providers to understand the factors that contribute to disease development prior to an intervention. Therefore, in order to ensure appropriate treatment and optimal care provision, healthcare providers, mainly physicians, require the basic and applied

DOI: 10.4324/9781003094487-3

knowledge of epidemiology. With this trajectory, care provision, namely treatment, must be based on an appropriate epidemiological design, such as a randomized placebo-controlled clinical trial utilized in the assessment of a given therapeutic agent. Furthermore, optimal preventive care services are required to ensure that disease relapse and patient readmissions are marginalized. Since clinical care involves preventive health services, clinical medicine must embrace epidemiologic principles in disease distributions and determinants, implying the utilization of epidemiologic findings in disease control and prevention.

2.2   History and Goal of Public Health

Public health evolves from health contemplation. Historically, health was linked with sanitation, personal hygiene, nutrition and lifestyle. Earlier in 1500 BC, the Mosaic Law reflected on the fundamental human responsibility of saving human lives. During the 4th century, the founding fathers of modern medicine, including Hippocrates, clearly observed that the pathway to curing any disease depends on the knowledge of its underlying cause. With this notion of the knowledge of the underlying cause of disease and the ancient society's application of sanitation, personal hygiene, healthful nutrients and physical fitness, the human society has an obligation to improve and control the health of the society, implying public health today.

Currently, public health involves disease causation at the community level, implying the utilization of this knowledge by public health organizations and agencies in disease control and health promotion practices. For example, during the 20th century, pioneers of public health, such as Lillian Wald, introduced public health nursing that allowed for the nursing care provision at the homes of the sick as well as the poor immigrants in New York City in the United States. Today public health evolves community outreach, home health or care, and community healthcare services.

While the founding fathers of modern medicine, namely Hippocrates of ancient Greek medicine, anticipated cure that is dependent on causation, this initiative serves as the building block of basic and clinical medicine as well as enhances the application of epidemiologic data or scientific evidence discovery in disease intervention, implying treatment and prevention. Historically, sanitation has remained an effective measure in disease prevention. The epidemiologic role in public health preventive measures was observed through Lind's investigation of scurvy and the discovery of vaccination by Dr. Jenner for smallpox prevention. Additionally, the cholera investigation by Dr. John Snow in 1845 provided public health with a scientific methodology for disease causation and mortality.

With the investigations of disease and mortality, the concept of assessment of health and health-related issues emerged as a core function of public health, implying epidemiology as the basic and applied science in disease prevention and control as well as health promotion practices as the goal of public health. Since optimal health is dependent on social, psychological, physical, mental and economic perspectives, the nexus between these attributes is required for enhancing and improving public health. Additionally, the application of basic medical sciences to the understanding of morbidity and mortality at the population or community level remains a feasible pathway to disease control and prevention. Currently, the application of immunology, virology, microbiology, pharmacology, genomics, epigenomics, genetics, epigenetics, sociology, psychology, behavioral sciences, policy and management science, environmental science and toxicology in the assessment components of the core function of public health, namely epidemiology, allows for enhanced public health improvement. As scientific data become available in the basic and applied sciences, namely epigenomics, public health and clinical medicine, efforts continue to be made to improve the health and well-being of the society.

2.2.1 History of Epidemiology and Current Trajectory

Epidemiology as a profession, not merely a discipline, emerges from the Greek notion of the assessment, examination or study of what is upon people. Literally, "epi" means upon, "demos" means people and "logos" means study. Simply, epidemiology implies the assessment of exposures or occurrences that are beyond normal at the human population level. As the basic and applied science of public health, the role of epidemiology in disease control and prevention remains that of assessing the distribution and determinants of disease and health-related events at the specific population level and utilizing these data in intervention mapping.

Between 1978 and 2017, the term "epidemiology" served as a discipline in characterizing the application of the terms "problems," "knowledge," "public health," "population," "study," "disease," "health" and "distribution" in societal health conditions such as morbidity and mortality. With these terms, epidemiology is basically the study of disease and health-related events or phenomena such as pregnancy, well-child visit and immunization at the population level. Specifically, with this notion and the application of "science," epidemiology reflects a scientific approach in the assessment of the distribution and determinants of disease, health-related events and mortality at the specific population level.

2.2.2 Modern Epidemiology and Disease Trajectory

With scientific inquiry utilizing dynamic and not static data in clinical and public health decision-making, the notion and concept of epidemiology remain transitional. The early 2000s human genome project (HGP) facilitated whole-genome sequencing (WGS) that provided information on global genomic sequencing in disease causation, implying risk/predisposing factors and etiology. The implication of genomic sequencing in the disease process allows for the reading and interpretation of genetic information in deoxyribonucleic acid (DNA) or RNA. For example, the current COVID-19 pandemic allows for genomic sequencing of SARS-CoV2 with respect to mutants, strains and variants of origin.

The DNA variations outside the exons influence gene expression and protein synthesis, which adversely affects entire or complete exome sequencing, termed WGS. This sequencing method WGS allows for the determination of the variations in an individual's nucleotides within the DNA. This process facilitates the DNA sequencing methods, namely clone preparation with entire genome of a species and clone DNA sequencing collection. The WGS allows for mutation detection by observing single nucleotide polymorphisms (SNPs) and several mutants.

2.3   Translational and Epigenomic Epidemiology Concepts and Application

Epigenomic epidemiology (EE) is the distribution and determinants of disease and health-related events driven by gene and environment interaction at a specific population level, and the application of these findings in intervention mapping with a specific focus on the environment such as endogenous, exogenous, physical, chemical, stress, isolation, structural and systemic racism, socioeconomic status, educational level, food insecurity, air pollutants, toxic waste and unsafe neighborhoods. With the current implication of environmental alteration of genes in disease causation, prognosis and survival, a process termed epigenomic modulation requires substantial understanding in epidemiologic investigation and critical appraisal.

While genomic sequences implicate DNA alteration, epigenomic modulation reflects alteration in genes activities and expression, resulting in dysfunctional protein synthesis and cellular dysfunctionality. Aberrant epigenomic modulation may lead to abnormal cell differentiation and proliferation, implying abnormal cellular proliferation characterized as malignant neoplasm [2, 3]. With this observation, epidemiologic investigation is required for aberrant epigenomic modulation such as malignant neoplasm, chronic renal disease, essential hypertension (HTN) and cardiovascular disease (CVDs) at the specific population level for intervention mapping, thus achieving the goal of public health, namely disease control and prevention as well as health promotion practices [4]. For example, the application of whole-genome bisulfite sequencing (WGBS) in the DNA methylation of the CpG region of the gene allows for the observation of aberrant epigenomic modulation, resulting in specific risk characterization and induction therapy prior to the standard of care. This initiative enhances the role of epidemiology in disease determinants and the application of such data in disease control and optimal preventive services.

Epidemiology today remains translational and epigenomic, implying translational EE in meeting the assessment core function of public health as well as individual patient therapeutics. While public health reflects what we as a society could do to remain healthy, implying optimal preventive care survives, clinical medicine requires disease and health intervention. With epidemiology as a basic and applied science in medicine, healthcare providers, mainly physicians, require training in this field to prevent disease recurrence in individual patients. Subsequently, while disease treatment remains the main focus of care in clinical medicine, healthcare providers' understanding of the environment of individual patients and the impact of such an environment on disease causation, association, etiology, prognosis and mortality remains a feasible pathway in disease control and prevention at the specific population level [5].

2.3.1 Genetic, Epigenetic, Genomic and Epigenomic Epidemiology

Genetic epidemiology emerged as an attempt to associate disease predisposition with genetic inheritance and heritability and the environment. *The application of environment in environmental epidemiology is very broad and involves in utero exposure, social determinants of health, physical and social exposures (exogenous), and endogenous exposure (hormones—testosterone and prostate cancer, estrogen and breast cancer).* The process by which disease is claimed to run in families opened the window for traditional epidemiologic studies on the familial origin of disease. For example, phenylketonuria, an inborn error of metabolism that involves a deficiency in the enzyme phenylalanine hydroxylase, influences the metabolism of an essential amino acid, phenylalanine, which is associated with mental retardation. This inborn error of metabolism requires an environmental factor prior to the development of mental retardation, the related phenotype. Environmental factors interact with genes to predispose to disease manifestation, such as in gene-environment interactions. In effect, the current epidemiologic approach to epigenetic and epigenomic modifications reflects a departure from the traditional model of investigation, namely: (a) family aggregation studies, (b) twin/adoption/half-sibling/migrant studies, (c) segregation analysis, (d) linkage analysis and (e) association studies.

In a broad sense, epigenetics is the study of heritable changes in gene expression, implying the examination of active versus inactive genes that do not involve changes to the underlying DNA sequence. Simply, it implies a change in phenotype without a change in genotype, but it affects how cells read the genes. While epigenetic change is a regular (ongoing) and natural occurrence, these changes are also influenced by multiple factors such as age, environment, lifestyle and disease status. Epigenetic modifications can manifest as mild and physiologic or normal, involving cell differentiation in skin, liver and brain cells. Additionally, epigenetic change can have more damaging effects, resulting in disease development. Currently, these systems include, though not limited to, DNA methylation, histone modification and non-coding RNA (ncRNA) that are associated with gene silencing and are involved in initiating and sustaining epigenetic changes (Figure 2.1).

While genetic studies in epidemiology reflect the contribution of individual genes, such as specific chromosomal abnormalities, to a disease process, as observed in 9p deletion in acute lymphoblastic leukemia (ALL) and p15 and p16 inactivation in ALL relapses, epigenetic studies characterize the environmental interaction with the individual genes, implying processes resulting in heritable changes or modulation in gene expression without alterations in the DNA sequence per se. The epigenetic investigation considers the processes affecting gene expression during cell division, such as the promoter or gene enhancer, as well as chromatin (*"DNA residence"*) modification, a dynamic nucleoprotein complex that regulates the DNA access for replication into single-strand DNA and the subsequent translation into mRNA. Specifically, epigenetic investigation in epidemiology involves the assessment of heritable phenotype that is not associated with DNA sequence alteration or modulation. Epigenomic modulation reflects these epigenetic modulations involving the entire or whole genome level in a cell or organism. Simply, epigenomics characterizes the epigenetics assessment of multiple genes within the cell or entire organism [6–8] (Figure 2.2).

Epigenetic changes underlie developmental and age-related biology. Genetic epidemiology implicates epigenetics in disease risk and progression, and suggests that epigenetic status depends on environmental risks as well as genetic predisposition. Epigenetic epidemiology represents a mechanistic link between environmental exposures, or genetics, and disease development and prognosis, and attempts to provide a quantitative biomarker for exposure or disease in areas of epidemiology currently lacking such measures.

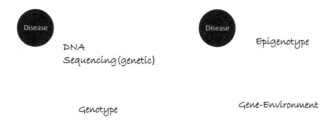

FIGURE 2.1   Epigenetic modification with the environment and epigenotype leading to disease.

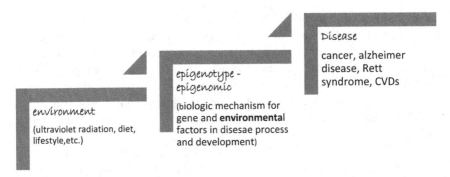

FIGURE 2.2 Epigenetic/epigenomic mechanism for gene and environment interaction.

Specifically, epigenetic or EE provides an added understanding of the biologic mechanism involved in disease causation and severity or survival. Therefore, epigenetic modifications allow for the examination of disease causality through: (a) a direct link or effect on disease risk characterization, (b) risk modifications implying impact on exploring disease association via epigenetic alterations, (c) disease and environment biomarkers, and (d) mechanisms for transgenerational effects or impacts. In terms of the direct link with disease, epigenetic studies have demonstrated that Rett syndrome is due to genetic mutations (genotype) caused by an epigenetic mechanism as a result of spontaneous mutations in the methyl-CpG-binding protein 2 (MECP2) gene on the X chromosome [2] Specifically, MECP2 is relevant for identifying epigenetic modifications that control gene expression. Additionally, mutated MECP2 has been observed to alter the expression of other genes that are usually regulated by epigenetic alterations. Another example has been illustrated by a SNP in the COMT gene, which is associated with a new CpG site and correlates with lifetime stress level and memory and the methylation level of the variant allele [3, 9–12]. Epigenetic alterations may serve as biomarkers of disease, implying no role in the mechanistic process of the disease. Such biomarkers could serve as prognostic factors that drive severity and survival, implying their role in patients' responses to a given therapeutic agent. For example, epigenomic epidemiologic data have observed tumor hypermethylation of the DNA repair enzyme O^6-methylguanine-DNA methyltransferase (MGMT) to be associated with increased favorable response, increasing survival [13, 14] (Figure 2.3).

2.3.2 Epigenomic Mechanism in Disease Causation

Malignant neoplasm is a condition that is highly influenced by epigenomic lesions due to the impact of mutation, whether heritable (germ cell) or environmental in nature. Epigenomic alterations in malignancies refer to the

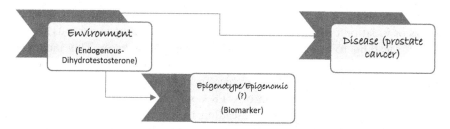

FIGURE 2.3   Epigenetic/epigenomic role as biomarker.

social, psychological, physical, chemical and occupational environments with genes and predispositions to impaired cell growth, differentiation and maturation. Specifically, social isolation, sustained social adversity and social stressors have been implicated in social signal transduction (SST) involving the sympathetic nervous system (SNS) and beta-adrenergic receptors, resulting in the upregulation and downregulation of some genes involved in inflammation and metastatic neoplasm.

While gene and physico-chemical interaction and disease outcome observation remain valid and accurate, we are beginning to experience more than ever before the role played by social isolation, low socio-economic status, discrimination, unstable social hierarchies, repeated social threats and unstable social status, which results in chronic stress, depression, chronic diseases, CVD and cancer. In effect, social environments comparing individuals who are isolated versus those who are not isolated have been shown to result in differences in pro-inflammatory gene expression, such as IL6, antibodies (immunoglobulins) and interferon gamma (IFN-γ). Specifically, repeated social threats or social isolation induces increased expression of pro-inflammatory genes, resulting in increased production of pro-inflammatory cytokines, namely IL-6, while inhibiting gene expression in antibody synthesis (response to pathogenic microbes) and IFN-γ (innate response to viral pathogens). This observation very clearly indicates a decreased elaboration of antibody synthesis, such as immunoglobulin G (IgG), and an increased elaboration of IFN-γ as a result of the increased response of the conserved transcriptional response to adversity (CTRA) gene. When comparing those isolated with those not isolated, available studies have indicated that there is an estimated 5% difference in the specific genes involved with this condition. However, in terms of the gene and environment, more than a 50% difference has been observed comparing individuals who are isolated versus those who are not isolated [4–6, 13–15]. These studies very clearly affirm the role played by genes and the environment in disease development.

Consequently, it is not the gene per se that indicates the differences in the outcome of isolation, but the gene in environment interaction, termed epigenomic. Specifically, social conditions play a substantial role in human gene expression which has been previously observed in animal models. Simply, stress or isolation evokes the SNS response within the central nervous system (CNS), leading to increased expression of the CTRA gene. This increased response of the CTRA gene has been observed in leukocytes due to repeated social threats, unstable social hierarchies and low social status. The observed alterations in the SNS activation of CTRA gene upregulation are due to the beta-adrenergic receptor response, leading to the elaboration of some transcription factors such as nuclear factor kappa-light chain enhancer of activated B-cells (NF-kB) and CAMP response element-binding (CREB) protein [5, 6]. These cascades result in a selective increase in pro-inflammatory gene expression such as interleukin 6 (IL-6), IL-1A, IL-1B and tumor necrosis factor (TNF) and a downregulation of the transcription factor responsible for INF-γ gene expression [7, 16, 17].

Additionally, the CTRA is involved in transcriptional regulation of the human immune system cells via transcriptional shifts in myeloid cells, namely monocytes and dendritic cells. Simply, the SNS response to stress or social isolation can upregulate pro-inflammatory monocyte elaboration via alteration of the hematopoietic process in the bone marrow. Furthermore, beta-adrenergic signaling has been shown to upregulate the transcription of the myelopoietic growth factor granulocyte-macrophage colony-stimulating factor, influencing monocyte development, differentiation and maturation. In effect, social threats or adversity has the potential to upregulate CTRA gene expression in the human immune system, leading to a chronic inflammatory response and excess malignant neoplasm, diabetes and chronic disease [3, 13, 14]. Substantial data support the implication between psychological, neural and endocrine processes in cancer patients and gene expression; however, cautious interpretation of these data to avoid reverse causation is required since malignant neoplasm may induce an inflammatory process with subsequent effects on the CNS, SNS and beta-adrenergic receptor-mediated SST and impaired gene expression (Figure 2.4).

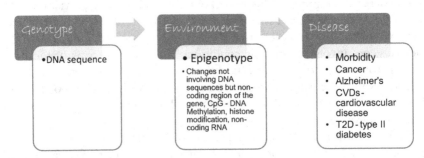

FIGURE 2.4 Epigenomic modulation and disease causation.

Genomic and epigenomic processes that involve specific gene expression reflect the inherent ability of humans to respond to sporadic and transient threats, creating cellular plasticity. For instance, the CTRA gene expression occurs as a result of stressful environments, such as objective and subjective isolation, and results in a molecular-level adaptive process. However, when the stressful circumstance becomes chronic and sustained over time, there emerged a pro-inflammatory response with the potential for type 2 diabetes, atherosclerosis, HTN, neurodegeneration, malignant neoplasm, etc. Additionally, sustained expression of the CTRA gene compromises immune responsiveness through antibody synthesis inhibition (IgG) as well as decreased elaboration of IFN-γ, as an innate response to viral pathogens [13].

To understand epigenomic, implying the interaction between the social, spiritual, economic and physical environment, such as toxins and pollutants, there is a need to understand the specifics of heredity material as we evolve as humans, mainly genes. The hereditary material, or gene, comprises a DNA molecule, which is present in all cells in the human body, and resembles a coiled ladder. Scientifically termed a double helix that contains all the information that constitutes individual characteristics. The DNA consists of four nucleotides—namely, adenine, cytosine, guanine and thymine—along with phosphate and sugar molecules. The combination of these nucleotides forms the codes that are required for the synthesis of amino acid, which are the building blocks of protein molecules. The process by which the protein molecules are developed for continued molecular and cellular function is based on the dogma of molecular biology that begins with the replication of the DNA, the transcription of the DNA into RNA and the subsequent translation of the messenger RNA into protein synthesis: Replication (R) → Transcription (T) → Translation (T).

The interaction between the gene and indigenous, exogenous, social, psychological, environment and the gene is an ongoing process occurring every moment and every instant of human existence. This process is termed epigenomic modulation, meaning above the gene, and reflects changes outside the coding region of the gene, but does not involve the DNA sequence. The normal changes or modulation in this direction reflects the stability of the genome and the normal regulation of everyday activities and health outcomes. In contrast, when there is an insult in this modulation, there occur poor health outcomes, including increased incidence of disease, poor prognostic and excess mortality. Specifically, epigenomic modulation begins with cell signal transduction that involves transcriptome factors and the subsequent utilization of these factors, which are protein molecules in gene expression. The epigenomic mechanistic process has been observed to affect DNA methylation, histone acetylation (ACH), hydroxyl-methylation (OH-CH$_3$) and other mechanisms, not required in this basic explanation. However, of this mechanistic process, the most fundamentally utilized is DNA methylation. This process begins at the promoter region of the gene, or the gene enhancer region, which is populated with cytosine and guanine residue (CpG island). While normal epigenomic modulation involves the DNA methyltransferase recruitment of the CH_3 molecules to the CpG island, aberrant epigenomic modulation involves dense DNA methylation, also termed DNA hypermethylation, that results in the inhibition of the transcriptome and the subsequent impairment in gene expression, adversely affecting protein synthesis and cellular function. Consequently, the methylation of the cytosine residue, resulting in dense DNA methylation at the CpG region, influences gene expression, inducing cellular dysfunctionality (Figure 2.5).

The available literature on social isolation or stress as associated with SST and changes in the SNS clearly indicates how stress signals the fight or flight emotions and reactions that eventually result in alterations that affect how the gene expresses itself. Specifically, the involvement of the SNS results in the elaboration or production of the beta-adrenergic response and the subsequent increase in the receptors associated with this elaboration. Social context involving stress, loneliness and social threats includes the tendency to provoke the hypothalamus-pituitary-adrenal (HPA) axis response, resulting in cortisol elaboration in response to stressful conditions. This response that involves the glucocorticoid receptor gene plays a protective function,

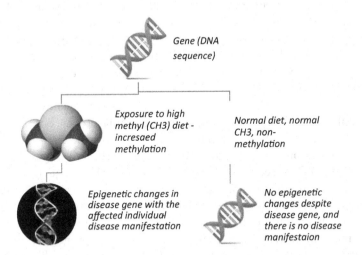

FIGURE 2.5 Aberrant epigenomic mechanistic process in disease manifestation.

Notes: The process of epigenetic changes or alteration in this diagram illustrates the possibilities of changes in a disease-relevant gene (for example, androgen receptor gene in prostate cancer). The exposure to a high-methylated diet results in aberrant epigenomic modulation, implying hypermethylated individuals manifesting diseases such as HTN, breast cancer and prostate cancer. The gene modification or changes in the methylation status lead to the differential expression of the disease gene, implying the development of prostate cancer and other diseases.

enhancing inflammatory recovery. However, chronic stress has been shown to downregulate this response, leading to chronic diseases, metastatic cancer and metabolic syndromes, indicative of the loss of cellular plasticity and the subsequent cellular damage and delayed response to damage, impairing cellular repair and restoration.

Epigenomic modulation, which is the gene and environment interaction, primarily involved a methylation process (CH_3), resulting in DNA methylation as mainly hypermethylation, implying adverse gene expression and downregulation. As stress, isolation and racial/ethnic discrimination impact the SST, this process results in the binding of the CH_3 at the non-coding region of the gene termed the CpG to the cytosine, leading to Methyl cytosine (CH_3-C). With the elaboration of CH_3-C, there remains an impaired transcriptome, leading to inverse gene expression, protein synthesis downregulation, marginalized drug receptors and cellular dysfunctionality as abnormal cellular proliferation [3, 5, 6]. The US subpopulations with aberrant epigenomic modulations, such as racial/ethnic minorities, are more predisposed to increase disease incidence, poor prognosis, excess mortality and marginalized survival.

The environmental alteration driven by CO_2 emissions, air pollutants and particulates, toxic waste and climate warming adversely affects animals and the human animal biologic system. Clinical medicine recognized from its inception the genetic as well as the environmental predisposition to disease and prognosis. However, if there is a genetic predisposition to a given disease, such manifestations have a higher incidence among families with defective genes relative to those without such a hereditary implication. Additionally, among those with a family history of such conditions, namely essential HTN, and stressful environments such as isolation and subordination at employment, this risk of HTN remains higher [4, 5]. This observation clearly implicates aberrant genomic modulations in this predisposition; however, in this clinical presentation, such disease progression is not reversible (aberrant genomics), although transgenerational. With respect to aberrant epigenomic modulation that reflects hyper- or hypo-DNA methylation at the non-coding but enhancer region of the gene, this mechanistic process that alters gene expression remains transgenerational although reversible.

EE is the study of the distribution and determinants of aberrant epigenomic modulation at the specific population level, and the application of these data in specific risk characterization and treatment induction prior to the standard of care, as well as optimal preventive care services, thus addressing the incidence of disease involved in epigenomic modulation as gene expression dysregulation. Epidemiology, in order to assist clinical medicine and public health, must focus on gene and environment interaction mechanistic processes in disease incidence reduction as well as environmental modification with respect to DNA methylation of the candidate genes in impaired gene expression and marginalized transcriptomes, adversely affecting drug response due to the unavailability of protein molecules as drug receptors. Additionally, given the multifactorial nature of disease etiology, epidemiology requires the application of translational as well as transdisciplinary trajectories in the assessment of disease determinants for feasible and effective intervention mapping.

2.4 Public Health and Epidemiology Integration

As observed earlier in this chapter, epidemiology is a basic and applied science of clinical medicine and public health, implying its role in the core function of public health, namely the assessment of health, disease, injury, disabilities, natural disasters, pandemics and health-related phenomena at a specific population level. The core function of public health reflects the assessment of health and health-related phenomena and the application of scientific evidence discovery in data-driven health policy and assurance, implying essential health services at the community level. In meeting the assessment (A) component of the public health core functions (Assessment (A) Policy (P) Assurance (A)), epidemiology is utilized in addressing the understanding of disease spectrum as observed in infectious and chronic disease, natural history of disease, subpopulations/community diagnosis and screening, disease risk and predisposing factors, identification of disease precursors, effectiveness of intervention, epidemics, endemics and pandemics investigation for disease control and preventive strategies and the assessment of the effectiveness of public health intentions.

The integrative role of EE in public health requires the societal identification of several environments that determine the social gradient: physical, chemical, physio-chemical, exogenous and endogenous in disease etiology. With these specific environments, EE remains necessary to enable the understanding of how these environments adversely influence gene expression, resulting in gene dysregulation, cellular dysfunctionality and disease development and progression at the specific population level. For example, the assessment of DNA methylation of the angiotensin converting enzyme (ACE) gene in a specific population with environmental differentials such as zip codes allows for the understanding of aberrant epigenomic modulation at such a geographic locale and the mapping of intervention involving environmental transformation, induction therapy following specific risk characterization and standard anti-hypertensive therapeutics.

2.5 Summary

Epidemiology, as a scientific discipline and profession, is characterized by the assessment of disease, injury, trauma, disabilities, natural disasters and health-related distributions and determinants at specific human and animal levels. With public health being what we as a society require to do to remain healthy and health reflecting not a mere absence of a physical disease process but a complete and total state of social, psychological, economic and mental well-being, the epidemiologic role in public health is to address the core functions of public health, namely assessment, policy and assurance (APA).

While epidemiology has transitioned and transformed its investigative initiatives since its modern onset, especially between 1978 and 2018, EE is an essential and very feasible perspective and trajectory today in addressing predisposing and causal factors in disease development, prognosis, survival and mortality. The understanding of the epigenomic mechanistic process in gene expression allows for specific risk characterization, induction therapy such as demethylase in DNA hyper-methylation and gene dysregulation. This epigenomic approach with reliable epigenomic study designs remains necessary to address disease incidence and mortality at specific population levels.

Simply, the understating of epigenomic modulations, implies the assessment of how environment interacts with human gene as DNA sequencing. Human gene as DNA sequence comprises a DNA molecule. This DNA molecule is structured as a double helix that contains all the information that constitutes individual characteristics, namely, 4 nucleotides: adenine, cytosine, guanine and thymine—along with phosphate and sugar molecules. Specifically, the combination of these nucleotides forms the codes that are required for the synthesis of amino acid, which are the building blocks of protein molecules. While protein molecules are vital to human existence and health, the process upon which the protein molecules are developed for continued molecular and cellular function reflects the dogma of molecular biology. This dogma implies the DNA replication as a primary process, the transcription of the DNA into RNA and the subsequent translation of the messenger RNA into protein synthesis: Replication (R) → Transcription (T) → Translation (T).

2.6 Questions for Review

1 Diseases do not occur in a vacuum or randomly but there is a pattern of distribution. What is epidemiology and how is this notion applicable to clinical medicine, patient care and public health disease control and preventive measures?
2 Describe public health and explain its core function.
3 Describe the relationship between public health and epidemiology.
4 Examine the contributory effect of aberrant epigenomic modulation on disease causation. Determine whether or not DNA methylation and/or histone modification predispose to cancer development and a poor prognosis from cancer chemotherapy.
5 What is epigenomic epidemiology? Describe the role of this aspect of epidemiology in: (a) cancer causality and (b) cancer disease control and preventive measures.

References

1 "Epidemiology: the foundation of public health." http://www.ph.ucla.edu/epi/faculty/detels/PH150/Detels_Epidemiology.pdf [Accessed 9 Mar. 2022].

2 Holmes L Jr, Opara F. *Concise Epidemiologic Principles and Concepts: Guidelines for Clinicians and Biomedical Researchers.* (Author House, 2013).

3 Holmes L Jr, Lim A, Okundaye O et al. DNA Methylation of candidate genes (ACE II, IFN-γ, AGTR 1, CKG, ADD1, SCNN1B and TLR2) in essential hypertension: A systematic review and quantitative evidence synthesis. *Int. J. Environ. Res. Public Health.* 2019;16(23):4829. doi: 10.3390/ijerph16234829.

4 Berger SL, Kouzarides T, Shiekhattar R et al. An operational definition of epigenetics. *Genes Dev.* 2009;23:781–783.

5 Rodenhiser D, Mann M. Epigenetics and human disease: Translating basic biology into clinical applications. *CMAJ.* 2006;174:341–348.

6 Ducasse M, Brown MA. Epigenetic aberrations and cancer. *Mol. Cancer.* 2006;5:60.

7 Robertson KD. DNA methylation and human disease. *Nat. Rev. Genet.* 2005;6:597–610.

8 Bogdanovic O, Veenstra GJ. DNA methylation and methyl-CpG binding proteins: Developmental requirements and function. *Chromosoma.* 2009;118:549–565.

9 Dehan P, Kustermans G, Guenin S et al. DNA methylation and cancer diagnosis: New methods and applications. *Expert Rev. Mol. Diagn.* 2009;9:651–657.

10 Cedar H, Bergman Y. Linking DNA methylation and histone modification: Patterns and paradigms. Nat Rev Genet. 2009;10:295–304.

11 Suganuma T, Workman JL. Signals and combinatorial functions of histone modifications. *Annu. Rev. Biochem.* 2011;80:473–499.

12 Kouzarides T. Chromatin modifications and their function. *Cell.* 2007;128:693–705.

13 Holmes L Jr, Shutman E, Chinaka C, Deepika K, Pelaez L, Dabney KW. Aberrant epigenomic modulation of glucocorticoid receptor gene (NR3C1) in early life stress and major depressive disorder correlation: Systematic review and quantitative evidence synthesis. *Int. J. Environ. Res. Public Health.* 2019;16(21):4280. doi: 10.3390/ijerph16214280.

14 Holmes L, Chinaka C, Elmi H, Deepika K, Pelaez L, Enwere M, Akinola OT, Dabney KW. Implication of spiritual network support system in epigenomic modulation and health trajectory. *Int. J. Environ. Res. Public Health.* 2019;16(21):4123. doi: 10.3390/ijerph16214123.

15 Holmes L Jr. *Applied Epidemiologic Principles and Concepts Clinicians' Guide to Study Design and Conduct.* (Boca Raton, FL: Taylor & Francis, 2018).

16 Bogdanovic O, Veenstra GJ. DNA methylation and methyl-CpG binding proteins: Developmental requirements and function. *Chromosoma.* 2009;118:549–565.

17 Chen H, Taylor NP, Sotamaa KM, et al. Evidence for heritable predisposition to epigenetic silencing of MLH1. *Int. J. Cancer.* 2007;120:1684–1688.

3

SCIENTIFIC RESEARCH CONCEPT AND APPLICATION

Public Health, Clinical Medicine and Epigenomic Epidemiology Studies

3.1 Introduction

Scientific research is a systematic, controlled, empirical and critical investigation of natural phenomena guided by theories and hypotheses about the presumed relations among them [1–3]. Consequently, research implies an organized and systematic way of finding solutions to questions. This attempt requires that solutions to the postulated questions be approached when they are feasible, interesting, novel, ethical and relevant. Clinical research thus involves three basic elements: (a) conceptualization, (b) design process and (c) statistical inference. As anticipated in this text, fundamental thinking in clinical and translational research involves these elements: (a) biologic relevance, (b) clinical and biological importance and (c) statistical stability.

Specifically, statistical inference allows conclusions to be drawn from data because the entire population is never assessed nor examined prior to generalizability [1, 4–6]. The combination of this tripartite approach to evidence discovery from the data remains the cornerstone of generating valid and reliable findings in clinical studies, as well as their cautious interpretation in the attempt to improve patient care.

Conducting research involves planning, which requires the measurement and quantification of the variables in the study, the careful administration of well-designed instruments, data collection, appropriate analysis and the interpretation of results [1]. Depending on the research question and the type of design, this process could be very time consuming and complex. For example, in clinical trials, an elaborate protocol for participants' enrollment, randomization and treatment administration is utilized to ensure appropriate documentation of events, such as drug safety, during the trial.

DOI: 10.4324/9781003094487-4

The materials in this chapter will enable readers to understand research conceptualization and the distinction between clinical medicine and epidemiology, as well as their implications for epidemiologic/population-based clinical and biomedical research. This chapter, as a brief overview of research processes, focuses on the description of terms applied in research conceptualization and provides practical examples, namely: (a) research conduct, (b) research objectives/purpose of research, (c) research questions, (d) hypotheses and (e) description of clinical and population medicine within a research context.

3.2   Structure and Function of Research

Research conduct involves several processes.

A scientific evidence discovery involves a meaningful and accurate as well as reliable application of research methodology [1, 7–9]. This initiative utilizes a basic understanding of research question, background and significance, materials and methods, data gathering and processing, analysis, tabulation, interpretation, discussion, limitations and inference (conclusion).

3.2.1   Research Question

A well-defined problem statement, research questions, purposes and potential benefits of the study to science, society and humanity are essential in a study. For example, epidemiologists or scholars in this field may formulate a research question on the implication of aberrant epigenomic modulation on pediatric acute lymphoblastic leukemia (ALL) survival. An appropriate scientific question involves the "PEICO" acronym, implying P=population; E=exposure; I=intervention; C=comparison and O=outcome. With this direction an accurate research question remains: *Does aberrant epigenomic modulation of the p53 gene downregulate programmed cell death, resulting in increased tumor incidence, poor prognosis and survival disadvantage?* Clinicians and biomedical researchers should realize that research questions are not study topics, since such topics are generally broad and research questions must be very specific as reflected by PEICO. Specifically, research questions should be formulated in such a way that they can be answered by observable evidence. Therefore, unless the research question is feasible, it cannot answer the question posed in a measurable manner.

3.2.2   Background/Significance

The background reflects the identification of the theory and assumptions and a search of background literature to address the magnitude of the problem [10–13]. Such a literature review is aimed at identifying what has been done in terms of previous research, the gap in literature, and what the proposed study intends to add to or contribute to the existing body of knowledge in the field. It is a common mistake made by novice researchers to avoid the intensive literature review of the subject of their interest until the research question and study designs are formulated. We caution against such an approach since there is a possibility that such questions have already been answered. It may lead to a study that is not novel and, hence, has very little to offer science in medicine.

3.2.3   Hypothesis and Variable Ascertainment—Measurement of Variables and Statement of Researchable Hypotheses

Research is simply an exercise in measurement, which is always subject to errors. In effect, an accurate research aims at minimizing measurement error, thus reducing variability in the ascertainment of a measured variable [12].

3.2.4   Materials and Methods (MM)

MM requires the identification of the appropriate study design and methodology to fit the research question or hypothesis. For example, as indicated above in the hypothetical research question on aberrant epigenomic modulation of p53 as a tumor suppressor gene in pediatric ALL, the selected design involved the utilization of the blood sample as specimens and the application of next-generation sequencing (NGS) in gene expression as an inverse among those with DNA hypermethylation. The design remains nested case-control or cross-sectional.

3.2.5   Conduct/Data Gathering

Development of an instrument for data gathering and identifying an appropriate sampling technique (Figure 3.1). Since the generalization of findings requires probability sampling of study subjects prior to baseline or cross-sectional data collection, the sample must be drawn from the population of patients with the same condition. Practically, every sample in the study must have a nonzero probability of being selected for the study [1, 3, 11–13].

3.2.6   Data Processing/Analysis

Selection of data analysis tools or statistical techniques to test the hypothesis or answer the research question and presentation of results and interpretation. For example, in the illustration with ALL, the null hypothesis may be that p53 aberrant epigenomic modulation is not associated with pediatric ALL survival and mortality. In testing this hypothesis, one analysis of variance (ANOVA) was performed if two or more than two measurement times were used and the outcome was measured on a continuous scale or correlation coefficient [12].

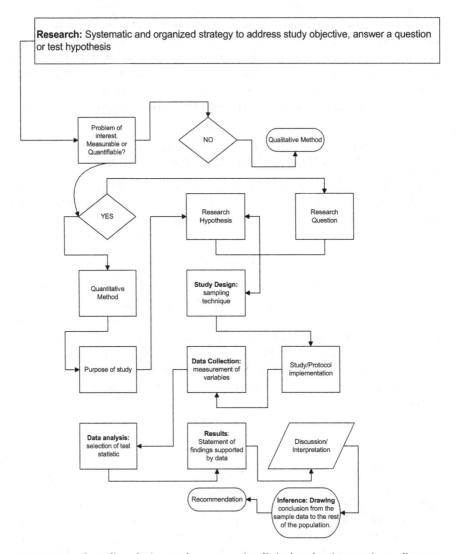

FIGURE 3.1 Sampling design and structure in clinical and epigenomic studies.

3.2.7 Inference/Generalizability

Offering conclusions that are based on the data as well as what the data suggests and recommendations (Figure 3.2).

3.3 Objective of Study/Research Purpose

Research conceptualization begins with the purpose of the study, which is a statement that describes the intent and direction of the study [1, 12–14]. The purpose statement or purpose of a study is the rationale behind the study,

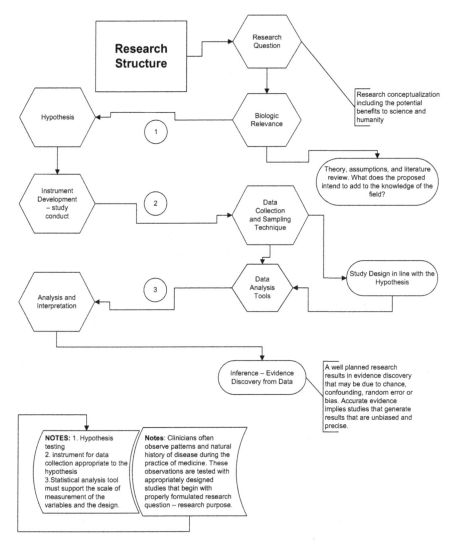

FIGURE 3.2   Research structure and direction.

which requires clarity in the research conduct or study protocol. Although the purpose of the study is often used interchangeably with the research question or the problem statement, they are distinct entities and should be clearly differentiated during the proposal development and manuscript preparation phases of the study. Simply, the purpose of the study describes the objectives, intent and aims of the study. The research question based on "PEICO" therefore remains a specific statement that needs to be answered, following the hypothesis testing in any quantitative research.

In clinical, epidemiologic, public health or biomedical research, the purpose of a study is the statement of the overall objective of the study. This statement identifies the independent and response variables, as well as how the variables will be measured and the design to be used to achieve the expected relationship, nexus, correlation or association. In published articles, we often use words and phrases such as relationship, mean comparison, effectiveness, efficacy and association to express the nexus or link between the response, outcome, or dependent variable and the independent, predictor, explanatory or antecedent variable [12–14].

For example, in the previous illustration, the purpose of the study was "To assess the DNA methylation (CH_3-C, Methyl Cytosine) as inverse gene expression differentials by subpopulation in pediatric ALL." The objective of a study is a concise statement describing the intent of the research. Such objectives can be evaluated from several standpoints or dimensions. For example, if the objective of a study is to assess the implication of sex hormone binding globulin (SHBG) in prostatic adenocarcinoma incidence and DNA methylation based on NGS cannot be measured but the plasma level of SHBG is utilized, hyper-DNA methylation remains an indirect measure termed "proxy." Then it is not an accurate or reliable objective. Therefore, in clinical, experimental and non-experimental studies, an accurate and valid study objective is that which is measurable. For example, if the objective of a study was to examine the DNA methylation of angiotensin-converting enzyme (ACE) II correlation in hypertension (HTn) severity and poor prognosis, the measurement of this aberrant epigenomic modulation of the ACE II gene as inverse gene expression (DNA hypermethylation) will be less severe and better prognosis, while the hypomethylation of ACE II implies more severity and poor HTn prognosis. Specifically, the conversion of ACE I to ACE II is indicative of increased peripheral resistance, hence elevated blood pressure (BP) and hypertension (HTn).

In practice, while the purpose of the study may not be easily differentiated from the objective, the research question remains a concise statement about the study objective. A research question's purpose is to imply what issue the research will address. Similarly, the purpose of the study is a broad scope of what the study intends to accomplish in terms of benefits to society, public health, medicine and science.

3.3.1 Purpose of Research or Study Objective

Study Objective/Research Purpose

- Purpose of study—why the study was conducted (completed study) or will be conducted (proposal)
- Intent of the study—the motivation for the study
- Expression of the main idea or concept behind the study
- Identification of independent and dependent variables in biomedical and epidemiologic studies

- **Hypothetical Example**: The purpose of the study was to determine the DNA methylation of the p27 gene in hepatocellular carcinoma relapses, with relapses as an outcome/response/dependent variable associated with the p27 DNA methylation as an independent/predictor/explanatory variable following the NGS among patients with remission and those with relapse (case-comparison design). This approach reflects the last paragraph of the introduction section of original articles in published manuscripts (Figure 3.3).

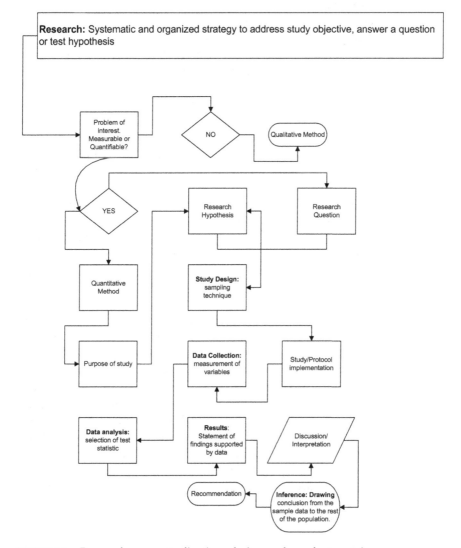

FIGURE 3.3 Research conceptualization, design and conduct matrix.

3.4 Research Questions and Study Hypotheses

3.4.1 Research Questions

Fundamental to clinical research is a clear statement of the question that is proposed to be answered. This question should be carefully selected and clearly defined prior to beginning to conduct research. For example, a research question may be framed in the context of trying to determine whether a new treatment, compared with the current or standard treatment, reduces the risk of coronary heart disease (CHD). Research questions could be primary or secondary. The primary question refers to the main outcome of the study. For example, "Does angiotensin-converting enzyme (ACE) inhibitor reduce the incidence of Hypertension?" A secondary research question aimed at a secondary outcome may assess physical activities in response to an ACE inhibitor such as Fosinopril. For example, the secondary research question may be stated as, "Are there racial/ethnic differences in improved HTn prognosis following ACE inhibitor use?" Additionally, another primary research question is: "Does Androgen Deprivation Therapy (ADT) prolong the survival of elderly men diagnosed with prostate cancer?" and the secondary question may be, "Are there racial differences in CaP survival in elderly men diagnosed with loco-regional disease and followed for the disease?"

Depending on the research question, participants may be randomly assigned to different treatments or procedures. This approach, which is called a human experiment or clinical trial, will be discussed at some length in the upcoming section on design. If a clinical trial is not feasible (ethical considerations), the researcher may collect data on participants (independent, dependent, or response variables and confounding) and conduct a non-experimental study. The information on the confounding variables is collected in order to control for the influence of the confounding on the response, dependent, or outcome variable since non-experimental studies' findings may be influenced by selection biases and confounding if not minimized and controlled for appropriately [12, 14, 15]. If the intent is to generalize from the research participants to a larger population, as is often the case in epidemiologic (non-experimental) and experimental studies, the investigator/epidemiologist will utilize probability sampling to select participants (sampling technique). This approach gives every study subject the same probability of being selected from the general population for inclusion in the study sample, and the variables to be studied are termed "random variables," which is required in inferential studies. In such a situation, statistical inference can then be applied to the study, implying the generalization of the findings beyond the sample studied to a larger or targeted population (Figure 3.4).

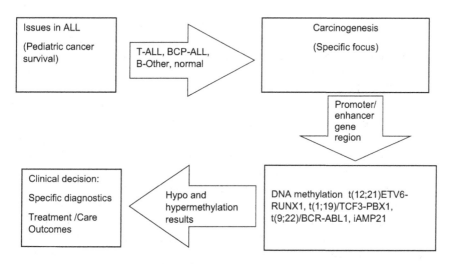

FIGURE 3.4   Research rationale and conceptualization—DNA methylation of ALL subtypes in survival differentials in pediatric ALL.

3.4.2   Study Hypothesis

Hypothesis testing is essential in quantitative study designs. The hypothesis of a study is a statement that provides the basis for the examination of the significance of the findings. Whenever an investigator wishes to make a statement beyond the sample data (descriptive statistics) or simply draw an inference from the data, hypothesis testing is required. A hypothesis is a statement about the population or simply the universe/world that is testable. An example of a hypothesis statement could be, "Selenium in combination with vitamin D decreases the risk of prostate cancer." To assess this association, the investigator needs to examine the data for evidence against the null hypothesis. If the data provide evidence against the null hypothesis (no association), the null hypothesis is rejected; in contrast, if the data fail to provide evidence against the null hypothesis, the null hypothesis is not rejected, thus negating any inclination to the alternative hypothesis of association between the response and the independent variable. While hypotheses will be described more in this text's companion, the biostatistics, it serves to note here that hypothesis testing includes the following:

a generation of the study hypothesis and the definition of the null hypothesis,
b determination of the level below which results are considered statistically significant, implying α level of 0.05, and
c identification and selection of the appropriate statistical test for determining whether to accept or reject the null hypothesis.

In determining whether or not an association exists, the investigator must first assume that the null hypothesis is true and then determine how likely the data collected from selenium with vitamin D are. Generally, if the data from selenium and Vitamin D in relation to prostate cancer are extremely unlikely should the null hypothesis be true, then there is evidence against the null hypothesis; in contrast, if the data in question are not unlikely if the null hypothesis were true, then there is no evidence against the null hypothesis. While hypotheses in medical and clinical sciences are often stated as alternative hypotheses, the testing of a hypothesis assumes the null—no difference. For example, there is no difference in prostate cancer risk among men who take selenium combined with vitamin D compared to those who do not. In clinical sciences, hypothesis testing involves single-group as well as two- and multiple-group comparison. Examples of such tests are single-group means using a single or one-sample t-test, population proportion using z-statistics (testing the difference between the sample proportion and hypothesized population proportion), differences between population proportions and differences between population means. The appropriate statistics and their assumptions are an essential part of these materials and are presented in detail in subsequent chapters.

Study Objective/Research. Purpose
Below are the basic descriptions of study purpose as well as the study intent:

- Purpose of study—why the study was conducted (completed study) or will be conducted (proposal)
- Intent of the study—the motivation for the study
- Expression of the main idea or concept behind the study
- Identification of independent and dependent variables in biomedical and epidemiologic studies

  - **Hypothetical Example:** The purpose of the study was to determine the risk of deep wound infection (outcome/response/dependent variable) associated with the intraoperative cell server (independent/predictor/explanatory variable) following spine fusion in children with cerebral palsy, using a retrospective cohort design (case only).

3.4.3   *Primary versus Secondary Outcomes*

The primary outcomes represent what the investigators intend to measure to answer their questions. This outcome is measured by the primary response variable. A primary response variable may be the incidence of a disease, disease severity, a biochemical end-point (such as prostate specific antigen (PSA) level) or a biomarker (such as for prostate cancer diagnosis). As an example, in a diabetes mellitus (DM) study, if the primary outcome is disease incidence, the response variable may be the blood-glucose ascertainment in a follow-up study of overweight and normal-weight adults until the diagnosis of DM is confirmed by well-defined clinical and laboratory measures.

Specifically, if the outcome is DM severity, the response variable may be measured by assessing retinopathy, the need for lower extremity amputation, erectile dysfunction in men, vascular stenosis and/or the occurrence of co-morbidities during the study period. With mortality as the primary outcome, death from all causes or from a given disease remains a clear, feasible and reliable measure of the outcome. For example, the effectiveness of androgen-deprivation therapy in the treatment of locoregional prostate cancer may be measured by the number of deaths due to prostate cancer or cause-nonspecific mortality occurring in the treatment arm (ADT) versus the control arm (non-ADT). These variables (response and independent) may be measured on a continuous, nominal or discrete scale, as will be illustrated in detail in the upcoming chapters. A study may also be conducted to assess other outcomes, which are not primary to the research question, termed secondary outcomes and measured by secondary variables. In this case, care should be taken to consider secondary outcomes that are more relevant to the primary research questions, since the more secondary outcome measures selected, the greater the likelihood that one will encounter a non-significant result as well as in-consistent and conflicting findings. A secondary response variable may be a biochemical failure, in which the primary response is death from the tumor. For example, if a study is conducted to examine the effectiveness of Tamoxifen in prolonging the survival of older women with nonoperable breast cancer, tumor grade/size may represent a secondary outcome measure, while mortal-ity remains the primary outcome measure.

3.4.4   Scales of Measurement of Variables

A continuous scale for the outcome measure (granted that it is clinically rel-evant, such as PSA level or blood-glucose level) carries an advantage of utiliz-ing a reduced sample size to show a difference between the treatment and control groups, should such an effect really exist, and facilitates the use of a more powerful test statistic, termed parametric (normality assumed). In con-trast, if the primary outcome measure is not death and the study population represents senior or older old adults with higher mortality risk, then there may be a sample size issue that may under-power the study, leading to type II error. These concepts are clearly described in upcoming chapters.

3.4.5   Clinical versus Population-Based Research

Clinical medicine focuses on individual patients. It is not evidenced-based un-less it is population-based. Population medicine, which may be used inter-changeably with population or public health, remains the collective effort of the society to remain healthy. To fulfill this task, public health utilizes sound research principles to conduct research into disease control and prevention at the population level. The management of individual patients in clinical medicine is based on the best available research data, which is derived from well-defined and measured evidence. Whereas population medicine or public health may represent the notion of preventive health practices at the population level, implying what the population does to remain healthy, clinical medicine is diagnostic and therapeutic.

In practice, there is an interrelationship between population and clinical medicine. The practice of clinical medicine or patient care is dependent on population-based data. For example, the use of antihistamines (H2 blockers) in gastric hyperacidity or anti-hypertensive drugs, such as beta-blockers, to control HTn in individual patients is based on data from clinical trials on the efficacy and community-based routine use of such agents and their effectiveness in the population. Consequently, the decision to place a patient on a chemoprophylactic agent for the prevention of cerebrovascular accidents is based on what is known about the agent at the population level and the probability that the individual patient may represent the population and therefore be responsive to the agent if administered in a comparable manner as in a clinical trial or non-experimental prospective studies (this is the basis of routine patient treatment).

3.6   Epidemiologic (Population-Based) Research

Epidemiologic research is not as simple as clinicians and researchers might assume. In the physical sciences, results hold the same under similar physical circumstances; however, epidemiologic investigation involves humans in specific populations, and since humans are genetically and psychosocially heterogeneous, the results could be paralyzed by confounding factors, rendering the findings nonfactual [11–13, 15]. Epidemiology is considered the basic and core science of public health and is simply defined as the study of the distribution and determinants of disease, disabilities, injuries and health-related events at the population level. With this definition, epidemiologic methods are not simple in terms of application, requiring basic education and training in some concepts like incidence rate involving person-time, incidence density, confounding, effect measure modifiers, causation and causal inference, association, random error quantification and the p-value function. It is because of this need to inform clinicians and biomedical researchers on the appropriate application of these concepts in the design and inference processes of research that this book was conceived. To illustrate the complexities of epidemiologic principles, let us consider two groups of patients. The average age of death for patients with infantile scoliosis (A) is 1.5 years, while the average age of death for patients with adolescent scoliosis (B) is 14 years. Does this mean that those in group A have a greater risk of dying? The age of death in this comparison does not reflect the risk of death but merely characterizes those who die. Thus, to maintain that one group is at a higher risk relative to the other without controlling for the age distribution of these two groups prior to comparison is epidemiologically fallacious. Second, the age at the onset of death does not account for the proportion of those who died. The materials in subsequent chapters will allow us to avoid such errors or fallacies in the interpretation of our results and to draw appropriate inferences.

Epidemiologic designs are generally used to estimate risk and measure incidence rate/density as well as prevalence. More complex designs are used to compare measures of disease occurrence, leading to causal prediction as well as the impact of disease in a defined human population. Epidemiologic designs or methods include ecological, cross-sectional (prevalence studies), case-control, cohort and hybrid.

3.7 Summary

The goal of clinical and population-based research in general is to provide useful data or information on the observed phenomenon, which is usually achieved through a methodical approach to answering the research question/s and testing the hypothesis. This goal is expressed in the attempt to draw inferences from the study results regarding the truth of the universe or targeted population. With this as the goal of research, investigators begin with research questions, formulate hypotheses (null and alternative), perform the test and answer the research questions. Clinical research is a systematic, empirical, critical and sometimes controlled investigation of phenomena in patients' settings (diagnostic, therapeutic and preventive). The approach could be divided into these categories: (1) research conceptualization, (2) design process and (3) statistical inference.

This process of scientific research conduct involves a well-defined problem statement, research questions, purposes, and potential benefits of the study to science and humanity; identification of the theory and assumptions; a search of background literature; measurement of variables; statement of researchable hypotheses; presentation of operational definitions and measurement; and selection of the appropriate study design. In addition, it requires determination of the methodology to fit the research question or hypothesis, development of an instrument or tools for data gathering, identification of an appropriate sampling technique, selection of a data analysis tool or statistical technique to test the hypothesis or answer the research question, and presentation of the results with interpretation and conclusions based on the data, as well as what the data suggests and recommendations for clinical research.

The purpose of a study is the statement of the overall objective of the study and identifies the independent (predictor or explanatory) and response (outcome or dependent) variables, as well as how the variables will be measured and the design to be used to achieve the expected relationship or association. The objective of the study describes the intent. Research questions and hypotheses are two basic ways of assessing the relationship or association between study variables. In quantitative studies, hypothesis testing is essential in drawing an inference or in making a statement beyond the sample data. Simply, hypothesis refers to a statement about the population or simply the universe/world that is testable.

The evidence from clinical research is dependent on how well the data has been interpreted regarding these elements:

1 biologic relevance of the findings
2 clinical importance of the observed data
3 statistical stability, which is the measure of how representative the sample is relative to the population; it is measured by the 95% confidence interval, as well as the p-value.

3.8   Questions for Review

1. Suppose that drug X is an established antimicrobial agent against postoperative deep wound infection after spine fusion in children with neuromuscular scoliosis. Investigators wish to study drug Y, a newly manufactured antimicrobial agent.

   a What is the research question and the purpose of the study? State the hypothesis to be tested.
   b What is the outcome variable, and what is an appropriate scale of measurement?
   c Which design or designs will be feasible in this study?
   d Would it be a good idea to have a placebo group in this study and compare three groups instead of two?

2 Suppose we wish to examine the relationship between breast cancer incidence and parity.

   a What would the hypothesis be?
   b How will the study population be selected?
   c Suppose you wish to compare the incidence rate of breast cancer between the exposed and the unexposed subjects, what would be an appropriate study design?
   d How should we assess the relationship between the outcome and independent variable in this example?

3 Consider a group of children aged 2–14 years with a high cholesterol level; you wish to see if there is familial aggregation of cholesterol levels.

   a Which study design would be adequate in examining the hypothesis in this context?
   b What is the hypothesis?
   c What other factors would you consider in assessing this relationship?

4 Assuming you are required to conduct a study on the decreased response of Nifedipine or Fosinopril, as anti-hypertensive agents, among African Americans with hypertension in the United States, and an aberrant epigenomic study is required:

   a What is the research question?
   b What sort of gene-specific alleles are required?
   c What is the specific epigenomic modulation mechanistic process required in this study?
   d What sort of analysis could be applied to determine inverse gene expression or downregulation of the transcriptome?

5 Discuss the scientific approach in epigenomic studies that results in induction-therapy recommendations prior to standard of care in the treatment of renal cell carcinoma or chronic myeloid leukemia (CML).

References

1 Hulley SB, Cummings SR, Browner WS et al. *Designing Clinical Research*, 2nd ed. (Philadelphia, PA: Lippincott, Williams & Wilkins, 2001).
2 Creswell JW. *Research Design: Qualitative, Quantitative and Mixed Methods Approaches*, 2nd ed. (Thousand Oaks, CA: Sage Publication, 2003).
3 Keppel G. *Design and Analysis: A Researcher's Handbook*, 3rd ed. (New York: Guilford, 1998).
4 Leventhal BG, Wittes RE. *Research Methods in Clinical Oncology*. (New York: Raven Press, 1988).
5 Friedman LM, Furberg CD, DeMets DL. *Fundamentals of Clinical Trials*, 3rd ed. (New York: Springer, 1988).
6 DuPont WD. *Statistical Modeling for Biomedical Researchers*. (Cambridge: Cambridge University Press, 2003).
7 Braitman LE. Statistical estimates and clinical trials. *J. Biopharm. Stat.* 1993;3:249–256.
8 Swinscow TDV, Campbell MJ. *Statistics at Square One*, 9th ed. (London: BMJ Books, 2002).
9 Altman DG. Statistics in medical journals. *Stat. Med.* 1982;1:59–71.
10 Rosner B. *Fundamentals of Biostatistics*, 5th ed. (Belmont, CA: Duxbury Press, 2000).
11 Holmes L Jr. *Applied Epidemiologic Principles and Concepts*. (Boca Raton, FL: Taylor & Francis Publisher, 2018).

12 Holmes L Jr. *Applied Biostatistical Principles & Concepts.* (Boca Raton, FL: Taylor & Francis Publisher, 2018).

13 Sackett DL, Richardson WS, Rosenberg W, Haynes RB. *Evidence-Based Medicine: How to Practice and Teach Evidence-Based Medicine*, 2nd ed. (Edinburg: Churchill Livingstone, 2000)

14 Katz DL. *Clinical Epidemiology & Evidence-Based Medicine: Fundamental Principles of Clinical Reasoning & Research.* (Thousand Oaks, CA: Sage, 2001).

15 Rothman K. *Epidemiology: An Introduction.* (New York: Oxford University Press, 2002).

4

DISEASE ASCERTAINMENT—
DIAGNOSTIC AND SCREENING TEST

4.1   Introduction

Medicine remains an inexact science, implying some amount of uncertainty in how we screen and diagnose disease, and the same applies to inference from clinical research data, given the genetic heterogeneity and aberrant epigenomic modulations of the patients we treat, observe and study. Clinical, medical and population health research also involve designs that examine the effect of a test on disease prognosis and outcome. Simply, a screening or diagnostic test is beneficial if survival is prolonged among those screened for the disease compared to those who are not screened. For example, the female breast cancer racial/ethnic survival outcome reflects the early stage at which the tumor is diagnosed. While the female breast cancer incidence is higher among whites, the survival disadvantage is higher among blacks/AA, which is explained in part by the late state at diagnosis given marginalized screening in blacks/AA population. Remarkably, the outcome of a diagnostic test is not the mere diagnosis, disease stage or grade of tumor, as in the Gleason Score used in prostate cancer (CaP) clinical assessment, but the mortality or morbidity that could be prevented among those who tested positive for the disease and were treated appropriately for the diagnosed condition.

The benefit of a diagnostic test depends on whether or not there are procedures and treatments in place to follow up on the true positives (patients or individuals with the symptoms who test positive for the disease). For example, to determine whether or not screening for prostate-specific antigen (PSA) prolongs survival or reduces the risk related to CaP, investigators may compare the rates of PSA among patients who died of CaP with controls who did not.

DOI: 10.4324/9781003094487-5

Medicine is a conservative science, and the practice of clinical medicine involves both art and science. The process by which clinical diagnosis is achieved remains complex, involving history, a review of the system, physical examination, laboratory data and neuroimaging, as well as probability reasoning. A screening test is performed on individuals who do not have the symptoms or signs of a disease or a specific health condition; for example, the use of PSA in asymptomatic (showing no signs or symptoms of CaP) African American men, 40–45 years of age, to assess the presence or absence of CaP in this population. A diagnostic test is performed in clinical medicine to acquire data on the presence (+ve) or absence (–ve) of a specific condition [1–3].

Specifically, epigenomic screening and disease confirmation, although not currently in place, will require sample assays to determine aberrant epigenomic modulation for disease. Epigenetic and epigenomic laboratory procedures involve the application of several laboratory techniques, depending on the nature and process of aberrant epigenomic modulation. The approach involves the following: (a) DNA immunoprecipitation-sequencing (DIP-seq), (b) chromatin immunoprecipitation-sequencing (ChIP-seq), (c) an assay for transposase-accessible chromatin using sequencing (ATAC-seq), (d) single-cell ATAC-seq (scATAC-seq) and single-cell multiome.

4.2   Diagnostic Test and Clinical Assessment

To address clearly and simply a diagnostic test approach, the following questions need to be addressed:

4.2.1   Why Conduct a Diagnostic Test?

A diagnostic test is performed to confirm the presence of a disease following the appearance of symptoms of an illness. For example, a 21-year-old white female presents with a mild fever and frequent and painful urination that is relieved after voiding the bladder. The physician suspects cystitis and recommends urinalysis for bacterial pathogen isolation. The test confirmed *E. coli* (gram-negative bacterial pathogen). The above example is illustrative of a diagnostic test, which simply confirms the diagnosis of bacterial cystitis in this hypothetical illustration. Additionally, if a male patient presents with CaP and is not responding to chemotherapy, the drug response needs to be examined through epigenomic diagnostics, reflecting DNA methylation (mDNA) and implying gene expression and protein synthesis as the specific drug receptors. The delay in such a diagnostic test could result in chemotherapy overdose, chemotoxicity and survival disadvantage. However, currently, such a test is univariable, requiring biomedical and clinical input in proceeding in this direction for enhanced therapeutics.

4.2.2   When is a Diagnostic Test Performed?

A diagnostic test could also be performed to:

1 Provide prognostic information in patients with a confirmed diagnosis of a disease, such as diabetes mellitus (DM), for example, a blood-glucose level. Additionally, it can be used to examine molecular sequencing and determine tumor subtypes, such as ependymoma, a cancer of the lining of the fourth ventricle of the brain, which has a poor prognosis without molecular sequencing and subtypes.
2 Monitor therapy to assess benefits or side effects, for example, to assess pseudoarthrosis among patients with adolescent idiopathic scoliosis (AIS) who underwent spine fusion to correct curve deformities.
3 Confirm that a person or patient is free from a disease. For example, though not a very reliable marker of CaP prognosis, the PSA level can be used to assess CaP remission in men diagnosed with locoregional CaP and treated for the disease with radical prostatectomy and radiation therapy (Figure 4.1).

4.2.3   What is a Screening Test, and What Are the Possible Results?

Screening is an effort to detect disease that is not readily apparent or risk factors for a disease in an at-risk segment of the population [3, 4]. This test can yield four possible outcomes or results:

1 true positive—positive test with the presence of disease
2 false positive—positive test in the absence of disease
3 false negative—negative test in the presence of disease
4 true negative—negative test in the absence of disease.

Diagnostic tests, results and implications of screening depend on both the prevalence of the disease and test performance. For example, rare diseases are associated with relatively frequent false-positives compared to true negatives, and common diseases are associated with relatively frequent false-negatives compared to true negatives. A screening test is generally inappropriate when the disease is either exceedingly rare or extremely common.

4.2.4   What Are the Measures of the Diagnostic Value of a Screening or Test?

Measures of the diagnostic value of a test are its sensitivity and specificity [1, 2]. These parameters have important implications for screening and clinical guidelines (Table 4.1).

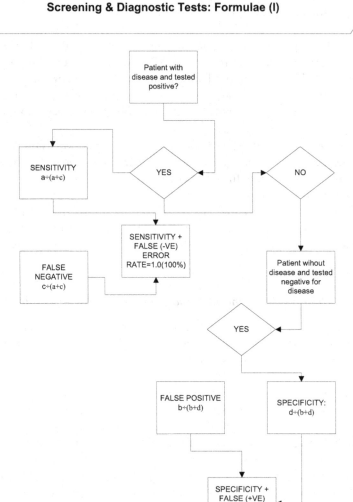

FIGURE 4.1 Diagnostic and screening test.

Notes and abbreviations: a = true positive, b = false positive, c = false negative and d = true negative. Sensitivity = a/a + c; specificity = d/b + d; positive predictive value (PPV) = a/a + b; negative predictive value = d/c + d; false positive rate = c/a + c and false negative rate = b/b + d.

TABLE 4.1 A 2 × 2 Contingent Table Illustrating Diagnostic Test Results

Test result	Population (target)	
	Disease	Non-disease or disease-free
Positive	a	b
Negative	c	d

Abbreviations and notes: a = true positive, b = false positive, c= false negative and d = true negative. Sensitivity = a/a + c; specificity = d/b + d; positive predictive value (PPV) = a/a + b; negative predictive value = d/c + d; false-positive rate = c/a + c and false-negative rate = b/b + d.

Sensitivity refers to the ability of a test to detect a disease when it is present. This measures the proportion of those with the disease who are correctly classified as diseased by the test.

Sensitivity = $a/(a + c)$

This implies subjects with true-positive test results (a)/(subjects with true-positive results + subjects with false-negative test results (a + c)). A test that is not sensitive is likely to generate a false-negative result (c). The false-negative error rate is given by the following: False-Negative Error Rate $=\Pr(T-\mid D+)$ $=c \div (a + c)$. This is otherwise termed beta error rate or a type II error. There is a relationship between sensitivity and false-negative error rate:

Sensitivity $[a/(a + c)]$ + False Negative Error Rate $= \Pr(T-\mid D+) =$ $[c \div (a + c)] = 1.0 (100\%)$

Specificity refers to the ability of test to indicate non-disease (disease-free) when no disease is present.

This is the measure of the proportion of those without disease who are correctly classified as disease-free by the test. Specificity is derived by:

Specificity $= d/(b + d)$

This implies subjects with true-negative test results (d)/(Subjects with true-negative result + Subjects with false-positive (b + d)). A test that is not specific is likely to generate false-positive results (b). False-positive error rate is calculated as follows:

False-Positive Error Rate $= \Pr(T+\mid D-) = b \div (b + d)$

There is a relationship between specificity and a false-positive error rate:

Specificity (d/b + d) + False Positive Error Rate (b/b + d) = 1.0 (100%)

4.2.5 What Are Predictive Values?

Predictive values refer to the probability of having the disease being tested for if the test result is positive and the probability of not having the disease being tested for if the result is negative [4, 5].

4.2.6 What Are the Types of Predictive Values?

There are two types of predictive values used in diagnostic/screening tests:

1 **Positive predictive value (PPV):** the probability of a test being positive given that the disease is present.
   Mathematically, **PPV** is given by the following equation:

   $$PD + \text{ or } PPV = a/\{a + [(pT+ \mid D-)pD-)]\} = a/\{a + b\}$$

   where PD+ = True positives/{True positives + False positives}. Using Bayes' theorem, PPV is the probability that an individual with a positive test result truly has the disease, which is the proportion of all positives (true and false) that are classified as true positives. PPV is thus the probability that a positive test result truly indicates the presence of disease.

2 **Negative predictive value (NPV),** or PD–, is the probability of disease absence following a negative test result. Mathematically, a NPV is given by the following equation:

   $$NPV = \text{True negatives}/\{\text{True negatives} + \text{False negatives}\} \rightarrow d/(d + b)$$

   Using Bayesian theorem:

   $$PD- = [\text{Specificity} \times (1 - \text{Prevalence})]/\{[\text{Specificity} \times (1 - \text{Prevalence})] + [\text{Prevalence} \times (1 - \text{Sensitivity})]\}$$

4.2.7 What is Disease Prevalence, and How is It Related to Positive Predictive Value?

Prevalence is the probability of the disease, while sensitivity, in comparison, is the probability of a positive test in those with the disease.

4.2.8   Relationship between Disease Prevalence, Sensitivity, Specificity and Predictive Value

- There is a relationship between disease prevalence, sensitivity, specificity and predictive values.
- The prevalence simply means the probability of the condition before performing the test (i.e., pretest probability).
- The predictive values refer to the probability of the disease being present or absent after obtaining the results of the test.
- Using the 2 × 2 table, PPV is the proportion of those with a positive test who have the disease $(a/(a + b))$, while the NPV is the proportion of those with a negative test who do not have the disease $(d/(c + d))$.
- The predictive values will vary with the prevalence of the disease or condition being tested for.
- Therefore, the probability of the disease before (prevalence) and the probability of the disease after (predictive value) will be interrelated, with the differences in predictive values driven by the differences in the prevalence of the disease.

4.2.9   What is Disease Prevalence, and How is It Related to Positive Predictive Value?

Prevalence is the probability of the disease, while sensitivity, in comparison, is the probability of a positive test in those with the disease.

Using Bayesian theorem: PD+ = (Sensitivity × Prevalence)/{[Sensitivity × Prevalence] + [(1 − Specificity)(1 − Prevalence)]}. Remember that sensitivity remains the probability of a positive test in those with the disease—$\{a/a = c\}$.

4.2.10   What Are Likelihood Ratios?

The likelihood ratio (LR) is the probability of a particular test result for an individual with the disease of interest divided by the probability of that test result for an individual without the disease of interest. There are two types of LRs: (1) LR positive (LR+) refers to the ratio of the sensitivity of a test to the false-positive error rate of the test. Here, it is mathematically given as follows:

LR+ = [a/(a + c)]/[b/(b + d)]
The LR+ = Sensitivity/(1 − Specificity).

The LR negative (LR−) refers to the ratio of false-negative error rate to the specificity of the test. Here it is mathematically given as follows:

LR– = {c/(a + c)}/{d/(b + d)}

The LR– = (1 – Sensitivity)/Specificity.

- What is the measure of the separation between positive and negative tests?

The ratio of LR+ to LR– refers to the measure of separation between the positive and negative test. Here it is mathematically given as follows:

LR+ to LR– ratio = LR+/LR–

This is an approximation of the odds ratio, OR = ad/bc, using the 2 × 2 contingent table. The odds ratio is the ratio of the odds of exposure in the disease to the odds of exposure in the non-disease. The odds of disease (lung cancer) = Probability that lung cancer will occur (P)/Probability that it will not occur (1 – P).

VIGNETTE 4.1

Consider 160 persons appearing in a deep vein thrombosis (DVT) clinic for a lower extremity Doppler ultrasound study. If 24 out of 40 subjects with DVT tested positive for DVT, and 114 out of 120 without DVT tested negative, calculate the following:

(1) sensitivity, (2) specificity, (3) false-positive error rate, (4) false-negative error rate, (5) PPV, (6) NPV, (7) LR positive, (8) LR negative, (9) ratio of LR+ to LR– and (10) prevalence of DVT.

Generate a 2 × 2 contingent table and perform the computation.

Computation: (1) Sensitivity = 24/40 = 0.6 (60%); (2) Specificity = 0.95 (95%); (3) FP error rate = b/(b + d) = 6/120 = 0.05 (5%); (4) FN error rate = c/(a + c) = 16/40 = 0.4 (40%); (5) PPV = 24(a)/30(a + b) = 0.8(80%); (6) NPV = 114(d)/130(c + d) = 0.88 (88%); (7) LR+ = {a/(a + c)} = Sensitivity/{b/(b + b)} (False-positive error rate) → 0.6/0.05 = 12.0; (8) LR– = False-negative error rate {(c/(a +c)/Specificity {d/(d + b)} → 0.4/0.95 = 0.42; (9) LR+ to LR– ratio = LR+/LR– = 12/0.42 = 28.57 and (10) Prevalence of DVT = (a +c)/(a + b + c + d) → 40/160 = 0.25 (25%).

False-positive error rate (alpha error rate or type I error rate) simply refers to an error committed by asserting that a proposition is true when it is indeed not true (false). If a test is not specific, this will lead to the test falsely indicating the presence of a disease in non-disease subjects (cell B; see accompanying table). The rate at which this occurs is termed the false-positive error rate and is mathematically given by B/(B + D). False-positive error rate is related to specificity: FP rate + Specificity = 1.0(100%).

4.2.11   What is Multiple or Sequential Testing?

Multiple or sequential testing refers to the following:
Parallel testing (ordering tests together)—the rationale is to increase sensitivity, but specificity is compromised. There are four possible outcomes in parallel testing:

1 T1+ T2+ (disease is present)
2 T1+ T2– (further testing)
3 T1– T2+ (further testing)
4 T1– T2– (disease is absent).

1 Sensitivity (net) = (Sensitivity T1 + Sensitivity T2) – Sensitivity T1 × Sensitivity T2.
2 Specificity (net) = Specificity T1 × Specificity T2.
3 Individual tested positive on either test is classified as positive.
4 Appropriate when false negative is main concern.

Serial testing refers to using two tests in a series, with test 2 performed only on those individuals who are positive on test 1 (Tables 4.2 and 4.3).

4.2.12   Disease Screening: Principles, Advantages and Limitations

Population screening refers to early screening and treatment in large groups in order to reduce morbidity or mortality from the specified disease among the screened. Screening for the purpose of disease control or mortality reduction involves the examination of asymptomatic or preclinical cases for the purpose of correctly classifying the diseased as positive and the non-diseased as negative [1–3].

4.2.13   Diagnostic or Screening Test Accuracy/Validity

Diagnostic or screening test accuracy/validity refers to the ability of the test to accurately distinguish those who do and do not have a specific disease. Sensitivity and specificity are traditionally used to determine the validity of a diagnostic test. Sensitivity is the ability of the test to classify correctly those who have the disease or specific/targeted disorder. Sensitivity is represented by $a/(a + c)$ in a 2 × 2 contingent table. "SnNout" is used to describe sensitivity, meaning that when "sen"sitivity is high, an "n"egative result rules "out" diagnosis. Specificity is the ability of the test to classify correctly those without the disease as non-diseased. Specificity is represented by $d/(b + d)$. "SpPin," which is used to describe specificity, implies that a very high specificity with a positive result effectively rules in the diagnosis.

The predictive value of the test addresses its effectiveness in accurately identifying those with the disease and those without. The PPV of the test addresses

TABLE 4.2 Screening and Diagnostic Test

Test Parameters	Estimation	Interpretation
True positive (TP)	A (2 × 2 table)	Number of individuals with the disease who have a positive test result
True negative (TN)	D (2 × 2 table)	Number of individuals without the disease who have a negative test result
False positive (FP)	C (2 × 2 table)	Number of individuals without the disease who have a positive test result
False negative (FN)	B (2 × 2 table)	Number of individuals with the disease who have a negative test result
Sensitivity = True positive rate (TPR)	TP/(TP + FN)	The proportion of individuals with the disease who have a positive test result
1 – Specificity = False-positive rate (FPR)	FN/(TP + FN)	The proportion of individuals with the disease who have a negative test result
Specificity = True negative rate (TNR)	TN/(TN + FP)	The proportion of individuals without the disease who have a negative test result
1 – Specificity = False-positive rate (FPR)	FP/(TN + FP)	The proportion of individuals without the disease who have a positive test result
Positive predictive value	TP/(TP + FP)	The probability that a patient with a positive test result will have the disease
Negative predictive value	TN/(TN + FN)	The probability that a patient with a negative test result will not have the disease
Likelihood ratio of a positive test result (LR+)	Sensitivity/(1 – Specificity)	The increase in the odds of having the disease after a positive test result
Likelihood ratio of a negative test result (LR–)	(1 – Sensitivity)/Specificity	The decrease in the odds of having the disease after a negative test result

Notes and abbreviations: This table is based on the following 2 × 2 contingency table, where the disease is represented in the column and the test results are on the row. *Bayes' theorem* refers to posttest odds, which are estimated by Pretest Odds × Likelihood Ratio (the odds of having or not having the disease after testing). *Accuracy of the test* is measured by (TP + TN)/(TP + TN + FP + FN) and is the probability that the results of a test will accurately predict the presence or absence of disease. Abbreviations: true positive (TP), false positive (FP), false negative (FN), true negative (TN).

TABLE 4.3 A 2 × 2 Contingency Table on Disease Sensitivity and Positivity

	Disease (+)	*Disease (−)*
Test (+)	(A) TP	(B) FP
Test (−)	(C) FP	(D) TN

Notes and abbreviations: a = true positive, b = false positive, c= false negative and d = true negative. True positive (TP), false positive (FP), false negative (FN) and true negative (TN).

the question: if the test result is positive in an individual, what is the probability that such an individual had the disease? This is estimated as follows: $a/(a + b)$. The NPV addresses the probability of an individual with a negative test being disease-free. This is estimated by $d/(c + d)$. The false-positive error rate is estimated by $1 - \text{specificity} = b/(b + d)$. The false-negative error rate is estimated by $1 - \text{sensitivity} = c/(a + c)$. Prevalence $= (a + c)/(a + b + c + d)$. LR+, which is the LR for a positive test, is estimated by Sensitivity$/(1 - \text{specificity})$. LR−, which is the LR for a negative test, is estimated as follows: $(1 - \text{Sensitivity})/\text{Specificity}$. The posttest probability is estimated by posttest odds$/(\text{posttest odds} + 1)$, where pretest odds are estimated by Prevalence$/(1 - \text{Prevalence})$ and posttest odds by Pretest odds × LR.

VIGNETTE 4.2

Consider a population of 2,000 people of whom 200 have unicameral bone cysts and 1,800 do not. If 160 with the disease were correctly identified as positive by the test, 40 were not. Of the 1,800 who did not have the disease, 1,600 were correctly classified as negative. Calculate (1) sensitivity, (2) specificity, (3) PPV and (4) NPV.

Solution: (1) Sensitivity $= a/(a + c)$; substituting: $160 \div 200 = 80\%$; (2) Specificity $= d(d + b) = 1,600 \div 1,800 = 89\%$; (3) PPV $= a/(a + b) = 160 \div 360 = 44.4\%$ and (4) NPV $= d/(c + d) = 1,600 \div 1,640 = 97.6\%$.

4.3   What is a Receiver Operating Characteristic (ROC) Curve?

The receiver operating characteristic (ROC), which is derived from electronics, was used to measure the ability of the radar operators to differentiate signals from noise. The ROC curve is a graphic approach to illustrating the relationship between the cutoff point that differentiates positive and normal results in a screening test and the influence of this cutoff point on the sensitivity and specificity of a test. This curve is constructed by selecting several cutoff points and using them to determine the sensitivity and specificity of the test. The graph is then constructed by plotting the sensitivity (true positive) on the Y-axis as a function of 1 – specificity (false-positive rate/proportion) on the X-axis [sensitivity versus (1 – specificity)]. The area under the ROC curve provides some measure of the accuracy of the test and is useful in comparing the accuracy of two or more tests. Simply, the larger area, the better or more accurate the test. In interpreting the area under the ROC curve (0.5–1.0), a value of 1.0 is indicative of a perfect test, while 0.5 represents a poor test; this implies that an ideal test is that which reaches the upper left corner of the graph (all true positive without false-positive results).

What is the relationship between disease prevalence and predictive value? There is a positive relationship between disease prevalence and predictive values; thus, the higher the prevalence in the population at risk or screened population, the higher the PPV.

4.3.1 Advantages and Disadvantages of Screening

Screening is most productive and efficient if it is directed at a high-risk population. It may motivate participants to follow a recommendation after the screening and seek medical services given positive test results. In terms of disadvantages of screening, if the entire population is screened and the condition is infrequent (low prevalence), this will imply a waste of resources, yielding few detected cases compared to the effort invested in the screening.

4.3.1.1 Early Disease Detection: Issues

What are the benefits of screening?

Early disease detection: The natural history of a disease involves the following stages:

a a preclinical phase, which is the phase that may be termed the biologic or psychological onset, but the symptoms have not yet occurred;
b a clinical phase, which is the period after which the symptoms occurred;
c a detectable preclinical phase, which is the natural stage of the disease where the disease is detected by screening;
d lead time, which is the interval by which the time of diagnosis is advanced by screening and early detection of disease relative to the usual time of diagnosis and
e a critical point, which refers to a point in the natural history of the disease in which the condition is potentially curable, implying optimal treatment potential. The inability to identify a critical point in the natural history of a disease through screening and early detection calls into question the benefit of screening.

4.3.1.2   Effectiveness and Benefits of Screening

a mortality reduction in the high-risk population screened
b reduction in case fatality
c increase in the percent of asymptomatic cases
d minimized complications
e reduction in recurrent cases or malignancies
f improvement in the quality of life.

The issues in screening include these elements: (1) sensitivity and specificity of the screening test as well as the predictive values, (2) false-positive test results, (3) cost of early detection, (4) emotional and physical adverse effects of screening, and (5) benefit of screening.

4.3.2   Biases in Disease Screening and Detection

1 referral bias, also referred to as volunteer bias
2 length-biased sampling associated with prognostic selection—this bias refers to a selection bias in which screening involves the selection of cases of disease with better prognosis
3 lead-time bias
4 over-diagnosis bias

4.3.3   What is Lead-Time Bias?

Lead-time bias refers to the apparent increase in survival time after diagnosis resulting from an earlier time of diagnosis rather than a later time of death.

4.3.4   What is Length Bias?

This is a form of selection bias and refers to the tendency, in a population screening effort, to detect preferentially the longer, more indolent cases of any particular disease.

VIGNETTE 4.3

Consider a new screening program for pediatric chronic myeloid leukemia (CML) in Delaware State, USA. The CML screening program used a test that is effective in screening for early stage ALL. Assume that there is no effective treatment for CML, and, as such, the screening results do not change the natural history or course of CML. Second, assume that the rates observed are based on all known cases of CML, and that there are no changes in the quality of death certification for CML. With these assumptions, a What will be the influence of this screening test on incidence and prevalence proportion during the first year of this program?

b What will be the implication of this screening on the case-fatality and mortality rate of CML during the first year of CML screening?

Solutions: (a) There will be an increase in both incidence rate and prevalence proportion. (b) There will be a decrease in the case-fatality rate while the mortality rate will remain constant because of the assumption that changes were not observed with respect to the quality of death certification.

4.4 Disease Screening: Diagnostic Tests and Clinical Reasoning

4.4.1 What is Clinical Reasoning?

The process by which clinicians channel their thinking toward a probable diagnosis is classically thought of as a mixture of pattern recognition and "hypothetic-deductive" reasoning. The reasoning process depends on medical knowledge in areas such as disease prevalence and pathophysiological mechanisms. Teaching on the process of reasoning, as diagnostic tests provide new information, has included modifications of Bayes' theorem in an attempt to get clinicians to think constructively about pretest and posttest possibilities.

Clinical decision-making is guided, by and large, by statistical and epidemiologic principles, as well as biologic and clinical reasoning. The understanding of the former is the purpose of this book, which is not intended to place statistical stability in results interpretation over sound biologic theories and clinical judgment in clinical research conceptualization, design, conduct and interpretation of results. A sound clinical judgment comes with experience, but such experience, in order not to be biased, ought to be guided by some statistical and epidemiologic principles, including but not limited to probability concepts (sensitivity, specificity and predictive value), Bayes' theorem, risk and predisposition to disease. Therefore, since clinical decision-making involves some risk acceptance, an understanding of probability serves to guide alternatives to treatment while assessing the risk and benefit of therapeutics.

VIGNETTE 4.4

A 68-year-old American Indian woman presents with a hip fracture. She has a history of metabolic fracture and was previously diagnosed with osteoporosis. The clinical scenario involves the estimation of the probability of hip fracture in this individual, and the clinical impression from previous cases indicates a common presentation of this condition in this subpopulation of age with a concurrent diagnosis of osteoporosis. The probability of response to treatment is dependent on the response of similar patients in the past, which is indicative of statistical reasoning. Although not a very good example to illustrate the application of diagnostic testing, the risk inherent in this case could be seen in the diagnosis of a hip fracture resulting in a false-positive or false-negative test result. Also the natural history of hip fracture may influence the clinical judgment in terms of the planned therapeutics. Clinical reasoning is also brought to question when considering alternative treatment.

As sound clinical reasoning (avoiding biases) continues to shape therapeutics, there remains the necessity of clinicians being able to appraise clinical and scientific literature for evidence, and the volumes of clinical and epidemiologic studies become the basis of clinical decision-making. Clinicians must understand how outcome studies are conducted and how the results obtained from these studies can be used in clinical decision-making involving care improvement and patient safety. The intent is not to train physicians or clinicians to become statisticians but to refine the already available skills in order to provide evidence-based care that is optimal through the utilization of results from internally (biases, confounding, random error) and externally (generalizability) valid studies.

4.4.1.1 Balancing Benefits and Harmful Effects in Medicine

Clinicians are interested in knowing the impact of treatment or intervention on individual patients. A large impact, relative to a small one, is of interest to both the clinician and his or her patient. The relative risk (RR) and absolute risk (AR) are two concepts that are extrapolated to determine risk in individual patients. The AR reduction is used to assess whether the benefit of treatment outweighs the adverse effects.

We present these concepts in detail in the chapter on the measure of disease association and effect, but here it suffices to provide a basic understanding of RR reduction (RRR), AR reduction (ARR), number needed to treat (NNT) and number needed to harm (NNH). Simply, the RRR refers to the difference in event rates between two groups, implying a proportion of event rate in the control (ERC) or untreated group. Suppose 40 patients had recurrent cystitis out of 100 patients treated initially with erythromycin (control group), and 30 patients had recurrent cystitis out of 100 patients treated initially with erythromycin plus amoxicillin (treatment group). What is the RRR? The RRR is the AR difference (40–30%) divided by the ERC group (40%).

The RRR = AR difference (ARD)/ERC, where Absolute rate difference (ARD) = ERC – Event rate in the treatment group, substituting 40 – 30/40 = 25%. This means that recurrent cystitis was 25% lower in the treatment group compared to the control. What is the ARR? Also termed risk difference, it is the arithmetic difference between two event rates expressed as the ERC minus the event in the treatment (ERT). Substituting, ARR = ERC – ERT = 40% – 30% = 10%.

The NNT simply reflects the consequences of treating or not treating patients, given a specified therapy. NNT may be described as the number of patients who would have to be treated for one of them to benefit. Mathematically, NNT is estimated by dividing 100 by the ARR expressed as a percentage (100/ARR). NNT could also be expressed as a proportion: 1/ARR. As ARR increases, NNT decreases, and inversely, as ARR decreases, NNT increases.

VIGNETTE 4.5

If the risk of stroke is 1.5 among hypertensive patients treated for the disease with a diuretic and 2.5 among the controls, how many hypertensive patients are needed to be treated (NNT)? What is the estimated ARR and NNT?

Solution: ARR = ERC – ERT. Substituting: 2.5 – 1.5 = 1.0. NNT = 1/ARR, substituting 100/1.0. Therefore, to prevent one incident of stroke, we need to treat 100 cases of hypertension.

The NNH is expressed as the inverse of the AR increase (1/ARI). The NNH represents the number of patients required to be treated for one of them to experience an adverse effect. Mathematically, NNH is estimated as 100/ARI, expressed as a percentage. NNT could also be expressed as a proportion: 1/ARI.

VIGNETTE 4.6

If the risk of developing postoperative infection in cerebral palsy children with scoliosis is 2.9 among those with rod instrumentation and 1.9 among those who received spinal fusion without instrumentation, examine the risk associated with unit rod instrumentation. What is the estimated ARI and the NNH?

Solution: ARI = Risk in cases (exposed) – Risk in control (unexposed) – Re – Ru. Substituting: 2.9 – 1.9=1.0. NNH = 100/ARI = 100/1.0. Consequently, we need to treat 100 patients (spinal fusion) in order for one patient to develop postoperative infection.

4.5 Detection and Ascertainment of Epigenomic Modulations: Clinical and Laboratory Approach

Epigenetic and epigenomic laboratory procedures involved the application of several laboratory techniques depending on the nature and process of aberrant epigenomic modulation. The approach involves the following: (a) DIP-seq, (b) ChIP-seq), (c) an ATAC using sequencing (ATAC-seq, (d) single-cell ATAC-seq (scATAC-seq) and single-cell multiome. These processes basically involved the main epigenomic modulation mechanisms, mainly, mDNA, histone acetylation, phosphorylation, non-coding RNA, chromatin, etc. [6].

4.5.1 DNA Immunoprecipitation-Sequencing (DIP-Seq)

DIP-seq is an antibody-based technology to profile the genome-wide distribution of DNA-associated epigenetic marks such as 5-methylcytosine (5mC), 5-hydroxymethylcytosine (5hmC), 5-formylcytosine (5fC) and 5-carboxylcytosine (5caC). The Epigenomics Development Laboratory and Recharge Center offers DIP-seq services using genomic DNA (2.5–10 µg) isolated from cell lines, fluorescence-activated cell sorting (FACS)-purified cells, buffy coat samples, tissues and FFPE-archived tissues [6–8].

4.5.2 Chromatin Immunoprecipitation-Sequencing (ChIP-Seq)

ChIP-seq is a valuable and widely used epigenetic approach for studying genome-wide protein-DNA interactions in cells and tissues. The Epigenomics Development Laboratory and Recharge Center offers standard or Tn5 transposase-based ChIP-seq services, depending on sample size (50,000 to 10 million cells). Suitable samples include cell lines, FACS-purified cells, whole blood, buffy coat samples, peripheral blood mononuclear cells (PBMC), frozen tissues, formalin-fixed, paraffin-embedded (FFPE) tissues and spike-in normalization.

4.5.3 Assay for Transposase-Accessible Chromatin Using Sequencing (ATAC-Seq)

The ATAC-seq provides information about open and accessible regions of chromatin that are indicative of active regulatory regions. Sample types suitable for this assay are around 50,000 cells or equivalent and include cell lines, buffy coat samples, sorted cells and frozen tissues.

4.5.4 Single-Cell ATAC-Seq (scATAC-Seq) and Single-Cell Multiome

The scATAC-seq provides information about genome-wide chromatin accessibility of thousands of individual cells in parallel, allowing identification of subpopulations of cells within a heterogeneous population that would otherwise be lost in standard bulk ATAC-seq. Sample types suitable for this assay include cell lines and sorted cells, requiring approximately 50,000–100,000 cells. The single-cell multiome combines scATAC-seq and scRNA-seq assays to accomplish simultaneous profiling of gene expression and chromatin accessibility from the same cell. Sample types suitable for this assay include cell lines and sorted cells, requiring approximately 50,000–100,000 cells.

4.5.5 Malignant Neoplasm and Epigenomic Detection and Screening

Epigenomic modulations, which reflect the cellular ability to respond to injury or insult, vary across race as well as sex and therefore may explain in part the survival disadvantage of black children relative to whites with acute lymphoblastic leukemia (ALL). These epigenomic changes begin very early in life, commencing at gametogenesis, in utero and postnatally, and reflect every day circumstances that result in the gene and environment interactions [8–10]. Epigenomic lesions have been observed to be several and most prevalent in T Cell-ALL relative to B Cell-ALL. Specifically, the gene and social-environment interaction that introduces methylation of the DNA and influences transcription factors and protein synthesis may result in abnormal cellular proliferation, implying leukomogenesis. In addition, the histone protein modification by acetylation process may result in a mutation that reflects an abnormal protein synthesis, either structural or regulatory, which is implicated in leukomogenesis by restricting DNA access and the subsequent transcriptome impairment [11]. The understanding of epigenomic modulations and the mechanistic process in gene and environment interaction in leukemic genes may facilitate specific risk characterization and induction therapy with demethylase building blocks prior to primary therapies in the treatment of pediatric ALL, thus narrowing the black-white risk differences in ALL mortality.

Available data on relapsed and remission T-ALL mDNA and mRNA sequencing inverse correlation and the stratification of such aberrant epigenomic modulation of the candidate genes involved in leukemic transformation (STAT5, MLL11, RB1, PTEN, IL-7R, KRAS, TLX1, TLX3, NKX2-1, LYL1, IL-7R, JAK1, JAK3, etc.) by sex and race will provide a further and more comprehensive explanation of the observed racial disparities in ALL survival, implicative of aberrant epigenomic screening and detection in ALL studies and mortality variances or disparities reduction. Specifically, epigenomic modulation reflects the gene and environment interaction involving the CpG island at the enhancer-promoter gene region but does not involve DNA sequence (mutational alteration in the underlying DNA) as stated earlier. The detection of aberrant modulation requires systematic analysis of mDNA and histone modifications such as acetylation and the correlated gene expression via mRNA sequencing [12, 13]. Such initiatives will lead to specific risk characterization, induction therapy through the demethylation process, transcription factors or protein accessibility, gene expression or upregulation, and the required biomolecules as chemotherapeutic agent receptors and subsequent treatment responses, minimizing dose escalation and chemotoxicity. Subsequently, given the restricted explanatory model of T-ALL in black-white differences in pediatric ALL survival, urgent epigenomic investigation of T-ALL relapse cases is required, which will involve candidate signaling pathway genes such as NOTCH1 and cell cycle regulator genes (CDKN2A (p16) and

CDKN2B (p15), bisulfite pyrosequencing, mRNA sequencing for mDNA and inverse gene expression correlation via next-generation sequencing (NGS). Therefore, to provide further explanation for the observed survival advantage of black and male children with ALL, the mDNA analysis implying the detection of epigenetic marks will require subpopulation samples, namely race/ethnicity and sex [12].

Normal hematopoietic cell development, differentiation and maturation require tightly controlled regulation of mDNA, histone modification and non-coding RNA expression: mDNA → epigenomic modulation → (1) gene expression, (2) genomic stability maintenance and (3) cellular differentiation [13]. Studies have implicated aberrant epigenomic modification/modulation in ALL pathogenesis (carcinogenesis). However, studies are lacking on subpopulation investigations, such as race and sex, on specific risk characterization in prognostic prediction and therapeutic decision-making in pediatric ALL.

Cancer epigenetics/epigenomic research is in an exciting phase of translational epigenomics, where novel epigenome therapeutics such as induction therapy are being developed for application in clinical settings [12, 13]. A range of different epigenetic "marks" or "signatures" can activate or repress gene expression. While aberrant epigenomic alterations are associated with most clinical conditions, epigenetic dysregulation have a substantial and significant causal role in ALL etiology, prognosis, relapses and survival. Specifically, epigenetically disrupted stem or progenitor cells have an early role in neoplastic transformations, while lesions or aberrations of epigenetic regulatory mechanisms controlling gene expression in cancer remain a contributing factor in ALL prognosis and mortality. The reversibility of epigenetic marks provides the possibility that the activity of key cancer genes and pathways can be regulated as a therapeutic approach. The growing availability of a range of chemical agents which can affect epigenome functioning has led to a range of epigenetic-therapeutic approaches for cancer and intense interest in the development of second-generation epigenetic drugs such as "Demethylase" agents as induction therapy, implying greater specificity and efficacy in clinical settings, thus enhancing precision medicine initiatives and optimizing care across all subpopulations of children with ALL, especially blacks and males. In effect, subpopulation differences in these lesions or aberrations remain a future prospect in rendering pediatric ALL racial and sex disparities in survival a history.

4.5.6   *Aberrant Epigenomic Mechanistic Process*

mDNA remains the most widely examined or assessed epigenetic mechanistic process. Specifically, the most commonly utilized mDNA pattern, 5mC, reflects the transfer of a methyl group (CH_3) to the C5 position of cytosine within CpG dinucleotides through an enzymatic process carried out by a group of DNA methyltransferases (DNMTs) [14]. Several CpG dinucleotides are often clustered together in a certain regulatory region, such as the promoter or enhancer gene region (CpG islands), which frequently participates in gene transcriptional regulation [15]. mDNA plays a substantial role in regulating various physiological and pathological processes, while aberrant mDNA is often associated with multiple disease developments, especially malignant neoplasms and CVDs.

Specifically, the most common way to influence biological procedures through mDNA is through gene expression control via dynamic regulation of the methylation status of CpG islands in the regulatory region of a specific gene [16, 17]. Hypermethylation of CpG islands in the gene regulatory region such as the promoter is normally associated with a compacted or closed chromatin structure, resulting in transcriptional silencing of the affiliated gene. By contrast, hypomethylation of CpG islands leads to an open chromatin structure, which is generally associated with gene transcriptional activation. Moreover, mDNA is also important in modulating various biological processes such as embryonic development, genomic imprinting, X inactivation, cellular differentiation and proliferation [17, 18]. Thus, aberrations of mDNA occurring within the promoter regions of critical tumor-related genes could result in dysregulation of gene expression such as tumor suppressor gene silencing and/or oncogenic activation, ultimately leading to tumorigenesis. Therefore, a precise and efficient method for detecting the exact mDNA contents is critical to elucidate the essential roles of mDNA in biological procedures and to enhance the development of novel diagnostic and therapeutic targets.

In addition to mDNA, chromatin modification is considered another important epigenetic mechanism that plays a key role in controlling gene transcription. Chromatin remodeling regulates gene expression through posttranslational modifications of histone proteins by a number of chemical processes, including, but not limited to, acetylation and methylation, which typically occur on specific lysine residues of core histone tails. Different from mDNA and histone modification convey a unique identity to the nucleosome that regulates transcriptional activity in a more robust and dynamic pathway during different biological stages. For example, increased histone acetylation is correlated with transcriptional activation, whereas histone deacetylation (HDACs) normally leads to gene transcription silencing. Histone methylation-induced gene transcriptional regulation is more complicated, showing both site-specific and methylation pattern-dependent indices. For instance, methylation of lysine residue K4 of histone H3 results in the transcriptional activation of chromatin regions, whereas methylation of lysine residue K9 of histone H3 usually leads to transcriptional repression [18].

The mechanisms by which histone modifications regulate gene transcription have been well documented. The most acceptable concept is that chromatin structure changes caused by histone modifications can directly change the spatial conformation of the DNA polymer, leading to accessibility changes of key transcriptional factors and/or epigenetic modulators to the core gene regulatory region of DNA and subsequently altering transcriptional activity. Multiple enzymes have been reported to actively catalyze the processes of histone modifications, such as the histone acetyltransferases (HATs), HDACs and histone methyltransferases (HMTs) [8]. These enzymes play major roles not only in regulating histone modification patterns through reversible enzymatic activities but also in maintaining chromatin configurations that allow faithful epigenetic inheritance. With the epigenetics field rapidly expanding, exploration of novel and advanced technologies for better illumination of biological consequences of individual epigenetic traits will be revolutionary in this advancing scientific area. However, reliability in the interpretation of these epigenomic data requires examining the possible confounding factors in the nexus between aberrant epigenomic modulations, such as mDNA as hypo- or hypermethylation, histone modification and non-coding RNA, in disease causation, prognosis and survival [19].

4.6   Summary

Clinical research is conducted primarily to improve therapeutics and prevent disease occurrence in clinical settings in contrast to population-based research. This effort involves adequate conceptualization, design process and conduct, analysis and accurate interpretation of the results, which are achieved through a joint effort of clinician and biostatistician. The selection of patients depends on accurate ascertainment of disease, implying a screening/diagnostic test that is capable of classifying those with the disease as test-positive (sensitivity) and those without it as test-negative (specificity). Screening is a particular form of disease detection test which is applied to a population at risk for developing a disease, such as CaP (PSA for older men, 50 years and older), in an attempt to diagnose CaP earlier than the natural history would manifest it. The intent is to diagnose CaP early where it is treatable and curable. Diagnostic tests are performed to confirm the presence of a disease following the appearance of symptoms of an illness.

The prevalence of disease simply means the probability of the condition before performing the test, meaning pretest probability. The predictive values refer to the probability of the disease being present or absent after obtaining the results of the test. Using the 2 × 2 table, the PPV is the proportion of those with a positive test who have the disease $[a/(a + b)]$, while the NPV is the proportion of those with a negative test who do not have the disease $[d/(c + d)]$. The predictive values will vary with the prevalence of the disease or condition being tested for. Therefore, the probability of the disease before (prevalence) and the probability of the disease after (predictive value) will be interrelated, with the differences in predictive values driven by the differences in the prevalence of the disease. Sensitivity and specificity are properties of a diagnostic test and should be consistent when the test is used in similar patients and in similar settings. Predictive values, although related to the sensitivity and specificity of the test, will vary with the prevalence of the condition or disease being tested. The difference in sensitivity and specificity of the test is most likely a result of it not being administered in similar conditions (patients and settings). The screening test should be highly sensitive (sensitivity) while the diagnostic test should be highly specific (specificity). As the cutoff point between positive and negative results changes, the sensitivity and specificity of the test will be influenced. This relationship is illustrated by the ROC curve, which assesses the extent to which a screening test can be used to discriminate between those with and without disease and to select the cutoff point to characterize normal and abnormal results.

The advantages and limitations of screening remind us of the balanced clinical judgment involved in recommending large-population screening tests. The common biases in screening include length-bias sampling, lead-time bias, over-diagnosis bias, and volunteer or referral bias (where those screened for the disease are healthier than the general population, thus influencing the conclusion regarding the benefit of screening). These systematic errors are all selection biases and, if not considered, have the tendency to affect the conclusions regarding the benefits of screening.

Often, clinicians may want to know the benefits or risks of treating a future or potential patient. In assessing the benefit-versus-risk ratio, the NNT and the NHH are practical alternatives to RRR or ARR in assessing the treatment effect. NNT remains a concise and clinically more useful way of presenting intervention effect. The NNT simply reflects the consequences of treating or not treating patients, given a specified therapy. The question remains about which NNT is clinically acceptable to clinicians and patients, which is termed the NNT threshold. To address this question, one must consider the cost of treatment, the severity of preventable outcomes, and the adverse or side effects of the treatment or intervention. NNT may be described as the number of patients who would need to be treated for one of them to benefit. The NNH is expressed as the inverse of the AR increase (1/ARI). The NNH represents the number of patients required to be treated for one of them to experience an adverse effect.

Aberrant epigenomic modulation detection in malignant neoplasms involves whole genome bisulfite sequencing (WGBS), reduced representation bisulfite sequencing (RRBS), NGS, etc. in detection, screening and diagnostics. The application of these data facilitates therapeutics via induction therapy prior to the standard of care. Specifically, the methylation level of individual CpG sites and non-CpG quantification on a given base C on the plus strand and the total number of C-carrying and T-carrying reads are estimated, with the methylated ratio assessed as $C/C + T$. Further, the methylation level is estimated by adding up the reads mapping to both strands.

4.7   Questions for Review

1 Suppose there is no good treatment for disease X such as pancreatic neoplasm.

   a What will be the advantages, if any, of performing a screening trial in this context?

   b What are the design issues in such a trial if you were to conduct one?

   c Survival is often seen as a definitive outcome measure in screening trials; would you consider population incidence of advanced disease and stage shifts as possible outcome measures?

   d Early detection induces a bias in the comparison of survival times that artificially makes screen-detected cases appear to live longer. What is this biased term, and how would you correct this in order to estimate the true benefit of screening?

2 Suppose that disease A is potentially detectable by screening during a window of time between its onset and the time when it would ordinarily become clinically manifest.

   a What is lead-time bias?

   b Would people with a longer window due to person-to-person variability in disease manifestation be more likely to be screened in the window?

   c Would you expect the "window of screening" to result in length-time bias?

3 Suppose that 82% of those with hypertension and 25% of those without hypertension are classified as hypertensive by an automated blood pressure machine.

   a Estimate the predictive value positive and predictive value negative of this machine, assuming that 34.5% of the adult US population has high blood pressure. Hints: Sensitivity = 0.82, specificity = $1 - 0.25 = 0.75$. Using Bayes' Theorem: PV+ = (sen × prevalence)/(sen × prevalence) + (specificity × prevalence). Comment on these results and state which is more predictive, positive or negative?

4 Suppose 8 out of 1,000 cerebral palsy children operated on for scoliosis developed a deep wound infection and 992 did not, while 10 out of 1,000 children who were not treated with surgery developed a deep wound infection. What is the RR of deep wound infection associated with surgery? Estimate the relative risk reduction (RRR). What is the ARR, also termed the AR difference? What is NNT? Hints: RR = (a/a + b)/(c/c + d); ARR = (c/c + d) − (a/a + b); NNT = 1/(c/c + d) − (a/a + b). What is the 95% CI for ARR and NNT? Hint: CI for NNT = 1/UCI − 1/LCI of ARR. Hints: 95% CI for ARR = + 1.96 [CER × (1 − CER)/number of control patients + EER × (1 − EER)/number of experimental or treatment patients].

5 Suppose a patient is diagnosed with essential hypertension and placed on Fosinopril and is not responding to this agent, while the family history is indicative of several family members with a similar condition and responding to this anti-hypertensive agent. What is a possible explanation for this non-response to this angiotensin converting enzyme (ACE) inhibitor? Could this be explained in part due to lack of drug receptors as transcriptomes?

   a Explain the application of DNA methylation target using Chip-seq, whole-genome bisulfite sequencing (WGBS) or reduced representation bisulfide sequencing (RRBS), and which method is more appropriate or considered gold standard in methylation profiling?

   b Is RRBS biased toward CpG-rich sites?

   c Does RRBS allow for rapid screening of patients?

   d Is RRBS cost-effective.

References

1 Alberg AJ, Park JW, Hager BW et al. The use of "overall accuracy" to evaluate the validity of screening or diagnostic tests. *JGIM.* 2004;19:460–465.

2 Maxim LD, Niebo R, Utell MJ. Screening tests: A review with examples. *Inhal. Toxicol.* 2014;26(13):811–828. doi: 10.3109/08958378.2014.955932.

3 Altman DG, Bland JM. Diagnostic tests 1: Sensitivity and specificity. *Br. Med. J.* 1994;308:1552.

4 Altman DG, Bland JM. Diagnostic tests 2: Predictive values. *Br. Med. J.* 1994;309:102.

5 Altman DG, Bland JM. Diagnostic tests 3: Receiver operating characteristic plots. *Br. Med. J.* 1994;309:188.

6 Kocher MS. Ultrasonographic screening for developmental dysplasia of the hip: An epidemiologic analysis (Part II). *Am. J. Orthop.* 2001;30:19–24.

7 MacLennan I. Autoimmunity: Deletion of autoreactive B cells. *Curr. Biol.* 1995;5(2):103–106.

8 Holmes L Jr, Shutman E, Chinaka C, Deepika K, Pelaez L, Dabney KW. Aberrant epigenomic modulation of glucocorticoid receptor gene (NR3C1) in early life stress and major depressive disorder correlation: Systematic review and quantitative evidence synthesis. *Int. J. Environ. Res. Public Health.* 2019;16(21). pii: E4280. doi: 10.3390/ijerph16214280.

9 Wang S, Dorsey TH, Terunuma A et al. Relationship between tumor DNA methylation status and patient characteristics in African Americans and European American women with breast cancer. *PLos One.* 2012;7(5):e37928.

10 Zhong J, Colicino E, Lin X et al. cardiac autonomic dysfunction: Particular air pollution effects are modulated by epigenetic immunoregulation of Toll-like receptor 2 and dietary flavonoid intake. *J. Am. Heart Assoc.* 2015;4(1):e001423.

11 Shroeder JW, Conneely KN, Cubells JC et al. Neonatal DNA methylation patterns associated with gestational age. *Epigenetics.* 2011;6(12):1498–1504.

12 Turner RJ, Avison WR. Status variations in stress exposure: Implications for the interpretation of research on race, socioeconomic status, and gender. *J. Health Soc. Behav.* 2003;44(4):488–505.

13 Hatch SL, Dohrenwend BP. Distribution of traumatic and other stressful life events by race/ethnicity, gender, SES and age: A review of the research. *Am. J. Commun. Psychol.* 2007;40(3–4):313–332.

14 Pratt GC, Vadali ML, Kvale DL, Ellickson KM. Traffic, Air pollution, minority and socio-economic status: Addressing inequities in exposure and risk. *Int. J. Environ. Res. Public Health.* 2015;12:5355–5372.

15 Wang C, Chen R, Cai J et al. Personal exposure to fine particulate matter and blood pressure: A role of angiotensin converting enzyme and its DNA methylation. *Environ. Int.* 2016; 94:661–666

16 Parikh PV, Wei Y. PAHs and PM 2.5 emissions and female breast cancer incidence in metro Atlanta and rural Georgia. *Int. J. Environ. Health Res.* 2016;3123:1–9.

17 Ritz B, Yu F, Chapa G, Fruin S. Effect of air pollution on preterm birth among children born in Southern California between. *Epidemiology.* 2000;11(5):502–511.

18 Palma-Gudiel H, Córdova-Palomera A, Eixarch E, Deuschle M, Fañanás L. Maternal psychosocial stress during pregnancy alters the epigenetic signature of the glucocorticoid receptor gene promoter in their offspring: A meta-analysis. *Epigenetics.* 2015;10(10):893–902.

19 Holmes L, Chan W, Ziang Z, Du XL. Effectiveness of androgen deprivation therapy in prolonging survival of older men treated with locoregional prostate cancer. *Prostate Cancer Prostatic Dis.* 2007;10:388–395.

5

EPIGENOMIC EPIDEMIOLOGY

Disease Association, Etiology, Prognosis and Outcomes

5.1 Introduction

deoxyribonucleic acid (DNA) modifications that do not change or alter DNA sequence can affect gene activities through the epigenome, meaning above the gene. Gene activities can be influenced by the addition of chemical compounds, thus regulating their activities; these modifications are termed epigenetic changes—gene and environment interaction. The epigenome reflects the chemical compounds added to one's DNA, which is the genome, by regulating the activity of all the genes within the genome (gene expression). These modifications remain as cells divide and, in some cases, can be inherited through the generations (transgenerational) and are reversible as well. For example, social conditions, diets, air pollutants, toxic waste, etc., impact the epigenome, which is indicative of aberrant epigenomic modulation. Gene and social environment interactions relate to socio-epigenomic modulation. Specifically, methylation or mDNA remains the most common process of epigenomic modulation.

Simply, every day encounter or daily interaction with the human environment affects the way in which human genes are expressed and the subsequent gene product as protein molecules. Basically, social conditions such as social isolation, discrimination, low socio-economic status (SES), social adversity (SA) and unemployment have the tendency to alter human gene expression in a negative direction, implying increased disease development, poor prognosis, survival disadvantage and excess mortality [1–4]. Genes remain hereditary materials acquired through 23 pairs of chromosomes and exert fundamental functions in cellular development, differentiation and maturation. Human proteins that serve as cell membranes, enzymes that catalyze biologic activities

DOI: 10.4324/9781003094487-6

and drug receptors which are molecules required for drug binding and response are all products of human gene expression [1]. Protein synthesis commences with the replication of the genetic material, termed DNA, followed by transcription and translation of the mRNA into protein, hence cellular function and adaptability. Meanwhile, gene-environment interaction is termed epigenomics, meaning above the gene are changes within the gene promoter or enhancer region that affect the transcription proteins (transcriptomes) and restrict gene expression, resulting in disease development, poor prognosis and survival disadvantage.

The gene-environment interaction may involve the social environment, diet, hormones, physical and chemical environment and in utero which may result in the recruitment of the methyl group (CH_3) to the prompter region where the dinucleotides CpG are located. The covalent binding of these CH_3 results in methylcytosine or the hydroxymethyl radical leading to hydroxymethylcytosine, both of which have different and opposing biologic functions and lead to impaired gene expression and protein synthesis, hence abnormal cellular function and impaired plasticity [2, 3].

Social signal transduction (SST) due to isolation, social stressors or discrimination reflects the fight or flight notion of the sympathetic nervous system (SNS) through the elaboration of norepinephrine (NE) and the activation of beta-adrenergic receptors. Specifically, adverse social environments serve as triggers of neural and endocrine responses, influencing the cellular response system and resulting in the activation of intracellular signal transduction pathways and the subsequent repression or activation of transcription factors that are involved in the transcription of gene-bearing response elements (GBRE).

The current initiative in precision medicine (PM) is due mainly to the constant observation of patient outcome differences resulting from individual treatment effect heterogeneity, rendering therapeutics ineffective and non-beneficial in some settings. Whereas attempts at understanding treatment effect heterogeneity have been made through sub-subpopulation analysis of treatment outcomes, there remains a feasible approach through epigenomic investigations for specific risk characterization and risk-adapted intervention mapping. Broadly, epigenetics refers to DNA and chromatin modulation due to environmental interaction, not explicitly affecting the DNA sequence. Specifically, these alterations or modifications reflect heritable, although reversible, changes in the gene and environment interaction that are not due to an alteration in DNA sequence but influence gene transcription and expression, nuclear organization, genomic instability, silencing and imprinting, resulting in changes in the developmental process, cellular differentiation and malignancies, among other pathologies [1]. The observed epigenetic changes are mediated by DNA postsynthetic modifications or alterations involving DNA and histone proteins, histone variants, non-coding RNAs and proteins regulating and interpreting the modifications [3]. Methylation as a process of biomolecular function is observed to modulate the positioning and phasing of the nucleosome DNA, altering the accessibility of DNA to regulatory proteins and the associated gene expression and function.

The purpose of this chapter is to provide researchers in epidemiology, health disparities epidemiology, biomedical sciences, as well as translational and clinical sciences a basic understanding of the perspectives and challenges surrounding the epigenomic mechanistic process in disease causality. It covers studies conducted and their applications in disease causal inference, prognosis and survival prolongation. The inherent approach is relatively basic and explains the challenges in epigenomic studies in the process of specific risk characterization and risk-adapted treatment in narrowing subpopulation prognostic and survival variances. Mention is made of the ongoing emphasis in PM today that reflects the challenges with current therapeutics in terms of individual response differences in therapeutics, mainly treatment effect heterogeneity or subpopulation variability in outcomes, driven in part by pharmaco-genetics and within-individual differences in gene expression or epigenetic alteration as a function of gene-environment interaction and gene function.

Epigenomic studies contribute to the mechanistic understanding of disease etiology and biomarkers of disease severity or prognosis, enabling specific risk characterization in defining the causal pathway and hence specificity in therapeutics and preselection treatment induction. Since the disease process is complex and multifactorial, neither genetic nor epigenetic studies per se are capable of providing data on meaningful disease etiology, requiring the need for epigenomic studies, especially gene interaction with social determinants of health and SA, namely socio-epigenomics, in reliable causal correlation investigation. This chapter aimed primarily to describe epigenetic alterations, study designs, analysis and challenges in translating the data from epigenomic studies to the PM initiative in addressing the persistent and reoccurrence treatment effect heterogeneity in disease management today.

5.2 Genomic and Epigenomic Epidemiology

Traditional epidemiology aimed at assessing the correlation or association between exposure and outcome, implying the risk factor that resulted in disease development or a health-related event [3]. However, despite the traditional epidemiologic investigation notion of non-causal association, this correlation has causal trajectory in terms of intervention mapping and therapeutics. Such traditional attempts focused less on cellular or molecular-level events or exposures without penetrating the "black box" of epidemiology. With molecular epidemiology, the interest shifted to molecular events such as disease and prognostic biomarkers—causal association through black box penetration. Additionally, the genetic predisposition to disease is traditionally assessed as single and polygene associations with disease process, as observed in conditions such as trisomy 21 (Down syndrome), XYY (Klinefelter syndrome) and phenylketonuria—an inborn error of metabolism associated with tyrosine hydroxylase enzyme deficiency and mental retardation.

With the challenges of treatment effect heterogeneity, multiple causal pathways in disease development and pharmaco-genetics, gene expression presents an added opportunity to explore disease processes, prognosis and survival. Specifically, early childhood trauma, social disadvantage and a disadvantaged neighborhood environment characterized by living conditions, SES and health inequity—as a systemic and unfair allocation of economic, social and environmental conditions related to health—have been observed to influence biologic processes resulting in disease development, progression and subpopulation survival differences. In effect, such influence has been implicated in gene-environment interactions resulting in epigenomic modifications of gene expression and disease propagation as well as severity, prognosis and survival. Consequently, disease propagation is driven by biologic, genetic, epigenetic, epigenomic, socio-epigenomic, behavioral, social, environmental and psychological predispositions. These complex predispositions including social inequity, social threats, SA, early life stress (ELS), and social determinants of health as well as culturally and linguistically competent care influence response to treatment, prognosis and survival [4].

5.2.1 Translational Epigenomic Epidemiology: Basic Notion and Application

While epigenomic epidemiology remains the investigation of the distribution and determinants of epigenomic modulations and aberrations in animal and human populations, along with the application of such data in disease control, prevention and health promotion practices, translational epigenomic epidemiology stresses the trans-disciplinary and team science approach in the conceptualization, design, conduct, the interpretation and applications of these findings. The team science approach in epigenomic epidemiology signals the limitations of a single field in meeting the scientific collaboration required in novel research and application at a translational level. This approach is complex, although adaptive, requiring a consensus on research objectives, conduct, analysis and integrated data interpretation for reliable and valid inference [5]. The translational epigenomic epidemiology investigative team requires a team with backgrounds in biological sciences, computational biology, molecular and genetic epidemiology, genomics and epigenomics, biostatistics, clinical medicine, behavioral/social sciences, computer programming and informatics. This composition reflects the integration of bioinformatics in the molecular and epigenomic investigation of disease development, prognosis and survival.

5.2.2 Epigenomics

Epigenomies characterize the unique transcriptional program of cells throughout the life course, from gametogenesis to aging, and refer to any process that alters gene activity without changing the DNA sequence and leads to modifications that can be transmitted to daughter cells but not without reversibility, implying transgenerational but reversible [6]. Simply, epigenetics controls genes, implying the switching on and off mechanism of the gene, and *genes are specific sequences of bases that provide instructions on proteins synthesis* (transcription to translation). Whereas the same or comparable DNA is expected to predispose to same functions and alterations in function, that is not the case given distinct gene expression due to different cell types for differential functional activities. Specifically, the changes in epigenome reflect the influence of environment, such as indicated earlier, namely stress, diet, drugs, exogenous environment, pharmacologic agents (treatment effect) on a defective or diseased gene that do not affect the DNA sequence but messenger RNA (mRNA) and gene expression. These alterations are implicated in developmental processes, cellular differentiation, disease susceptibility (cancer, depression, hypertension (HTN), diabetes, etc.), prognosis and survival, implying the understanding of epigenomic modifications for complex disease pathways and their implications in therapeutics [7].

5.2.3 DNA Molecule and Structure

A basic understanding of gene structure and function is required for epigenomic epidemiology with no background in molecular biology or biochemistry and allows for a reliable interpretation of the epigenetic signatures and mechanisms in various disease processes. With cells as the fundamental unit of life, understanding cell structure in relation to the genes which specify protein production is relevant to epigenomic epidemiology. Animal cells comprise the nucleus and cytoplasm, with the genetic material, the DNA, located in the chromosome within the nucleus, the molecular basis of hereditary.

Simply, DNA comprises sequences of base pairs such as four nucleotides—namely adenine (A), thymine (T), guanine (G) and cytosine (C)— along with sugar and phosphates. These compositions, termed the backbone or core of DNA molecule, allow for the understanding of epigenomic alterations induced by DNA methylation (mDNA). The basics of molecular genetics illustrate the organization of nuclear DNA into 46 chromosomes, implying 22 autosomes and one sex chromosome derived from each human animal parent. The synthesis of protein, either structural or regulatory, follows the central dogma of molecular biology, implying an information pathway or flow from DNA to mRNA and then the synthesis of protein, hence *replication (cells replicate as they divide into two identical strands of DNA: T-A, A-T, G-C, C-G), transcription* (a strand of RNA constructs using U instead of thymine) and *translation* (*mRNA is translated into amino acid (AA)* (***RTT***)). Therefore, since genes consist of the base sequences or dinucleotides that map the direction of the complimentary mRNA, the specific protein produced depends on this translation.

What is the DNA transcription process? Genes provide information for protein synthesis as polypeptides which involves transcription and translation. Transcription, also known as rewriting or transcribing, is the process that involves the copying or replication of the DNA sequence to generate an RNA molecule. In this process, the "T" from DNA is replaced by "U," transforming DNA into mRNA. What is translation? This is the process in which the RNA sequence is decoded into the AA of a polypeptide for protein synthesis—the mRNA codon is translated into an AA as a polypeptide, such as the AUG codon into methionine. Therefore, in protein synthesis, the protein-coding gene expresses information from DNA to mRNA using the dogma of molecular biology, namely replication, transcription and translation. The functionality of the synthesized protein in effect depends on the accuracy of such translation in the formation or development of a specific AA as the building block of proteins, which supports the role of mDNA in gene expression and the subsequent protein production, whether regulatory or structural. For example, 64 condons code for 20 AAs: UCG (ser), AUG (met) and AUC (Ile) as codons for AAs termed polypeptides, with protein as the sequence of AAs.

5.2.4   Human Gene, Chromatin, DNA, mRNA and Protein Synthesis

The basic appraisal of terms used in epigenomic modification is essential for mDNA processes such as promoter, enhancer, transcription factors and transcriptional control, as well as nucleosomes and chromatin. As indicated earlier, a gene is a component of DNA, and the bases or nucleotides that code for AA are organized into exons and blocks. The introns comprise bases that are not specific to AA and hence protein synthesis but may contain the control regions located between the exons [8].

The nucleosome is the subunit of all chromatin, and micrococcal nuclease releases individual nucleosomes from chromatin as 11S particles. A nucleosome contains ~200 bp of DNA, two copies of each core histone (H2A, H2B, H3 and H4) and one copy of H1. More than 95% of the DNA is recovered in nucleosomes or multimers when micrococcal nuclease cleaves DNA from chromatin [9]. The length of DNA per nucleosome varies for individual tissues in a range from 154 to 260 bp, and DNA is wrapped around the outside surface of the protein octamer. Nucleosomal DNA is divided into core DNA and linker DNA, depending on its susceptibility to micrococcal nuclease. Basically, the core DNA is the length of 146 bp that is found on the core particles produced by prolonged digestion with micrococcal nuclease [10].

In a typical gene, DNA strands have one side referred to as the 5' end while the other side is termed the 3' end. The promoter or enhancer region of the DNA strand is associated with the 5' end, and is enriched with cytosine (C) and guanine (G) bases [11]. The transcription process in the central dogma theorem involves the binding of this region, the 5' end, with the transcription factors, resulting in the synthesis of complementary mRNA thanks to RNA polymerase. Protein synthesis involves the new primary copy of the gene, the removal of introns, and binding or stitching together of exons [12]. As the process evolves, the ribosomes then utilize the mRNA as a template in the synthesis of the polypeptide chain as the basic structure for proteins, whether structural or regulatory. Histones or histone proteins play a role in epigenetic mechanisms and are the central DNA packing within the nucleosomes [13]. The aberrant modulation of histone protein modification results in limited access to DNA and, hence, impaired protein synthesis or abnormal cellular functionality.

5.2.5 Epigenomic Mechanistic Process: DNA Methylation (mDNA)—Covalent Binding of Methyl Group (CH3) to Gene Promoter Region (CpG)

mDNA is a process by which cells create epigenetic markers or signatures. As observed above, the promoter regions of genes contain sequences, namely cytosine (C), alternating with guanine (G), expressed as 5'-CG-3'(CpG). *What is the gene promoter or enhancer?* These are regions in the DNA that comprise C-G and T-A where the transcription factor binds as a result of RNA polymerase facilitation, commencing transcription. However, CpG is located in other areas besides the promoter region of the gene. The C of the CpG is predisposed to modification by the DNA methyltransferase; thus, a covalent reaction involving the addition of the methyl (CH_3) to this portion (C) results in the formation of 5'-methylcytosine [14]. *What is the cellular or physiologic consequence of this formation, 5'-methylcytosine?* Since the promoter region of the gene is involved in the transcription process, methylation of C, which is an enduring process, may result in the inability of this region to bind relevant transcription factors as observed above, thus inhibiting and stopping transcription. The large proportion of mDNA in vivo suggests a link between the physical properties of methylated and unmethylated DNA and the control of gene expression. Evidence observes the physical implications of mDNA in nucleosomal DNA, especially the preferred location with respect to the nucleosome core particle and the consequences of mDNA for the accessibility of the genetic materials [15]. Specifically, the detachment of DNA-binding proteins after methylation results in a spontaneous shift of the DNA's phase due to relaxation of the base steps toward more unfavorable positions, with this modification resulting in DNA inaccessibility and impaired DNA read-out mechanisms [15].

5.2.6   *Epigenome and Epigenomic Epidemiology*

Traditionally, modern epidemiology emerged from clinical medicine in an attempt to quantify the risk and predisposing factors in disease, implying the role of exposure in the causal pathway of disease despite the stress on association as the core of epidemiologic investigation. While exposure was traditionally and initially conceived at a non-cellular level, such as cigarette smoking in bronchial carcinoma risk, epidemiologic evidence indicated a factual association as well as a causal inference based on the magnitude of effect and dose-response explanation as implied in causal inference [3]. Epidemiologic investigation continues to evolve with the examination of cellular level exposure, namely biomarkers of disease, thus the penetration of the "black box" to the emergence of molecular epidemiology [3]. With the worldwide genomic project that opened the window for comprehensive gene study, the role of epigenetics in epidemiology has emerged, implying the exposure function of gene-environment interaction in disease predisposition, severity, prognosis, mortality and survival. For example, epigenomic modifications provide an understanding of how social conditions such as SA or ELS influence gene expression and subsequent disease processes, including carcinogenesis or tumorigenesis. Endocrine and neural regulation are observed in specific types of cells involved in tumorigenesis, progression and survival. Carcinogenesis initiation, progression and metastasis have been illustrated to correlate with beta-adrenergic signal transduction from the SNS and with upregulation of specific genes involved in tumorigenesis and survival [16]. Upregulation of the glucocorticoid receptor (GR) gene NR3C1 correlates with DNA repair inhibition in cancer cells, enhancing therapeutic resistance of a specific gene and gene product via mDNA [3]. Stressful events such as racial or gender discrimination have been shown to be less beneficial in terms of therapeutics, resulting in a poor prognosis, given epigenomic modification involving the hypothalamus, pituitary and adrenal (HPA) axis. Signal transduction is a set of events that translate extracellular biochemical signals, such as hormones or neurotransmitters (dopamine [DA], NE, serotonin or 5-hydroxytriptamine [5-HT]), into changes in gene expression through the activation of protein transcription factors which bind to DNA and flag it for transcription into RNA [17]. The social signal reflects upstream neural dynamics that translate social conditions into specific systematically distributed signaling molecules—glucocorticoids from the HPA-axis or catecholamine from the SNS. For instance, when NE is released from the SNS as a result of racial discrimination (social stressor), cells associated with beta-adrenergic receptors translate that signal into the activation of the transcription factor CAMP response element binding (CREB; cyclic, 3'-5' ADMP response element-binding protein) [18]. Activated CREB proteins upregulate hundreds of cellular genes and are determined by the nucleotide sequence of the gene's promoter or enhancer. Consequently, adverse social events (sexual abuse, child maltreatment, domestic violence, maternal separation, trauma, social stressors) initiate SST of neural and endocrine origin involving tumorigenesis and tumor and stromal cell responses to gene transcription [19, 20].

Prenatal and early childhood adverse events (ECAS) have been illustrated to modulate epigenomics, leading to increased risk of adult chronic disease, obesity, metabolic syndrome, cardiovascular disease, neurodegenerative disorders and cognitive impairment [21]. The observed epigenomic changes (epigenomic regulations of gene expression and cell functionality) reflect later life adverse health outcomes of prenatal malnourishment and ELS. Whereas animal studies applying "epidemiologic designs" are numerous and have clearly illustrated the contributions of epigenetic mechanisms in disease causal association and prognosis, comparable mechanistic processes of epigenomic modulation have been observed in human models, although few, especially in ELS and HTN, cardiovascular diseases, type II diabetes, major depressive disorders (MDDs), schizophrenia and malignancies [22–25]. For example, perinatal maternal stress due to violent neighborhood factors, including racial discrimination as a social stressor, asphyxia, thermic dysregulation, labor complications and maternal mortality resulting in early separation, and racial variation in perinatal care and labor, may result in neural and endocrine cellular malprogramming or dysregulation and the subsequent impaired rapid response to stress and cognitive impairment. The observed phenotypic response, including low birth weight, is indicative of the epigenomic mechanistic process involving excessive exogenous glucocorticoids or 11β-hydroxysteroid dehydrogenase type II, which reflects the HPA-axis, implying the excess accessibility of the fetal brain to maternal glucocorticoids (placental barrier dysfunction) [26]. The upregulation of GR and corticotrophin-releasing factors (CRF), along with increased corticosterone and adrenocorticotropic hormone (ACH), has been observed with reliable variance in ELS when comparing those with and without [27–29]. The observed neuroendocrine changes that influence cellular chemistry and function [30], resulting in these diseases in adult life, occur because of epigenomic changes and the accompanying gene expression without modification of the underlying DNA sequence [31].

5.2.7   Mechanisms of Epigenetic Programming or Regulation

Basically, epigenomic epidemiologic investigations involve the assessment of hereditable changes in gene expression that occur in the absence of underlying DNA sequence as observed in epigenetic regulators, namely mDNA (addition or removal of a methyl group (CH_3), predominantly where cytosine bases occur consecutively), histone modifications, prions, microRNA and DNA microarray [32]. Unlike DNA staticity during ontogeny, epigenomic codes or programming undergo dramatic modification during embryogenesis, reflecting differential patterns in gene expression and related tissue development and cellular function. Besides methylation, other processes could alter gene activities without affecting DNA sequence, such as acetylation, phosphorylation and ubiquitylation [33]. However, mDNA remains the most common mechanistic process for epigenomic modulation due to its relative stability with storage and several processes and technologies for analysis [34]. Simply, the mDNA process involves the insertion of a methyl group (CH_3) at the 5-carbon position of cytosine by specific enzymes termed DNA methyltransferase, leading to 5-methylcytosine. The mechanism, as indicated earlier, remains the most common pathway of epigenomic regulation and programming [35]. The mDNA study or assessment measures the percentage of methylated cytosine residues within CpG dinucleotides. The CpG-rich regions, also termed CpG islands, where cytosine nucleotides are accompanied by guanine nucleotides, are primarily associated with mDNA. Typically, this area is related to the transcription factor or the promoter or enhancer region of the gene. The histone protein modification which is a posttranslational process involves mainly acetylation but other epigenetic regulations of transcription and subsequent gene expression include methylation, phosphorylation and ubiquitination of histone tails [2]. The functionality of histone acetylation (ACH), a process where lysine residues bind to the amino-terminal tails of histone, reflects the neutralization of their positive charges, thus inhibiting their affinity for DNA and enhancing the accessibility of transcriptional regulatory proteins to chromatin templates. Like mDNA involving the DNA methyltransferase enzyme, the histone epigenomic regulatory mechanism involves histone acetyltransferase and deacetylases, enzymes that function to accelerate the insertion and deletion of the ACH group in transcriptional regulation.

The modulation of gene expression via non-coding RNAs ((ncRNAs) has been implicated in epigenetic regulation, and involves gene expression at both transcriptional and posttransactional stages. Epigenetic regulations with ncRNAs involve mDNA, histone modification, heterochromatin formation and silencing of the gene [36].

5.2.8   Epigenomic Role in Epidemiologic Investigation of Disease Etiology

In a broad sense, epigenomics is the study of heritable changes in gene expression, implying the examination of active versus inactive genes that does not involve changes to the underlying DNA sequence. Simply, it implies a change in phenotype without a change in genotype, but it affects how cells read the genes—gene expression and the associated cellular function. While epigenomic change is a regular (ongoing cellular process) and natural occurrence, these changes are also influenced by multiple factors such as age, environment, SA, SES, social threats, lifestyle, in utero environment and disease status (epigenetic prognostic biomarkers). Epigenomic modifications can manifest as mild and physiologic or normal, involving cell differentiation in skin, liver and brain cells [37]. Additionally, epigenomic change can have more damaging effects, resulting in disease development as well as severity and survival disadvantage. Currently, these systems include, though not limited to, mDNA, histone modification and non-coding RNA (ncRNA) that are associated with gene silencing and are involved in initiating and sustaining epigenetic change.

5.2.9   Genetic, Epigenetic, Genomic and Epigenomic Epidemiology

Genetic epidemiology emerged as an attempt to associate disease predisposition with genetic inheritance and heritability and the environment. *The application of environment in environmental epidemiology is very broad and involves in utero exposure, social determinants of health, physical and social exposures (exogenous), and endogenous exposure (hormones—testosterone and prostate cancer, estrogen and breast cancer).* The process by which disease is claimed to run in families opened the window for traditional epidemiologic studies on the familial origin of disease. For example, phenylketonuria, an inborn error of metabolism that involves a deficiency in the enzyme phenylalanine hydroxylase, influences the metabolism of an essential AA, phenylalanine, which is associated with mental retardation. This inborn error of metabolism requires an environmental factor prior to the development of mental retardation, the related phenotype. Environmental factors thus interact with genes to predispose to disease manifestation, such as in gene-environment interactions. In effect, the current epidemiologic approach to epigenetic and epigenomic modifications reflects a departure from the traditional model of investigation, namely: (a) family aggregation studies, (b) twin/adoption/half-sibling/migrant studies, (c) segregation analysis, (d) linkage analysis and (e) association studies.

While genetic studies in epidemiology reflect the contribution of individual genes, such as specific chromosomal abnormalities, to a disease process, as observed in 9p deletion in acute lymphoblastic leukemia (ALL) and p15 and p16 inactivation in ALL relapses, epigenetic studies characterize the environmental interaction with the individual genes, implying processes resulting in heritable changes or modulation in gene expression without alterations in the DNA sequence per se. The epigenetic investigation considers the processes affecting gene expression during cell division, such as the promoter or gene enhancer, as well as chromatin (*"DNA residence"*) modification, a dynamic nucleoprotein complex that regulates the DNA access for replication into single-strand DNA and the subsequent translation into mRNA. Specifically, epigenetic investigation in epidemiology involves the assessment of heritable phenotype that is not associated with DNA sequence alteration or modulation. Epigenomic modulation reflects these epigenetic modulations involving the entire or whole genome level in a cell or organism. Simply, epigenomics characterizes the epigenetics assessment of multiple genes within the cell or entire organism.

Epigenetic changes underlie developmental and age-related biology. Genetic epidemiology implicates epigenetics in disease risk and progression, and suggests that epigenetic status depends on environmental risks as well as genetic predisposition. Epigenetic epidemiology represents a mechanistic link between environmental exposures, or genetics, and disease development and prognosis, and attempts to provide a quantitative biomarker for exposure or disease in areas of epidemiology currently lacking such measures.

Specifically, epigenetic or epigenomic epidemiology provides an added understanding of the biologic mechanism involved in disease causation and severity or survival. Therefore, epigenetic modifications allow for the examination of disease causality through: (a) a direct link or effect on disease risk characterization, (b) risk modifications implying impact on exploring disease association via epigenetic alterations, (c) disease and environment biomarkers, and (d) mechanisms for transgenerational effects or impacts. In terms of the direct link with disease, epigenetic studies have demonstrated that Rett syndrome is due to genetic mutations (genotype) caused by an epigenetic mechanism as a result of spontaneous mutations in the methyl-CpG-binding protein 2 (MECP2) gene on the X chromosome [2]. Specifically, MECP2 is relevant for identifying epigenetic modifications that control gene expression. Additionally, mutated MECP2 has been observed to alter the expression of other genes that are usually regulated by epigenetic alterations. Another example has been illustrated by a single nucleotide polymorphism (SNP) in the COMT gene, which is associated with a new CpG site, and correlates with lifetime stress level and memory and the methylation level of the variant allele [15]. Epigenetic alterations may serve as biomarkers of disease, implying no role in the mechanistic process of the disease. Such biomarkers could serve as prognostic factors that drive severity and survival, implying their role in patients' responses to a given therapeutic agent. For example, epigenomic epidemiologic data have observed tumor hypermethylation of the DNA repair enzyme O^6-methylguannine-DNA methyltransferase (MGMT) to be associated with increased favorable response, increasing survival [3].

5.3   Applied Epigenomics—Cancer and Epigenomic Mechanism of Carcinogenesis

Malignant neoplasm is a condition that is highly influenced by epigenomic lesions due to the impact of mutation, whether heritable (germ cell) or environmental in nature. Epigenomic alterations in malignancies refer to the social, psychological, physical, chemical and occupational environments with genes and predispositions to impaired cell growth, differentiation and maturation. Specifically, social isolation, sustained SA and social stressors have been implicated in SST involving the SNS and beta-adrenergic receptors, resulting in the upregulation and downregulation of some genes involved in inflammation and metastatic neoplasm.

While gene and physico-chemical interaction and disease outcome observation remain valid and accurate, we are beginning to experience more than ever before the role played by social isolation, low SES, discrimination, unstable social hierarchies, repeated social threats and unstable social status, which results in chronic stress, depression, chronic diseases, cardiovascular disease and cancer [38–42]. In effect, social environments comparing individuals who are isolated versus those who are not isolated have been shown to result in differences in pro-inflammatory gene expression, such as IL6, antibodies (immunoglobulins) and interferon gamma. Specifically, repeated social threats or social isolation induces increased expression of pro-inflammatory genes, resulting in increased production of pro-inflammatory cytokines, namely IL-6, while inhibiting gene expression in antibody synthesis (response to pathogenic microbes) and interferon gamma (innate response to viral pathogens). This observation very clearly indicates a decreased elaboration of antibody synthesis, such as immunoglobulin G (IgG), and an increased elaboration of interferon gamma (IFN-γ) as a result of the increased response of the conserved transcriptional response to adversity (CTRA) gene. When comparing those isolated with those not isolated, available studies have indicated that there is an estimated 5% difference in the specific genes involved with this condition [43]. However, in terms of the gene and environment, more than a 50% difference has been observed comparing individuals who are isolated versus those who are not isolated [43]. These studies very clearly affirm the role played by genes and the environment in disease development.

Consequently, it is not the gene per se that indicates the differences in the outcome of isolation, but the gene in environment interaction, termed epigenomic. Specifically, social conditions play a substantial role in human gene expression which has been previously observed in animal models. Simply, stress or isolation evokes the SNS response within the central nervous system (CNS), leading to increased expression of the CTRA gene. This increased response of the CTRA gene has been observed in leukocytes due to repeated social threats, unstable social hierarchies and low social status [44]. The observed alterations in the SNS activation of CTRA gene upregulation are due to the beta-adrenergic receptor response, leading to the elaboration of some transcription factors such as nuclear factor kappa-light chain enhancer of activated B-cells (NF-kB) CREB protein. These cascades result in a selective increase in pro-inflammatory gene expression such as interleukin 6 (IL-6), IL-1A, IL-1B and tumor necrosis factor (TNF) and a downregulation of the transcription factor responsible for INF-γ gene expression.

Additionally, the CTRA is involved in transcriptional regulation of the human immune system cells via transcriptional shifts in myeloid cells, namely monocytes and dendritic cells. Simply, the SNS response to stress or social isolation can upregulate pro-inflammatory monocyte elaboration via alteration of the hematopoietic process in the bone marrow. Furthermore, beta-adrenergic signaling has been shown to upregulate the transcription of the myelopoietic growth factor granulocyte-macrophage colony-stimulating factor, influencing monocyte development, differentiation and maturation [45]. In effect, social threats or adversity has the potential to upregulate CTRA gene expression in the human immune system, leading to a chronic inflammatory response and excess malignant neoplasm, diabetes and chronic disease [46, 47]. Substantial data support the implication between psychological, neural and endocrine processes in cancer patients and gene expression; however, cautious interpretation of these data to avoid reverse causation is required since malignant neoplasms may induce an inflammatory process with subsequent effects on the CNS, SNS and beta-adrenergic receptor-mediated SST, leading to impaired gene expression.

Genomic and epigenomic processes that involve specific gene expression reflect the inherent ability of humans to respond to sporadic and transient threats, creating cellular plasticity. For instance, the CTRA gene expression occurs as a result of stressful environments, such as objective and subjective isolation, and results in a molecular-level adaptive process. However, when the stressful circumstance becomes chronic and sustained over time, there emerged a pro-inflammatory response with the potential for type 2 diabetes, atherosclerosis, HTN, neurodegeneration, malignant neoplasm, etc. Additionally, sustained expression of the CTRA gene compromises immune responsiveness through antibody synthesis inhibition (IgG) as well as decreased elaboration of IFN-γ, as an innate response to viral pathogens.

To understand epigenomic, implying the interaction between the social, spiritual, economic and physical environment, such as toxins and pollutants, there is a need to understand the specifics of heredity material as we evolve as humans, mainly genes. The hereditary material, or gene, comprises a DNA molecule, which is present in all cells in the human body, and resembles a coiled ladder. Scientifically termed a double helix that contains all the information that constitutes individual characteristics. The DNA consists of four nucleotides—namely, adenine, cytosine, guanine and thymine—along with phosphate and sugar molecules. The combination of these nucleotides forms the codes that are required for the synthesis of AA, which are the building blocks of protein molecules. The process by which protein molecules are developed for continued molecular and cellular function is based on the dogma of molecular biology that begins with the replication of the DNA, the transcription of the DNA into RNA and the subsequent translation of the mRNA into protein synthesis: Replication (R) $\rightarrow$ Transcription (T) $\rightarrow$ Translation (T).

The interaction between the gene and indigenous, exogenous, social, psychological, environment and the gene is an ongoing process occurring every moment and every instant of human existence. This process is termed epigenomic modulation, meaning above the gene, and reflects changes outside the coding region of the gene, but does not involve the DNA sequence. The normal changes or modulation in this direction reflects the stability of the genome and the normal regulation of everyday activities and health outcomes. In contrast, when there is an insult in this modulation, there occur poor health outcomes, including increased incidence of disease, poor prognostic and excess mortality. Specifically, epigenomic modulation begins with cell signal transduction that involves transcriptome factors and the subsequent utilization of these factors, which are protein molecules in gene expression.

The epigenomic mechanistic process has been observed to affect mDNA, ACH, hydroxyl-methylation ($OH-CH_3$) and other mechanisms, not required in this basic explanation. However, of this mechanistic process, the most fundamentally utilized is mDNA. This process begins at the promoter region of the gene, or the gene enhancer region, which is populated with cytosine and guanine residue (CpG island). While normal epigenomic modulation involves the DNA methyltransferase recruitment of the CH_3 molecules to the CpG island, aberrant epigenomic modulation involves dense mDNA, also termed DNA hypermethylation, that results in the inhibition of the transcriptome and the subsequent impairment in the gene expression, adversely affecting protein synthesis and cellular function. Consequently, the methylation of the cytosine residue, resulting in dense mDNA at the CpG region, influences gene expression, inducing cellular dysfunctionality.

The available literature on social isolation or stress as associated with SST and changes in the SNS clearly indicates how stress signals the fight or flight emotions and reactions that eventually result in alterations that affect how the gene expresses itself. Specifically, the involvement of the SNS results in the elaboration or production of the beta-adrenergic response and the subsequent increase in the receptors associated with this elaboration. Social context involving stress, loneliness and social threats includes the tendency to provoke the hypothalamus-pituitary-adrenal (HPA) axis response, resulting in cortisol elaboration in response to stressful conditions. This response that involves the GR gene plays a protective function, enhancing inflammatory recovery. However, chronic stress has been shown to downregulate this response, leading to chronic diseases, metastatic cancer and metabolic syndromes, indicative of the loss of cellular plasticity and the subsequent cellular damage and delayed response to damage, impairing cellular repair and restoration [43, 48].

5.3.1 Epigenomic Modulation Investigation: T-ALL and B-ALL Proliferation

Kinases have been implicated in increased cellular proliferation, a hallmark of malignancies. They are known to regulate a variety of cellular activities associated with cell homeostasis, which are commonly mutated in several malignancies [49]. Since IL-7 has been observed to enhance both T-ALL and B-ALL proliferation, the mDNA of the gene encoding for IL-7 represents aberrant epigenomic modulation in ALL immune phenotypes [50]. An epigenomic epidemiologic investigation requires examining promoter hypermethylation and repression of IL-7 in both B-ALL and T-ALL to determine the ALL differential progression. Additionally, because GATA4 and HOX genes are involved in hematopoiesis, epigenetic repression of these genes with respect to differentiation as a function of transcription factors requires an assessment.

5.3.2 Epigenetic Deregulation and T-ALL and B-ALL Risk Characterization

The knowledge of mDNA differences between ALL immunogenotypes allows for the identification of subtype-specific mDNA patterns correlated with B-ALL and T-ALL. Distinct mDNA profiles associated with B-ALL cytogenetic subtypes have been identified in epigenomic and early genome-scale mDNA studies. Further, epigenetic deregulation has been observed in B-cell subtypes, namely ETV6-RUN1I and hyperdiploid. Compared to other B-cell subtypes, DSC3 was observed to be hypomethylated in ETV6-RUNX115, while another study indicated DSC3 promoter hypermenthylation and simultaneous or concurrent downregulation of hyperdiploid and other B-cell ALL. The translocation in ETV6-RUNX1 has been shown to be the most frequently observed mutation in ALL, and is associated with cellular differentiation and apoptosis inhibition. Specifically, ETV6-RUNX1 by binding and activating EPOR, and hence leukomogenesis through the JAK2-STAT3 activation pathway.

Additionally, the cell surface molecule CD44, which is involved in angiogenesis, has been shown to be downregulated in ETV6-RUNX1, which is indicative of enhanced survival. The expression of asparaginase synthatase (ASNS) has been observed to be lower or downregulated in ETV6-RUNX1 and affects survival, given the role of L-asparginease in ALL induction therapy in enhancing a five-year event-free survival.

5.3.2.1 ALL Apoptotic Process and Mechanism

The activation and propagation of cAMP-mediated signals have been implicated in pre-B-cell apoptosis. Studies have shown that the repression of genes involved in cAMP-mediated signals provides protection against DNA damage-induced apoptosis in B-ALL. The epigenetic repression of adenylate cyclase and cAMP-specific phosphodiesterases that catalyze ATP-cAMP and CAMP-AMP respectively has been observed in B-ALL. Apoptosis dysfunction and abnormal cellular proliferation have been observed in the deregulation of calcium channels and transient receptor potential channels, as well as sustained potassium channel opening and efflux in apoptosis. While the latter has not been observed in the B-ALL apoptosis mechanism, the former has been illustrated. Since the identification of repressed plasma membrane-bound subunits that are associated with apoptotic transduction and cell signaling, especially in T-ALL, epigenomic epidemiology requires examining the potentials of the ALL cells to receive and propagate apoptotic signals with DNA methyltransferase inhibition, such as observed in up- or downregulation of the tumor suppressor gene, p53 receptor.

5.3.3   Epigenomic Epidemiology of Hypertension Causation

Epigenomic epidemiology requires assessing the implication of epigenomic modulation in HTN predisposing factors/causation. The investigation requires utilizing the biomarkers and the associated candidate gene, and applying the mDNA to examine the gene expression in this context—cellular function and plasticity—and assessing their association with elevated blood pressure based on the clinical understanding of essential HTN. With the conjoint effect of cardiac output as stroke volume and heart rate as well as peripheral HTN as an obstacle to the flow of blood, the biologic plausibility of mDNA in these pathophysiologic dimensions of HTN requires to be assessed in such studies. The ability to identify aberrant epigenomic modulation in HTN results in specific risk characterization and therapy induction, and hence HTN complications, comorbidities and mortality.

The HTN genes to be examined should include (1) Adducin1 gene (ADD1). Adducins are cytoskeletal proteins encoded by three genes, namely alpha, beta and gamma. Adducin binds with high affinity to Ca (2+)/Calmodulin. (2) Keratin 13 (KRT 13 gene) encodes for the production of keratin protein—a tough, fibrous protein that forms the structural framework of epithelial cells; the KRT13 gene partners with KRT4 to form intermediate filaments, which function by protecting the mucosa from being damaged by friction or everyday physical stress. (3) The Capping Actin Protein, Gelsolin-like (CAPG gene) encodes a member of the gelosin/villin family of actin regulatory proteins. The encoded protein reversibly blocks the barbed ends of F-actin filaments in a Ca^{2+}-dependent manner and hence contributes to the control of actin-based motility in non-muscle cells. (4) The Sodium Channel Epithelial 1 Alpha Subunit (SCNN1A gene) encodes for the epitheilal sodium channel (ENaC) complex. The ENaC transports sodium into cells and decreased ENaC may result in excess volume or fluid in some organs. The mutation (deletion, restriction-shortening) in this gene has been observed in psuedohypoaldesterionism type 1 (PHA1), characterized by hyponatremia (low Na level), hyperkalemia (high K level) and severe dehydration. (5) The Sodium Channel Epithelial 1 Beta Subunit (SCNN1B gene) plays a similar role to the alpha unit, with impairment in this beta unit associated with sodium channel disruption and fluid balance as well as impaired Na reabsorption and hyponatremia. (6) Angiotensin II receptor, type1 (AGTR1 gene), encodes for the angiotensin II receptor (AT1 receptor).

The AT1 receptor is a protein involved in the renin-angiotensin system that regulates BP, fluid and salt balance. This receptor binds with angiotensin II, stimulating chemical signals that result in vascular constriction and HTN. In addition, this binding results in aldosterone production, hence increased renal absorption of salt and water—increased extracellular fluid leads to BP elevation [7]. The toll-like receptor 2 gene, TLR2 (CD282, TIL4), encodes for the toll-like receptor (TLR) which is involved in pathogen recognition, and innate and non-adaptive immune response activation. Activation of TLRs by pathogen-associated molecular patterns (PAMPs) results in the upregulation of signaling pathways in modulating host's inflammatory response [8]. The ACE gene, which stands for angiotensin I converting enzyme, encodes for the angiotensin converting enzyme, which regulates BP and the balance of NaCl and H_2O.

This enzyme cleaves Angio I to Angio II, a potent vasoconstrictor, elevating BP. ACE cleaves bradykinin, a vasodilator, thus inactivating this molecule or protein and elevating BP and hence HTN. The protein encoded by this gene belongs to the angiotensin-converting enzyme family of dipeptidyl carboxy-dipeptidases and has considerable homology to the human angiotensin-1-converting enzyme. This secreted protein catalyzes the cleavage of angiotensin I into angiotensin II. The organ- and cell-specific expression of this gene suggests that it may play a role in the regulation of cardiovascular and renal function, as well as reproductive processes.

5.3.4 Epigenomic Epidemiology Investigation of Major Depressive Disorders (MDD): Aberrant Epigenomic Modulation in MDD Causation

An epigenomic epidemiologic investigation on the association between ELS as SA and MDD in adulthood requires the assessment of the candidate gene implicated in ELS, including child abuse and neglect, namely the nuclear receptor subfamily 3 group C member 1 (NR3C1), which encodes GRs, functions as a transcription factor (TF) and binds to the glucocorticoid response element (GRE) in the promoter region of glucocorticoid responsive genes to activate their transcription, mDNA, gene expression and gene product, enhancing cellular function and plasticity. The dysfunction of mutation associated with this gene involves generalized glucocorticoid resistance. The mDNA of this gene predisposes some population to chronic stress and depression, serving as potential explanation of subpopulation differences in MDD.

Epigenomic modifications provide an understanding of how social conditions such as adversity or ELS influence gene expression and subsequent disease processes, including MDD and carcinogenesis or tumorigenesis. Endocrine and neural regulation are observed in specific types of cells involved in tumorigenesis, progression and survival. Social signals involving the CTRA gene, NR3C1 (GR gene) and TLR2 gene methylation have been implicated in cellular proliferation and differentiation as well as impaired apoptosis (p53 gene transcription factor inhibition), resulting in carcinogenesis. Carcinogenesis initiation, progression and metastasis have been illustrated to correlate with beta-adrenergic signal transduction from the SNS and with upregulation of specific genes involved in tumorigenesis and survival, namely the GR gene.

The NR3C1 encodes GR, which functions as: (1) a transcription factor that binds to glucocorticoid response elements (GRE) in the promoters of glucocorticoid responsive genes (GRG) to activate their transcription, and (2) a regulator of other transcription factors. The GR is involved in inflammatory responses, cellular proliferation and differentiation in target tissues. Mutations in GR gene are associated with generalized glucocorticoid resistance.

Social stressors such as ELS have been illustrated in pre- and postnatal stress and maternal care insufficiencies associated with behavioral pathologies. Animal models with rodents demonstrated an inverse correlation between adequate postnatal maternal care and increased stress-reactivity, anxiety, and fear reactions. In general, the main neural substrates involved in epigenetic modulation of ELS and maternal care include HPA, amygdala, medial prefrontal cortex and hippocampal region of the brain. The observed phenotypes in the aberrant epigenomic modulation in ELS are explained by the NR3C1 gene's downregulation and decreased expression, a GR gene. The animal model in this context observed dense methylation of the CpG in the promoter region of NR3C1, increased activity of the HPA-axis and elevated serum glucocorticoids level. Additionally, animal models reveal increased stress reactivity, anxiety, impaired social interaction and depressive episodes associated with maternal separation. The observed manifestations correlated with genome-wide aberrant mDNA and brain neural pathway gene transcripts.

A prolonged activation of the HPA-axis, altered gene transcription and aberrant mDNA were observed in CNS and peripheral T lymphocytes among infants and juveniles deprived of maternal care. Aberrant epigenomic modulation (mDNA) and hydroxymethyl cytosine at the brain-derived neurotrophic factor (BDNF) locus, a member of the nerve growth factor family of neutrophils, have been observed in adolescence and adulthood distress associated with maternal maltreatment during neonatal nursing of offspring. Other neural changes include hippocampus, amygdala and medial prefrontal cortex.

Further studies observed increased expression of arginine vasopressin (Avp) and gene loci, a protein-coding gene for antidiuretic hormone (Vasopressin) associated with diabetes insipidus and DNA hypomethylation in the paraventricular nucleus of the hippocampus in ELS, due to maternal separation. Similarly, the overexpression of proopiomelanocortin (pomc) gene loci, which is involved in the production of adrenocorticotropic hormone (ACTH) and binds to melanocortin 2 receptor (MC2R), stimulating cortisol release, is observed in ELS associated with maternal separation. The overexpression of NR3C1 inversely correlates with corticotrophin-releasing hormone (CRH) transcription in chronic stress induced by ELS.

5.3.5 Precision Medicine and Epigenomic Implication

Precision, individualized, personalized or genomic medicine and therapeutics emerged from individual treatment effect heterogeneity and the subpopulation differences in treatment outcomes. With respect to the healthcare notion of PM, this approach involves treatment tailoring toward an individual patient based on the individual's genome and environment factors such as lifestyle. Whereas PM is a contrast to traditional or conventional clinical medicine, it remains a complement to traditional medicine by enhancing therapeutic initiative based on the molecular, genetic and genomic information of the individual patient in addressing specific risk characterization, treatment prediction, treatment, prognosis, survival and prevention.

Using ALL as an example, the PM initiative requires the immunophenotype characterization of T-ALL, B-ALL and others. Within this classification emerged cytogenetics such as the 9p deletion and NOTCH1 (T cell differentiation) in T-ALL, as well as CDKN2A/2B and RB1 as cell cycle modulators, PAX5, E2-2, IKZF1 and EBF in B-cell differentiation and ETV6 in B-cell transcription factor While advances in cytogenetics have indicated prognostic values in B-ALL, such values have not been achieved in T-ALL, implying poorer survival and increased relapses. With T-ALL having increasing epigenomic lesions relative to B-ALL, epigenomic epidemiology is challenged by assessing mDNA and chromatin modification in T-ALL cytogenetics with the intent to personalize care through PM initiatives geared toward specific transcriptome, gene expression, induction therapy and standard of care which will result in dose de-escalation and chemotoxicity reduction, enhancing remission and survival while decreasing T = ALL relapses.

5.4 Challenges in the Design, Conduct and Interpretation of Epigenomic Studies

The challenge in epigenetic epidemiology is the clarity and feasibility of study design, measurement tools, statistical methods, and biological, physiologic and clinical interpretation, as well as the scientific collaboration required in the design, conduct and interpretation of such findings. These aspects are required in this attempt to provide a causal inference on the pathway of epigenetic alteration as an exposure function of disease, severity, prognosis and survival.

Genome-wide association studies (GWAS) of conditions have identified hundreds of genomic regions containing variants robustly associated with disease. These variants have been shown to reside in large regions of strong linkage disequilibrium and most do not index coding variants involving or affecting protein structure. In effect, there is substantial uncertainty regarding the causal genes involved in disease and the way in which they are functionally regulated by associated risk variants. Therefore, in an attempt to localize the functional consequences of disease-associated variants, there is a need to characterize mDNA quantitative trait loci (mQTLs) in organ-system and relate these to genetic findings from clinical conditions and disorders.

While there is optimism in the field of epigenomic epidemiology for informing PM, the challenges are obvious given the differences between genetic epidemiology and epigenetic epidemiology. Primarily, the approach to epigenomic studies requires an understanding of the level of epigenome of interest, namely mDNA, histones and microRNA, which depends on the stability of the epigenetic marker as well as the sensitivity to changes in the external and internal environment.

Additionally, the location of the marker is important, given millions of epigenetic markers in a cell. For instance, the mDNA process places emphasis on CpG islands and CpG island shores, stressing inter-individual variability in epigenome. Since epidemiology is concerned with determining the differences, epigenomic investigation must examine between and within variance to gain a better understanding of epigenetic alterations that result in a disease or serve as a biomarker of disease severity or prognosis. For example, mDNA studies for epigenomic variation require cross-tissue (intra-individual and within subject) and cross-population (between subjects, inter-individual) assessment in determining the variability in methylation as a function of disease as well as the topography or location (spatial relationship). Very importantly, and a departure from genetic epidemiology, epigenomic epidemiology requires an understanding of the temporal variation or changes in the epigenome, implying dynamic changes and the timing of the sample collection and processing.

5.4.1 Quantitative Measures of DNA Methylation—Procedures Accuracies and Limitations

The data from mDNA, the most commonly utilized mechanistic process in epigenomic modulation, requires a reliable and valid quantitative analysis for gene expression in disease causation, prognosis and survival. The quantification requires the measurement of events or mDNA at the CpG island or shores of the genes involved in the postulated association or causation. Since an estimated 28–29 million CpG islands or shores, also termed sites, are targets of mDNA, the assessment of hypo- or hypermethylation processes requires specificity and reliability on a genome-wide scale. The hybridization microarrays and next-generation sequencing (NGS) are utilized in the detection of these methylation profiles or statuses which enable mDNA quantification and gene expression correlation via mRNA seq. The applicable method of mDNA requires the epigenomic epidemiologic assessment of: (a) the available DNA sample in terms of quantity, (b) the degree of genomic resolution and coverage, and (c) the potentials for mDNA quantification in terms of reliable detection and specific measurement with precision.

The methods of mDNA have evolved with time, with the three most commonly used methods implicating: (i) enrichment of methylated genomic positions, (ii) methylation-sensitive restriction enzyme digestion and (iii) application of sodium bisulfite treatment that enables the conversion of unmethylated cytosine residues into thymine (RNA nucleotide) while protecting the methylated cytosine from conversion. Therefore, while assessing studies on mDNA, the epidemiologic approach requires the assessment of the methods utilized in the approach prior to the application of the inferences from these studies (Figure 5.1).

The above-mentioned approaches to methylation analysis, namely island/shore enrichment and digestion of the methylation-sensitive restrictive enzymes and the subsequent application of hybridization microarrays in results reading, enable the estimation of the amount of the methylated cytosine (5'-methylcytosine) at any region of the genome as presented on the probes on the array. These methods are limited despite the observed strength in covering relatively large genomic regions. This DNA region enrichment approach, however, fails to provide single-base resolution of mDNA at individual CpG islands, requiring a mDNA approach with individual CpG sites single-base resolution provision. This limitation is addressed by the utilization of sodium bisulfite. These methods include (a) the MassArray system which applies robust quantification of methylated DNA levels at the targeted CpG sites, (b) Illumina assays such as the Golden Gate assay and Infinium BeadChip assays, (c) the Human Methylation 27 K BeadChip and 450 K, and (d) the Infinium MethylationEpic (850 K array). Despite the advantages of these methods, an estimated 3% of the 28 million CpG sites are targeted in the genome, requiring a complete genome-wide sequencing of bisulfite-treated DNA.

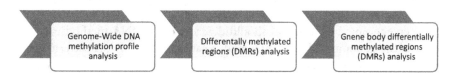

FIGURE 5.1   The DNA methylation analysis strategies: (a) genome-wide DNA methylation profiles, (b) differentially methylated regions and (c) gene body differentially methylated regions (DMRs).

The current approach to mDNA for aberrant epigenomic detection involves whole genome-wide bisulfite sequencing (WGBS). This method involves the development of WGBS libraries from genomic DNA, bisulfite conversion and NGS for mRNA seq. Although the WGBS approach provides an advantage in epigenomic data application in disease causation, prognosis and survival, there is a limitation by the bisulfite conversion failure to differentiate between 5′-methylcytosine (5mC) and 5′-hydroxymethyl cytosine (5hmc). Such limitations hinder the interpretation of epigenomic data given the contrasting biologic functions of 5mC and 5hmC, requiring the application of oxidation in the above method of bisulfite conversion [49].

The required approach in epigenomic epidemiology mDNA and chromatin modification needs to address the following areas: (a) assay description, (b) sample (controlled and case samples) and specific sample specification, (c) DNA quantity (determining the amount of genomic DNA not less than 1 μg), (d) BeadStudio software, which facilitates the analysis and ascertainment of the beta values of Cy3 and Cy5 intensities as well as the random error quantification (p-value) for sample and control probes. The BeadStudio also generates a heatmap for gene expression implying mDNA and mRNA seq correlation, (e) data analysis mDNA using yellowed or specified color pixels as well as methylated and unmethylated alleles data), (f) interpretation, (g) reproducibility and validity (duplicate sample assaying by mean correlation coefficient). The genomic location may vary the mDNA information, requiring method correlation (correlation coefficient) with an expected high correlation, r >7.0, as a high validity indicator, implying high concordance for beta values.

While the genome-wide mDNA method involving bisulfite-genome DNA sequencing of the selected regions is currently used, this procedure has some limitations, such as large sample requirements and bioinformatics labor intensiveness. In contrast, Illumina's Infinium Human Methylation BeadChip offers more advantage. This mDNA analysis, for example the HumanMethylation27 BeadChip, allows for the determination of 27,578 CpG dinucleotides from an estimated 14,495 genes with a very small DNA sample (1 μg of genomic DNA). With this high-thoroughput analysis of the Infinium platform, this method of mDNA provides accuracy in differentiating between normal and pathologic cells as well as increased sensitivity for mDNA biomarker identification or discovery [51].

An epigenomic investigation should describe the mDNA method used to conduct the genome-wide screening and isolation of the mDNA pattern, sample accommodation by single BeadChip, amount of DNA required for initial bisulfite conversion where unmethylated cytosine is chemically deaminated to uracil (U), while methylated cytosine remains as cytosine (C), and the process of conversion such as the thermocycling program, purification of the bisulfite DNA samples, application to the BeadChips and the hybridization implying the annealing of the WGA-DNA molecule to locus-specific DNA oligomers linked to individual bead types. Once the methylated and unmethylated types of beads are measured, the DNA methylated values, termed beta values, are obtained for each sample by the BeadStudio software. A quantitative scale of measurement, or measurement scale, is used for the mDNA beta values which ranges from 0 to 1 and reflects the ratio of the intensity of the methylated bead type to the combined locus intensity [52].

5.4.2   *Epigenomic Investigation Scientific Collaboration: Transdisciplinary and Translational Epigenomic*

An efficient team science implying transdisciplinary collaboration is required in the conduct of epigenomic studies, and requires molecular epidemiologists, genetic epidemiologists and, recently, epigenomic epidemiologists, clinicians and bioinformatics. Of significant relevance in the conceptualization of these studies by epidemiologists is the early onset consultation and interaction with the bioinformatics team that comprises computer scientists with programming backgrounds, and others with mathematical and statistical backgrounds and expertise.

Bioinformatics is the multidisciplinary or transdisciplinary effort involving biological sciences, computer science, information engineering, mathematics and statistics in the analysis and interpretation of biological and molecular biology data such as DNA sequence, RNA, gene expression, mDNA and ACH. Such investigations include, but are not limited to, candidate gene identification, SNPs, genomics, epigenomics and proteomics. The effectiveness of a transdisciplinary approach to epigenomic epidemiology investigation requires a functional bioinformatics core facility that can support the different components of the investigation, namely: (a) service consultancy, which provides information on specific specimen analysis techniques such as next-NGS for mRNA sequencing to correlate gene expression with methylation status; (b) research collaboration/connectome, which requires scientific collaboration beyond technical assistance on the interpretation and future implication of that mDNA and mRNA correlation data in a given disease, such as ALL malignant neoplasms; and (c) technical assistance, which entails activities such as specimen preparation and transfer to core facility, as well as bioinformatics analysis (Figure 5.2).

Gene expression involves several mechanisms in its regulation, which include transcription factor binding, interaction with non-protein-coding RNA, mDNA and histone modification. Specifically, transcription factors are proteins that recognize short DNA motifs in the genome and bind to the motifs associated with specific gene, resulting in up- or downregulation of the gene. This process is facilitated by mDNA and histone modification, explaining impaired gene expression or inverse expression given mDNA.

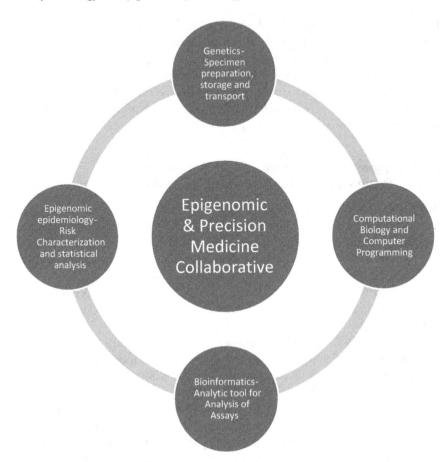

FIGURE 5.2 Epigenomic epidemiology and precision medicine connectome.

5.4.3 Epigenomic Investigation Study Design

The *study design* requires uniqueness relative to traditional epidemiologic or genetic epidemiology design, as mentioned earlier, implying differences in study timing, samples (frozen or fresh) and the type of epigenome. Samples must be collected in a manner that preserves the epigenetic mark of interest to the investigators, since these are dynamic exposures that can undergo changes or vary over a short period. In traditional epidemiology, if exposure and disease variables are collected simultaneously, it is difficult to establish causality, and the same applies to epigenetic markers or alterations. Similarly, the assumption that epigenetic markers are causal in the disease pathway requires attention to the timing of sample collection, namely at the disease state or pre-disease state, as well as the type of non-experimental or experimental epidemiologic design. Because of the stress on epigenomic investigation in addressing mechanistic processes in disease, genomic epidemiologic studies require prospective or longitudinal designs. Such designs that implicate repeated prospective epigenetic measures are highly likely to establish causal inference in epigenetic alterations and disease causation. Like in traditional epidemiologic risk studies, epigenomic epidemiologic studies can be used to characterize risk if samples are collected at the pre-disease or subclinical stage of disease manifestation. In addition, because epigenetic alterations may be influenced by aging, stratification by age remains an important approach in the design of epigenomic epidemiologic studies. While cross-sectional and case-control traditional epidemiologic designs are applicable in epigenomic studies, caution is required in the causal interpretation, thus avoiding reverse causation. Design, in this context, should be planned a priori in terms of disease causation or a biomarker of disease, given epigenetic alterations as the function of these outcomes (epigenetic as causal or biomarker of disease severity/prognosis).

5.4.4   Bio-Specimen and Analysis

Of interest to epigenomic studies is the ***availability of biosamples***. With specific reference to the method of examination of the epigenetic alterations, the sample storage method may not be appropriate. For example, histone modification and microRNA samples are considered unstable in frozen form while mDNA is not, implying the use of frozen samples for mDNA studies. The ***statistical approach*** to the analysis of epigenomic studies requires both a traditional inferential approach and reliable modeling of complex data. The cell type distribution with disease may serve as confounding, requiring stratification or a multivariable regression model once the cell types are identified and isolated. A reliable analytic approach to causal inference in epigenomic studies should conform to reality in the modeling of biomedical and epidemiologic research data by addressing issues arising from batch, normalization and confounding by cell type distribution. Currently, a statistical approach involves single-CpG statistical tests and region-based tests, also termed bump hunting. This technique derives information from neighboring sites and examines the correlation of methylation signals. While ***sample size and power estimations*** require a clinically meaningful effect size, which is difficult to estimate with epigenomic alteration studies, power and sample size estimations are needed in these studies. Additionally, since the absence of evidence does not imply evidence of absence and small studies are likely to yield a statistically insignificant finding, the probability value (p) is a function of sample or study size and not a measure of evidence which is provided by the parameter values or estimates.

Since many epigenetic marks are easily influenced by several factors, including external and internal milieu, epigenomic epidemiology remains an attempt to provide a mechanism for the interaction of the genome with environmental exposures, an essential pathway to disease etio-pathogenesis and prognosis.

Therefore, epigenomic epidemiology explores how disease-associated nutritional or dietary, chemical, physical and psychosocial factors mediate changes to the epigenome, specifically at the level of mDNA, implying the mediation of cellular responses to several environmental agents such as drugs, physical environmental chemical exposure such as pollutants, dietary exposure and lifestyle by epigenetic processes. In addition, socio-epigenomic epidemiology attempts to specifically examine the interaction between social determinants of health and health inequity factors with epigenetic processes involved in disease predisposition, causality, prognosis and mortality outcomes. As previously observed, the mDNA induced by diet, for example, results in the formation of 5'-methylcytosine that may halt the transcription process, affecting gene expression.

5.5   Challenges: Design, Conduct, Analysis and Interpretation

A feasible approach in epigenomic epidemiology is the use of prospective cohort studies that allow for the assessment of epigenetic changes over time and the ability to assess these patterns in relation to temporal changes in exposure and disease prevalence. The longitudinal analysis of epigenetic changes in a population cohort of monozygotic (MZ) twins is a strategy that can be particularly informative for understanding epigenetic variation and its causal association with disease. MZ twins share their DNA sequence, parents, birth date and sex, and are likely to have experienced a very similar prenatal environment. Therefore, epigenomic epidemiologic investigations involving twin cohorts serve to provide a direct understanding of the causal pathway from gene and environmental exposure to disease development.

While the epigenomic epidemiology endeavor remains to benefit clinical medicine and public health, this approach is translational in understanding the mechanistic basis of disease in humans or non-human animals. These challenges are obvious, including but not limited to collaboration, consortia, data sharing and dataset development and maintenance. Additionally, the sample and the context of the design are challenging since epigenetics may reflect biological decline with aging and not necessarily be a disease biomarker. A further challenge in this epidemiologic attempt at disease causal mechanisms with epigenetics is not only the location of the changes or differences but also the timing of the epigenetic changes during gametogenesis/embryogenesis and disease. With an epigenomic epidemiologic approach to the timing of epigenetic changes, intervention mapping is feasible if a time point sensitive to the epigenetic changes is identified, enhancing public health and clinical medicine intervention initiatives. Finally, epigenomic epidemiologic studies are challenged with the inherent interpretation regarding gene-epigene nexus, the impact of inherited genes relative to environment, aging as a decline in biologic function, random errors and false discovery rate (FDR) on epigenetic landscape.

Despite these limitations, epigenetic modifications have been shown to be beneficial in assessing causal mechanisms in certain cancers, neurodegenerative diseases such as Alzheimer's disease and twin studies. With respect to twin studies, there is a greater epigenetic difference across lifespan due in larger part to accumulated environmental stress (physiologic) and disease. The basis of precision (personalized) medicine today lies in the ability of collaborative and team science efforts in epidemiologic investigation of the role of epigenetics in disease causation. Genomic and epigenomic epidemiology is challenged in this context, requiring a meaningful and objective team science initiative, an assessment of reliable, factual and non-confounded data (minimized confoundability), and implying a causal association between epigenetics and disease development or prognosis. The data from these initiatives and epigenomic epidemiology remain a reliable source for clinical trials and translational clinical trials in testing therapeutics in PM.

5.6   Summary

Medicine remains imprecise and inexact due to individual treatment effect heterogeneity, necessitating precision or personalized medicine in patient care optimization and health equity transformation. This initiative, which is based on individual and subpopulation differences in outcome of treatment such as prognosis and survival, as well as the evolving data on pharmaco-genetics, requires specific-risk characterization and subsequent therapy induction. While the global genomic studies have facilitated the understanding of thousands of human gene functions, there remain limited specificities in complex causal pathways of disease and prognosis.

A feasible and more specific alternative is the effort to examine the gene-environment interaction in generating epigenomic and socio-epigenomic data for specific-risk characterization and care optimization, hence transforming health equality and equity. In an attempt to enhance PM initiative, we examined the epigenomic studies in disease causal pathways and prognosis, namely: (a) design, (b) specimen and methods, (c) analysis and interpretation, and (d) application. In addition, aberrant epigenomic signatures in HTN, ELS and MDDs were identified using an applied meta-analytic procedure, namely quantitative evidence synthesis (QES), for scientific statement and therapeutic application. This systematic review and the QES indicate design insufficiencies in terms of specimen timing and the design strategy, implying reverse causation. Specifically, epigenomic specimen collection and analysis or differentiation for mDNA from patients diagnosed with a condition cannot be used for causal inference but for association. However, such data are feasible for biomarkers of prognosis and survival and for specific prognostic or survival risk characterization. Causal association epigenomic studies require data on epigenomic signatures for mDNA and differential mDNA obtained in utero, gestationally and early postnatally, as well as postnatal data from disease-free individuals based on exposure (intrapartum stress versus no intrapartum stress) and repeated measures for aberrant epigenomic signatures and disease causation.

Epigenomic epidemiology presents the opportunity to understand the mechanistic process of disease via "extra-gene" and environment interaction, and remains instrumental in PM initiative that depends on specific risk characterization for risk-adapted treatment protocols. However, this initiative is challenged by design, analytic and interpretation issues in the appropriate transformation of such findings to therapeutics in enhancing PM initiative, thus addressing treatment effect heterogeneity, especially in malignancies, given the complex and several pathways of cellular proliferation, prognostic biomarkers and anti-apoptotic dynamics. The anticipated advances in PM initiative require team science and transdisciplinary approach in disease causal pathway, treatment, prognosis and prevention. Therefore, a translational epigenomic epidemiology approach to epigenomic investigation that places this profession in a strategic position remains a viable pathway in achieving reliable valid data in addressing individual and subpopulation treatment effect heterogeneity.

5.7 Questions for Review

1 Describe epigenomic epidemiologic principles in the understanding of gene expression and proteomics.
2 What are the epigenomic mechanistic processes and could this be applied to the understanding of abnormal cellular proliferation and malignant neoplasms?
3 Examine acute lymphoblastic leukemia (ALL) for T-ALL survival disadvantages with respect to aberrant epigenomic modulations of the candidate genes.
4 Discuss the next-generation sequencing (NGS) procedure in DNA methylation and histone acetylation if feasible.
5 What are the challenges of the current epigenomic laboratory techniques for reliable and accurate inverse gene expressions or inverse correlations of the mean methylation index in the DNA methylation process?

References

1 Yan H, Tlan S, Slager SL, Sun Z, Ordog T. Genome-wide epigenetic studies: A primer on-omic technologies. *Am. J. Epidemiol.* 2016;183(2):96–109.
2 Jirtle R, Skinner M. Environmental epigenomics and disease susceptibility. *Nat. Rev. Genet.* 2007;8(4):253–262. doi: 10.1038/nrg2045.
3 Holmes J. *Applied Epidemiologic Principles and Concepts*, 2nd ed. (Boca Raton, FL: Taylor and Francis, 2017).

4 Michele L, Lorenzo DS, Elia S. Social epigenetics and equality of opportunity. *Public Health Ethics.* 2013;6(2):142–153. doi: 10.1093/phe/pht019.

5 Relton CL, Davey SG. Epigenetic epidemiology of common complex disease: Prospects for prediction, prevention, and treatment. *PLoS Med.* 2010;7(10):100–356. doi: 10.1371/journal.pmed.1000356.

6 Sarda S, Hannenhalli S. Next-generation sequencing and epigenomics research: A hammer in search of nails. *Genomics Inform.* 2014;12(1):2. doi:10.5808/gi.2014.12.1.2.

7 Petronis A. Epigenetics as a unifying principle in the aetiology of complex traits and diseases. *Nature.* 2010;465(7299):721–727. doi: 10.1038/nature09230.

8 Robertson KD, Wolffe AP. DNA methylation in health and disease. *Nat. Rev. Genet.* 2000;1(1):11–19.

9 Joel M, Gottesfeld PJ, Butler G. Structure of transcriptionally-active chromatin subunits. *Nucleic Acids Res.* 1977;4(9):3155–3174. doi: 10.1093/nar/4.9.3155.

10 Louis J, Libertini E, Small W. Salt induced transitions of chromatin core particles studied by tyrosine fluorescence anisotropy. *Nucleic Acids Res.* 1980;8(16):3517–3534. doi: 10.1093/nar/8.16.3517.

11 Garieri M, Delaneau O, Santoni F et al. The effect of genetic variation on promoter usage and enhancer activity. *Nat. Commun.* 2017;8(1). doi: 10.1038/s41467-017-01467-7.

12 Russo VEA, Martienssen, RA, Riggs AD. *Epigenetic Mechanisms of Gene Regulation.* (Cold Spring Harbor, NY: Cold Spring Harbor Laboratory Press, 1996).

13 Pennings S, Allan J, Davey C. DNA methylation, nucleosome formation and positioning. *Brief. Funct. Genom.* 2005;3(4):351–361. doi: 10.1093/bfgp/3.4.351.

14 Spruijt CG, Gnerlich F, Smits AH, Pfaffeneder T, Jansen PW, Bauer C et al. Dynamic readers for 5-(hydroxy)methylcytosine and its oxidized derivatives. *Cell.* 2013;152(5):1146–1159.

15 Portella G, Battistini F, Orozco M. Understanding the connection between epigenetic DNA Methylation and nucleosome positioning from computer simulations. *PLoS Comput. Biol.* 2013;9(11):e1003354. doi: 10.1371/journal.pcbi.1003354.

16 Quốc LKV, Nguyễn LT. The roles of beta-adrenergic receptors in tumorigenesis and the possible use of beta-adrenergic blockers for cancer treatment: possible genetic and cell-signaling mechanisms. *Cancer Manag. Res.* 2012;4:431–445. doi: 10.2147/CMAR.S39153.

17 Robichaux WG 3rd, Cheng X. Intracellular cAMP sensor EPAC: Physiology, pathophysiology, and therapeutics development. *Physiol. Rev.* 2018;98(2):919–1053. doi: 10.1152/physrev.00025.2017.

18 Sanders V, Straub R. Norepinephrine, the β-adrenergic receptor, and immunity. *Brain Behav. Immun.* 2002;16(4):290–332. doi: 10.1006/brbi.2001.0639.

19 Mravec B, Gidron Y, Kukanova B, Bizik J, Kiss A, Hulin I. Neural–endocrine–immune complex in the central modulation of tumorigenesis: Facts, assumptions, and hypotheses. *J. Neuroimmunol.* 2006;180(1–2):104–116. doi: 10.1016/j.jneuroim.2006.07.003.

20 Garcia-Gomez A, Rodríguez-Ubreva J, Ballestar E. Epigenetic interplay between immune, stromal and cancer cells in the tumor microenvironment. *Clin. Immunol.* 2018;196:64–71. doi: 10.1016/j.clim.2018.02.013.

21 Tarantal A, Berglund L. Obesity and lifespan health—importance of the fetal environment. *Nutrients.* 2014;6(4):1725–1736. doi: 10.3390/nu6041725.

22 Lemche E. Early life stress and epigenetics in late-onset Alzheimer's dementia: A systematic review. *Curr. Genomics.* 2018;19(7):522–602. doi: 10.2174/1389202 919666171229145156.

23 Agorastos A, Pervanidou P, Chrousos GP, Baker DG. Developmental trajectories of early life stress and trauma: A narrative review on neurobiological aspects beyond stress system dysregulation. *Front. Psychiatry.* 2019;10:118. doi: 10.3389/fpsyt.2019.00118.

24 Ding X, Yang S, Li W et al. The potential biomarker panels for identification of Major Depressive Disorder (MDD) patients with and without early life stress (ELS) by metabonomic analysis. *PLoS One.* 2014;9(5):e97479. doi: 10.1371/journal. pone.0097479.

25 Çöpoğlu ÜS, Igci M, Bozgeyik E et al. DNA methylation of BDNF gene in schizophrenia. *Med. Sci. Monit.* 2016;22:397–402. doi: 10.12659/msm.895896.

26 Entringer S, Buss C, Wadhwa PD. Prenatal stress and developmental programming of human health and disease risk: concepts and integration of empirical findings. *Curr. Opin. Endocrinol. Diabetes Obes.* 2010;17(6):507–516. doi: 10.1097/MED.0b013e3283405921.

27 Lippmann S, Fuhrmann C, Waller A, Richardson D. Ambient temperature and emergency department visits for heat-related illness in North Carolina, 2007–2008. *Environ. Res.* 2013;124:35–42. doi: 10.1016/j.envres.2013.03.009.

28 Korosi A, Baram T. Plasticity of the stress response early in life: Mechanisms and significance. *Dev. Psychobiol.* 2010;52(7):661–670. doi: 10.1002/dev.20490.

29 Nishi M, Iwamura M, Kurosaka S, Fujita T, Matsumoto K, Yoshida K. Laparoscopic Anderson-Hynes pyeloplasty without symphysiotomy for hydronephrosis with horseshoe kidney. *Asian J. Endosc. Surg.* 2013;6(3):192–196. doi: 10.1111/ases.12038.

30 Champagne F. Early environments, glucocorticoid receptors, and behavioral epigenetics. *Behav. Neurosci.* 2013;127(5):628–636. doi: 10.1037/a0034186.

31 Hochberg Z, Feil R, Constancia M et al. Child health, developmental plasticity, and epigenetic programming. *Endocr. Rev.* 2010;32(2):159–224. doi: 10.1210/er.2009-0039.

32 Dwivedi S, Purohit P, Misra R, et al. Diseases and molecular diagnostics: A step closer to precision medicine. *Indian J. Clin. Biochem.* 2017;32(4):374–398. doi: 10.1007/s12291-017-0688-8.

33 Elia AE, Boardman AP, Wang DC et al. Quantitative proteomic atlas of ubiquitination and acetylation in the DNA damage response. *Mol. Cell.* 2015;59(5):867–881. doi: 10.1016/j.molcel.2015.05.006.

34 Day JJ. New approaches to manipulating the epigenome. *Dialogues Clin. Neurosci.* 2014;16(3):345–357.

35 Smith Z, Meissner A. DNA methylation: roles in mammalian development. *Nat. Rev. Genet.* 2013;14(3):204–220. doi: 10.1038/nrg3354.

36 Dogini DB, Pascoal VD, Avansini SH, Vieira AS, Pereira TC, Lopes-Cendes I. The new world of RNAs. *Genet. Mol. Biol.* 2014;37(1 Suppl):285–293.

37 Lu Y, Reyes J, Walter S et al. Characterization of basal gene expression trends over a diurnal cycle in Xiphophorus maculatus skin, brain and liver. *Comp. Biochem. Physiol. C Toxicol. Pharmacol.* 2018;208:2–11. doi: 10.1016/j.cbpc.2017.11.013.

38 Hermes GL, Delgado B, Tretiakova M, Cavigelli SA, Krausz T et al. Social isolation dysregulates endocrine and behavioral stress while increasing

malignant burden of spontaneous mammary tumors. *Proc. Natl. Acad. Sci. U. S. A.* 2009;106:22393–22398.

39 Miller GE, Chen E, Sze J, Marin T, Arevalo JM et al. A functional genomic fingerprint of chronic stress in humans: blunted glucocorticoid and increased NF-kappaB signaling. *Biol. Psychiatry.* 2008;64:266–272.

40 Volden PA, Wonder EL, Skor MN, Carmean CM, Patel FN et al. Chronic social isolation is associated with metabolic gene expression changes specific to mammary adipose tissue. *Cancer Prev. Res. (Phila).* 2013;6:634–645.

41 Feng Z, Liu L, Zhang C, Zheng T, Wang J, et al. Chronic restraint stress attenuates p53 function and promotes tumorigenesis. *Proc. Natl. Acad. Sci. U. S. A.* 2012;109:7013–7018.

42 Luca F, Kashyap S, Southard C, Zou M, Witonsky D et al. Adaptive variation regulates the expression of the human SGK1 gene in response to stress. *PLoS Genet.* 2009;5:e1000489.

43 Idaghdour Y, Czika W, Shianna KV, Lee SH, Visscher PM et al. Geographical genomics of human leukocyte gene expression variation in southern Morocco. *Nat. Genet.* 2010;42:62–67.

44 Antoni MH, Lutgendorf SK, Blomberg B, Stagl J, Carver CS et al. Transcriptional modulation of human leukocytes by cognitive-behavioral stress management in women undergoing treatment for breast cancer. *Biol Psychiatry.* 2012;71:366–372.

45 O'Donovan A, Sun B, Cole S, Rempel H, Lenoci M et al. Transcriptional control of monocyte gene expression in post-traumatic stress disorder. *Dis. Markers.* 2011;30:123–132.

46 Sloan EK, Priceman SJ, Cox BF, Yu S, Pimentel MA et al. The sympathetic nervous system induces a metastatic switch in primary breast cancer. *Cancer Res.* 2010;70:7042–7052.

47 Thaker PH, Han LY, Kamat AA, Arevalo JM, Takahashi R et al. Chronic stress promotes tumor growth and angiogenesis in a mouse model of ovarian carcinoma. *Nat. Med.* 2006;12:939–944.

48 Holt-Lunstad J, Smith TB, Layton JB. Social relationships and mortality risk: A meta-analytic review. *PLoS Med.* 2010;7:e1000316.

49 Holmes L, Vandenberg J, McClarin L, Dabney K. Epidemiologic, racial and healthographic mapping of delaware pediatric cancer: 2004–2014. *Int. J. Environ. Res. Public Health.* 2015;13(1):ijerph13010049. Published 2015 Dec 22. doi: 10.3390/ijerph13010049.

50 Seregard S, Lundell G, Svedberg H, Kivela T. Incidence of retinoblastoma from 1958 to 1998 in northern Europe: Advantages of birth cohort analysis. *Ophthalmology.* 2004;111:1228–1232. doi: 10.1016/j.ophtha.2003.10.023.

51 Upadhyay M, Samal J, Kandpal M et al. CpG dinucleotide frequencies reveal the role of host methylation capabilities in parvovirus evolution. *J. Virol.* 2013;87(24):13816–13824. doi: 10.1128/JVI.02515-13.

52 Micevic G, Theodosakis N, Bosenberg M. Aberrant DNA methylation in melanoma: Biomarker and therapeutic opportunities. *Clin. Epigenetics.* 2017;9:34. doi: 10.1186/s13148-017-0332-8.

PART 2

Traditional and Modern Epidemiologic Designs

6

MEASURES OF DISEASE OCCURRENCE AND EFFECT OR ASSOCIATION

6.1   Introduction

While epidemiology is primarily concerned with disease association [1], it implies the relationship between the disease and the potential risk factor or exposure (conceived to result in the disease). In considering the fundamental role of epidemiology in public health, epidemiologic investigations are directed at causation and the etiologic role of exposure in disease causation if the intervention mapping, which is intended to be risk-adapted, is to lead to the prevention and control of the disease. Causation refers to the process of an event (disease, disability or injury) occurring as a result of either intrinsic or extrinsic factors acting individually or collectively [2–4]. The causal action of exposure comes before the subsequent development of disease as a consequence of exposure. This is the basis of a longitudinal study in which exposure data or information refers to an earlier time than that of disease, disability or injury occurrence. The intrinsic factor in disease causation simply refers to the host factor (organism). Examples of this factor include the immune system as well as the personality, social class membership and race. The extrinsic factor refers to the environmental factors, which are identified as biologic, social and physical environments. Specifically, the combination of the external and internal environment signals environmental alteration of the biologic system, resulting in morbidity, prognosis and mortality.

The understanding of the measures of disease occurrence as frequency remains relevant in the basic knowledge of a specific exposure as environment, namely stress, isolation, loneliness, discrimination, structural and systemic racism, air pollutants, poor air quality, toxic waste, urbanicity,

DOI: 10.4324/9781003094487-8

socio-economic status, education, sexual orientation, sex, age, diet, physical activities, etc. [5, 6]. This knowledge of disease occurrence by prevalence or frequency in a specific population facilitates the pathway to the risk and the understanding of the determinants for a reliable intervention mapping.

Epidemiologic studies on aberrant epigenomic populations' tumor suppressor genes, p27 or p53 inactivation, result in excess malignant neoplasm in such populations, but the risk factors remain unknown, requiring an exposure assessment implying assertions, relationships, nexus or causal inference. Aberrant epigenomic modulation, implying the DNA methylation of a specific gene enhancer or promoter region and inverse gene expression as a specific gene downregulation, may facilitate causal inference in disease development [6, 7]. The measure of DNA methylation with respect to the inverse DNA methylation mean index facilitates the understanding of either DNA hypermethylation or hypermethylation as causal in morbidity, treatment, remission, relapse and survival [8–12].

6.2   Measures of Disease Frequency and Occurrence

In epidemiologic investigations, the occurrence of cases of disease is related to the "population at risk," which is the population that gave rise to the cases. Several measures of disease frequency are in common use. The measures of disease frequency, occurrence and association in epidemiology include prevalence, incidence, ratios, proportion and rates [12].

Rates as used in epidemiology involve incident rates, mortality rates, attack rates (AR) and fatality rates. The basic measures of disease frequency in epidemiology are incidence and prevalence. A ratio is expressed by dividing one number (X) by another (Y). For example, the sex of adults attending a blood pressure screening clinic could be compared in this way (e.g., male/female, male/male + female). Proportion is a type of ratio, but the numerator is included in the denominator. The distinction between a ratio and a proportion, therefore, implies that the proportion represents the relationship between X and Y.

6.2.1   Notion of Rate

Rate is a type of proportion and is a measure of the occurrence of events in a population over time. Time is, therefore, an integral part of the denominator in rate. Mathematically, this appears as follows:

Rate = Number of cases or events occurring during a given time period/ Population at risk during the same time period × $10n$.

VIGNETTE 6.1

During the first 12 months of Nostate's surveillance for AIDS malignancy (AM), the health department received 2,166 case reports that specified sex; 1,000 cases were in females, 1,166 in males. How will you calculate the female-to-male ratio for AM? In addition, how will you calculate the proportion of males with AM?

Ratio computation: Identify the number of AM cases of females (X) and the number of AM cases of males (Y). Compute the ratio by using the basic formula: X (cases in female)/Y (cases in males). Substituting for X and Y → 1,000/1,166 = 0.86:1. Therefore, there was less than one female patient for each male patient who reported for AM to the health department.

Proportion computation: Identify the number of AM cases of females (X) and the combined number of AM cases of females and males (Y). Compute the proportion by using the basic formula: (cases in females)/Y (cases in females and males). Substituting for X and Y → 1,000/2,166 = 0.46. Therefore, less than five out of every ten AM cases were in females. Ratios and proportions are used to characterize populations by age, sex, race, exposure, etc. Rates, ratios and proportions are used to describe morbidity, mortality and health outcomes in human conditions.

6.2.2 Measures of Disease Occurrence

The measure of disease occurrence in epidemiology compares disease frequency. These measures include risk, incidence rates (IR), period prevalence, cumulative incidence (CI) and prevalence proportion (PP). Risk refers to the probability that an individual or a group of persons will develop a specific disease. For example, if the total number of persons in a population (Notown) equals T, and D represents the number of people out of the T population who develop the disease (AM) during the period of time, the proportion D/T represents the average risk of developing AM in the population during that period.

6.2.3 Formula for Risk

The basic formula for risk computation is D/T = Number of subjects developing the disease or the event of interest during a time period/Number of subjects followed for that time period.

6.2.4 Average Risk or Cumulative Incidence

The average risk of a disease in a population is interchangeable with the incidence proportion as well as the CI of the disease. CI is the proportion of the population that becomes diseased or presents with the event of interest over a specified period of time.

6.2.5 Average Risk or Cumulative Incidence Computation

The average risk of getting a disease over a period of time, which is the probability of getting a disease, is an adequate measure when there are few or no losses to follow-up. The basic formula for CI is: Number of new cases of disease or event of interest or related health factor/Number in the population of interest, over a specific time period.

6.2.6 Incidence Rate or Incidence Density Computation

The IR is the measure of disease frequency that utilizes CI or average risk and ignores the concept of competing risk, thus underestimating the point estimate. Rates can be used to estimate risk only when the period of follow-up is short and the rate of the disease over that interval is relatively constant. IR takes into account the competing risk by modeling the disease occurrence with the person-time (P-T) of observation. The IR or incidence density (ID) is the occurrence of new cases of disease or events of interest that arise during P-T of observation.

6.2.7 How is Incidence Density or Incidence Rate Computed?

IR measures the incidence when the population at risk is roughly constant. The basic formula for IR is: Number of subjects developing the disease or events of interest (new cases)/Total time experienced by the subjects followed (person-time) of observation.

VIGNETTE 6.2

Consider that in Newcity, 35,000 women were at risk of postmenopausal breast cancer and contributed 250,000 person-years of follow-up. If there were 1,500 incident cases during the ten-year follow-up, what would be the ID for breast cancer in this population?

Computation: Identify the number of cases during the time period (A) and identify the total person-time of observation (follow-up) (B). Apply the basic formula, A/B. Substituting → 1,500/250,000 = 600.0 per 100,000 per year.

This formula measures incidence when the population is not constant, since the measure of incidence is complicated by changes in the population at risk during the period when cases are ascertained, for example, through births, deaths or migrations. This difficulty is overcome by relating the number of new cases to the person-years at risk. The denominator (person-years at risk) is calculated by adding together the periods during which each individual member of the population is at risk during the measurement period.

6.2.8   Cumulative Incidence Computation

The CI is related to IR by the formula CI = IR × T, where T is the specified period of time. Risk is related to IR and is mathematically given by: **Risk = IR × T.**

6.2.9   Prevalence Proportion

The PP measures the frequency of the existing disease (disease status). Two types of prevalence measures are common in epidemiology: point prevalence (proportion of the population that is diseased (new cases, current cases, old cases)) at a single point in time and period prevalence (proportion of the population that is diseased during a specified duration of time), for example, during the year 2006. The denominator for the point prevalence is the estimated population at the point in time, whereas the denominator for the period prevalence is the estimated population at mid-interval.

6.2.10   Factors Influencing Disease Prevalence

Prevalence is influenced by time. Therefore, the longer the duration of the disease, the greater the prevalence. Prevalence is also influenced by both IR and disease duration. The relationship between prevalence and IR is given by P = IR × D, where D is the duration of the disease or the event of interest (applicable to low disease prevalence, i.e., less than 10%).

When the prevalence of the disease is not low, the relationship between the prevalence and the IR is given by ID/1 + ID, where I = incidence and D = the duration of the disease.

Formula for point prevalence and period prevalence. The basic formula for **point prevalence** is given by the formula:

Number of existing cases of disease or event of interest/Number in total population, at the point in time.

Period prevalence is given by the formula:

Number of existing cases of disease or event of interest/Number in total population (estimated population at mid-interval).

6.2.11   Uses of Incidence and Prevalence Data

Epidemiology generates information for public health and clinical medicine decision-making. Information generated from prevalence studies, such as cross-sectional, is useful in program planning in public health services or quality assurance and training in clinical medicine settings for healthcare improvement. Similarly, incidence data that are generated from prospective cohorts or clinical trials point to the direction of factors that determine the observed effect and are primarily useful in assessing etiology (Table 6.1).

6.2.12   Limitations of Prevalence Data

Prevalence data tend to produce a biased picture of health-related events, such as disease, favoring the inclusion of chronic over acute diseases. Second, cause and

TABLE 6.1 Uses of Incidence and Prevalence Data in Public Health

Disease/Mortality Measures	Advantage	Disadvantage
Prevalence	Important and useful in the planning and monitoring of public health services (facilities, personnel, manpower) Expresses the burden of health-related events in a specified population Useful in determining the extent of the health-related events	Misclassification biases Reverse causal inference Simultaneous temporal trends on cause and effect
Point prevalence	Point prevalence is useful in tracking changes of health-related events in a population over time Substitution for the calculation of the impact of the health-related events in the absence of incidence data	Not an adequate estimator of incidence
Incidence	Important in estimating disease etiology Provides direct measure of disease/disability/injury rate or risk Allows for hypothesis testing on the magnitude of the effect of the risk factor(s) on the outcome of the health-related event (disease/disability/injury)	

effect are measured simultaneously. Third, they cannot be used for causal inference, and finally, the prevalence is determined from one survey, whereas incidence requires at least two sets of observations (records/data) of the same subject.

6.2.13   Proportionate Mortality and Morbidity

6.2.13.1   Proportionate Mortality (PM)

The PM refers to the fraction or proportion of deaths observed in a specified population over a specified period of time due to different causes. Mathematically, each cause is expressed as a percentage of all deaths, with the sum of causes approximated at 100%. This measure is useful in describing the burden of death in a population given a specific cause. Holmes Jr. et al. conducted a study to examine racial and ethnic disparities in in-hospital pediatric mortality in a specific population [6]. The proportionate mortality (PM) was used to assess specific causes of death among in-hospital mortality. This analysis used the total number of deaths as the denominator and deaths from specific causes as the numerator. The PM for respiratory diseases was estimated by using the number of children who died from any respiratory condition, such as respiratory failure, divided by the total number of in-hospital deaths and then multiplied by 1,000.

Mathematically proportionate mortality (PM) = specific cause of death/ in-hospital total number of deaths × 1,000.

As part of the results, 80 deaths (in-hospital) were observed over two years period, and using these, data, PM was computed which indicated the highest in-hospital proportionate mortalities in respiratory diseases (20/80; 25%, 250 per 1,000 deaths) and cardiovascular disorders (19/80; 23.8%, 238 per 1,000 deaths). The mortalities related to respiratory diseases were acute respiratory failure (8.8%, 88 per 1,000) and both acute and chronic respiratory failure (5%, 50 per 1,000), and the mortalities related to cardiovascular diseases were cardiac arrest (3.8%, 38 per 1,000) and ventricular septal defect (2.5%, 25 per 1,000). Gastrointestinal disorders, mainly necrotizing enterocolitis in newborn, were associated with 11.3% (113 per 1,000), and malignancy accounted for 8.8% (88 per 1,000). Other conditions included pneumonitis due to food inhalation (5%, 50 per 1,000), subdural hematoma (2.5%, 25 per 1,000), septicemia due to gram-negative pathogenic microbes (2.5%, 25 per 1000), complications of bone marrow transplant (2.5%, 25 per 1,000), epileptic grand mal seizures (3.8%, 38 per 1,000) and congenital anomalies (2.5%, 25 per 1,000).

Holmes et al. illustrated the use of PM in their study of pediatric cerebral palsy patients discovered dead during sleep between 1993 and 2011. Of the 177 patients who expired during this period, 19 were discovered dead during sleep (DDDS), resulting in a PM rate of 114.5 per 1,000. The study also indicated proportionate morbidity in the comorbidity associated with DDDS [4].

6.2.13.2 Proportionate Morbidity

Proportionate morbidity reflects the number of cases of a specific disease in a specified population divided by the total number of observed diseases over a specified period. PM has been used to characterize the number of cases in a subpopulation of cases of a specific disease divided by the total number of cases during a specified period of time. For example, suppose 5,250 adults were hospitalized during 2014 for several diseases in a comprehensive tertiary hospital. The hospitalization included asthma (650), chronic obstructive pulmonary disease (COPD) (450), CHF (300), pneumonia (550), metabolic disorders including diabetes mellitus (400), uncontrolled hypertension (414), cancer (800), stroke (900), infection (500), fractures (300), psychiatric conditions (195), substance and chemical dependency (105), and angina pectoris (86). The proportionate morbidity for uncontrolled hypertension during 2014 was $414/5,250 = 7.89\%$, implying that 8 out of every 100 patients were hospitalized for uncontrolled hypertension. The PM for stroke was $900/5,250 = 0.17 = 17.14\%$; stroke hospitalized in this hypothetical situation was 17 per 100 patients. Holmes et al. (2015) conducted a study on racial and ethnic disparities in pediatric asthma admission and readmission [6]. Using proportionate morbidity with subpopulation count divided by the total number of children admitted with asthma (n = 1,070) during 2010 and 2011, the highest proportionate morbidity was indicated to be highest among whites (40.9%) and blacks (40.5%), intermediate among others (16.7%) and lowest among Asians (0.6%), American Indian/Alaska Native (0.3%) and Hawaiian Native/Pacific Islander (0.3%) [6].

6.3 Measures of Disease Association or Effect

There are many steps in the epidemiologic investigation, one of which is determining the association between exposure and disease development. Measures of disease association include, but are not limited to, commonly used point estimates in epidemiologic research. These measures can be absolute or relative, such as risk difference and relative risk respectively. The application of such measures depends on multiple steps, which involve an association in the first place and the establishment of factual association by eliminating random error, confounding and effect measure modifier as possible explanations of such an association in the second. Commonly used measures of disease association include, but are not limited to, odds ratio, relative risk, risk ratio (RR), coefficient and hazard ratio.

6.3.1 Types of Rates (Crude, Specific, Adjusted)

6.3.1.1 Crude Rates

Crude rates are based on the actual number of events in a population over a given time period.

6.3.1.2 Crude Rates Computation

Examples of crude rates are birth rate, infant mortality rate, fetal death rate, maternal mortality rate, etc. Crude birth rate is computed by the basic formula: Number of live births within a given period/Population size at the middle of that period × 1,000 population.

VIGNETTE 6.3

Consider a population of Novelcountry to be 280,000,000 during 1996, and the number of babies born was 4,500,000 during the same period.

The crude birth rate will be: Number of live births (A)/Population size (B) × 1,000. Substituting for A and B → 4,500,000/280,000,000 × 1,000 = 16.07 per 1,000 (Table 6.2).

In epidemiology, the rate is often incorrectly used to refer to proportions or ratios, as in these illustrations.

TABLE 6.2 Crude Rates—Example and Basic Formula for Rate Estimation

Crude Rate	Formula	Interpretation
Birth rate	Number of live births within a given period/Population size at the middle of that period × 1,000 population	Affected by number of women of childbearing age Projects population changes
Infant mortality rate	Number of infant deaths among infants aged 0–365 days during the year/Number of live births during the year × 1,000 live births	Used for international comparison Low rates reflect balanced health needs
Post-neonatal mortality rate	Number of infant deaths from 28 to 365 days after birth/Number of live births minus neonatal deaths × 1,000 live births	Low rates reflect environmental events, infectious disease control and adequate nutrition

---

VIGNETTE 6.4

Consider a population of 200,000 people of whom 40 were diagnosed with pancreatic neoplasm (PN) in 2005, and during the same time period, 36 died from pancreatic neoplasm. How will you calculate the mortality rate in 2005 in this population, as well as the case fatality rate?

Computation: Mortality rate as a result of PN: 36/200,000 = 0.00018 (0.018%) or 18.0 per 100,000. Case fatality as a result of PN: 36/40 = 0.9 (90%).

6.3.1.3   Specific Rates

Specific rates refer to a particular subgroup of the population defined, such as age, sex, social class and race. An example of a specific rate is the age-specific rate. The age-specific rate refers to the number of cases per age group of population during a specified time period.

VIGNETTE 6.5

Consider that in no-county during 2006, there were 1,100 deaths due to bronchial carcinoma (BC) among the 55–74 age group, and there were 35,000,000 persons in the same age group. What will be the age-specific bronchial carcinoma death rate in this age group?

6.3.1.4   Specific Rate Computation

Computation: Using the formula Number of deaths (BC) among those aged 55–74 years (A)/Number of persons aged 55–74 years during 2006 (B) × 100,000. Substituting → A/B × 100,000; 1,100/35,000,000 × 100,000 = 3.14 per 100,000.

6.3.1.5   Adjusted Rate

An adjusted rate refers to summary measures of the rate of morbidity and mortality in a population in which statistical procedures have been applied to remove the effect of differences in the composition of the various populations, such as age, for the purpose of comparison. Two methods of rate adjustment are most commonly used in public health: the direct method is used if age-specific death rates in a population to be standardized are known and a suitable standard population is available. The indirect method, or standardized mortality ratio (SMR), is used when the age-specific death rates are unknown or unstable [5, 7, 8, 12].

6.3.1.6   Direct Method Computation

Direct method: Multiply the age-specific rate by the number of persons. Sum the expected number of deaths in each age group to determine the total number of expected deaths.

The age-adjusted rate is:

Total expected number of deaths/Number of deaths in the standardized or combined population × 100,000.

The result, the adjusted death rate, ensures that the observed differences in the death rates between the two populations compared are not due to age, gender or sex.

VIGNETTE 6.6

Using Table 6.3, consider the age group in years, the age-specific death rates per 100,000 in populations X and Y, and the number in the United States in 1998 (census population estimates). Determine which population has excess mortality.

Computation: Multiply A by C to obtain D, expected deaths for population X. Multiply B and C to obtain E, expected death for population Y. Obtain the age-adjusted rate for population X by summing the total in column D and dividing by the total in column C, then multiplying by 100,000. Repeat these steps for population Y as well. Subtract the rate in X (702.56 per 100,000) from Y (815.15 per 100.000). The excess age-adjusted mortality rate is 112.6 per 100,000.

6.3.1.7   Indirect Age-Adjusted Rate Computation

Indirect age-adjusted rate (SMR) is calculated by:

Observed number of deaths (A)/Expected number of deaths (B) × 100.

VIGNETTE 6.7

Consider the number of observed deaths in Notown from angina pectoris to be 1,200 during 2005. If the expected number of deaths is 2,000, what is the SMR?

Computation: SMR = A/B × 100. Substituting → 1,200/2,000 = 0.6 (60%).

TABLE 6.3 Age-Specific Mortality Rates for Populations X and Y

Age Group	Population X (age-specific rates per 100,000) (A)	Population Y (age-specific rates per 100,000) (B)	US Population (1998 census estimate) (C)	D (expected death for population (X))	E (expected death for population (Y))
<5 years	149.19	181.40			
5–19	43.44	36.78			
20–24	165.97	178.23			
45–64	521.18	725.04			
>65 years	4,011.94	4,517.68			
Total	417.91	1,060.94			

Source: Data from National Center for Health Statistics, Division of Data Services.

6.4   Measures of Disease Comparison

Measures of disease comparison are interchangeably used with measures of association or effect. We presented these measures by listing them earlier in this chapter. Next, we present the formula to enable clinicians to apply these crude measures of effect in understanding these basic epidemiologic approaches to disease association.

Absolute measure reflects the difference that is computed through subtraction. We can determine this by subtracting one number from the other. For example, if infant mortality in blacks is 11 per 1,000 live births and in whites is 4 per 1,000. The absolute risk difference in infant mortality comparing blacks to white children is 7 per 1,000 live births. This measure provides information about the public health impact of an exposure.

Relative measure reflects the difference that is computed through division. This measure is obtained by dividing one number from another. Using the above example, the relative risk for infant mortality comparing black to white children is 2.75, implying that black children are almost three times as likely to die before their first birth day compared to whites. This measure provides information about the strength of the relationship between exposure (independent variable) and outcome (disease, disabilities or injuries).

Absolute measures of comparison are risk difference, rate difference, IR difference, CI difference and prevalence difference.

Relative measures of comparison are RR, rate ratio, relative rate or relative risk, IR ratio, CI ratio and prevalence ratio.

6.4.1   Rate versus Risk

Risk is the accumulated effect of rate occurring during some specified time period. Risk has no time dimension, and the reference population in risk is the population unaffected at the beginning of the period of observation as well as the population with lower incidence or prevalence as the control.

AR, although not specifically a rate but a proportion, is the CI of a disease during an outbreak or transient epidemic.

AR = Diseased (exposed and developed an illness)/Diseased and Non-diseased (all exposed to the suspected agent of contamination) × (multiplier [100]) during a time period.

Secondary AR (SAR) is the proportion of individuals exposed to the primary case (primary cases), who themselves develop the disease (secondary case). SAR = Number of new cases in group minus initial case(s)/Number of susceptible persons in a group – Initial case(s).

VIGNETTE 6.8

Consider data on primary and secondary attack from salmonella pathogen. Is this a rate or ratio?

Solution: Because time is not involved in the denominator, this measure of disease is strictly not a rate but a risk (proportion).

6.4.2   Measures of Comparison/Association

The measures of disease association or comparison between the subpopulations of interest are assessed by: (a) rate or RR, (b) attributable proportion among total population, (c)

6.4.3   Rate or Risk Ratio (RR)

The rate or RR is calculated as RE/RU, where RE = risk or rate in the exposed and RU = risk or rate in the unexposed. This rate computation assesses or examines the strength of association between exposure (predictor as risk) and the disease (outcome).

6.4.4   Attributable Proportion among Total Population (APTP)

The APTP is computed by (RT − RU)/RT × 100, where RT = IR, CI or PP in the total population and RU is the IR, CI or PP in the unexposed population. The APTP measures the excess proportion of disease in the total population, assuming that the exposure is causal and implying that the proportion of disease in total population would be eliminated if the exposure were eliminated.

6.4.5   Attributable Proportion among the Exposed (APE)

The APE is computed by (RE – RU)/RE × 100. The APE measures the proportion of disease among the exposed, assuming that the exposure is causal and implying that the proportion of disease among the exposed will be eliminated if the exposure is eliminated [5, 12].

6.4.6   Population Rate Difference (PRD)

The PRD is computed by RT – RU or RD × PE, where RD = IR difference, CI difference or PP difference; and PE = proportion of population that is exposed, and RD = RE – RU. This PDR measures excess rate or risk of a disease or outcome in the total population.

6.4.7   Rate or Risk Difference (R-RD)

The R-RD is computed by RE – RU. This rate or risk difference measures rate or risk of disease or outcome among the exposed population.

6.4.8   Attack Rate (AR)

The AR is computed by ND/TP, where ND = number of people at risk for whom a certain outcome develops and TP = total number of people at risk. This AR compares the risk of outcome in groups with different exposure.

6.5   Sources of Epidemiologic Data

Data are available for epidemiologic studies, with sources ranging from vital statistics to NIH and other US Health and Human Services agencies. These preexisting data enable retrospective analysis of cross-sectional or prospectively collected data. The use of these data sources, while recommended, requires caution in the interpretation of their results. Therefore, like with most preexisting data, data validity and reliability remain an issue in terms of internal and external validity of the findings derived from these data sources.

Below are descriptions of the sources of epidemiologic data mainly:

Genomic/Epigenomic Data: The Epigenomics database is the current resource of the National Center for Biotechnology Information (NCBI) for a comprehensive public use of whole-genome epigenetic datasets (www. ncbi.nlm.nih.gov/epigenomics). The epigenetic Tools and Databases for Bioinformatic Analyses are located at https://epigenie.com/epigenetic-tools-and-databases. This tool involves the following dimensions, namely:

(a) **RNA**- nf-core/rnaseq: a bioinformatic analysis pipeline used for RNA sequencing data built using STAR: RNA-seq aligner that performs simultaneous; (b) **DNA** methylation involving: (i) pipelines and analyses (WGBS, RRBS, etc.), (ii) methylKit (single CpG statistics); (c) **Chromatin**: (i) nf-core/chipseq: a pipeline used for chromatin immunoprecipitation sequencing (ChIP-seq) data built using nextflow [13].

Vital statistics (VS): The VS provides information for births, deaths, marriages, divorces, etc.

US Census: It provides information on complete counts of US population every ten years. The types of information include race, sex, age and marital status (all samples) and income, education level, housing and occupation (representative samples).

National Health Interview Survey (NHIS): This survey provides data on major health problems, such as acute and chronic disease conditions, impairments and injuries, and the utilization of health services, such as dental care. The NHIS is useful in examining annual changes in disease and disability conditions.

National Health and Nutrition Examination Survey (NHANES): The NHANES provides information on the health and diet of the US population based on home interviews and nutritional examinations.

Behavioral Risk Factor Surveillance System (BRFSS): This is a survey of a random sample of the US population by phone interviews on behaviors affecting health and well-being (exercise, smoking, obesity, alcohol, automobile seat belt use and drinking and driving).

National Notifiable Diseases Surveillance System: This dataset provides information on most communicable diseases, including HIV/AIDS, botulism, gonorrhea, human and animal rabies, etc.

Surveillance, Epidemiology and End Results Program (SEER): This is the US National Institute of Health (NIH), National Cancer Institute (NCI) database that provides information on trends in cancer incidence, mortality and survival. The information provided includes patient demographics, primary cancer sites, pathology, first mode of therapy and severity of the disease.

World Health Statistics Annual: It provides information on international morbidity and mortality.

Cancer Incidence of Five Continents: This data source reflects the WHO's international agency for research and cancer that provides information on cancer incidence and mortality globally (estimated 170 cancer registries in 50 countries)

National Occupational Hazard Survey and National Occupational Exposure Survey: It provides data on workers exposed to chemical, physical and biologic agents.

Surveillance of AIDS and HIV Infection: This data source provides information on HIV/AIDS incidence and prevalence, as well as cumulative incidence.

6.6 Summary

Epidemiologic objectives remain the identification of populations at risk and the application of such knowledge to disease prevention and control. Clinical medicine is comparable given that the clinicians have an obligation to prevent death in the process of treating disease and prevent complications following treatment, thus maintaining health. Within this context, epidemiologic principles and methods are applied by clinicians in the process of minimizing therapeutic complications, prolonging survival and maintaining health.

The objective of clinical research is to provide valid and reliable evidence regarding therapeutics, screening, diagnostics and prevention, which depends on the design as well as the statistical methods used to generate these results. Clinical research designs are broadly classified as observational or epidemiologic and experimental or clinical trials if conducted in human populations, but this distinction remains inaccurate since experimental designs are also observational with respect to outcome or end-point. This (clinical) evidence is presented as measures of effects of disease, treatment, procedure, screening, etc. These effects are described as absolute or relative measures of comparison. Absolute measures of comparison describe and quantify the differences between two measures of disease frequency, while relative measures of comparison describe and quantify ratios of two measures of frequency, as well as the strength of association or relationship between exposure and the outcome of interest. For example, the rate difference measures the excess rate of outcome or disease among the exposed patient population, while the relative rate compares the rate of the exposed with the unexposed and indicates the strength of the relationship between the exposed and the disease or outcome. The rates of disease or outcome obtained from clinical studies may be compared across different study populations, but the reliability of such comparisons requires adjusted rates (for example, age-adjusted rates), also termed standardized rates.

Understanding the interpretation of these measures is essential to the application of the findings of clinical research to the improvement of patient care. Therefore, although sound statistical methods and inference are highly relevant to clinical results, it is important to give due consideration to the epidemiologic methods or the principles of the design of an investigation since valid evidence cannot be obtained unless the design is sound and accurate. Finally, because clinical research or epidemiologic studies are often entangled with confounding, caution is required in the interpretation of measures of disease occurrence or effects where these factors are not adjusted and illustrated in the crude or raw measures of association.

6.7 Questions for Review

1 Review a study by Holmes et al. (2019) on Aberrant epigenomic modulation of the glucocorticoid receptor gene (NR3C1) in early life stress (ELS) and major depressive disorder (MDD) correlation.

   a Examine the measure of the contributory effect of the gene, FKBP5 polymorphism, a gene that codes for protein that regulates the glucocorticoid complex, implicated in childhood trauma.
   b What percentage of DNA demethylation on itron 7 of this gene impacts childhood trauma?
   c Examine Table 1 and comment on the methylation index (MI) percentage of the 1F exon on the NR3C1 gene with respect to social adversity and major depressive disorders.
   d Examine Table 2 and discuss MI % in the mDNA of the NR3C1 gene.

2 Suppose you are conducting a study on the incidence of cerebral palsies in children (aged 0–4 years) exposed to maternal can beverage consumption during gestation, and a similar study is conducted in a different center with children (aged 12–21 years).

   a What is the measure of effect of can beverage consumption?
   b What is the problem in comparing these two incidence rates?
   c How will you perform a valid comparison in this case?
   d Is the association in this case causal?

3 One way to measure the effect of disease is by relative risk or odds ratio. What is the distinction between these two measures? Comment on the advantage of one over the other in determining the direct association between exposure and disease.

4 In a hypothetical study of the relationship between polycystic ovarian syndrome (POS) and endometrial carcinoma, 80 out of 280 with POS had developed endometrial carcinoma, compared with 600 out of 4,000 control women, who had endometrial carcinoma at some time in their lives.

   a Compute the odds ratio in favor of never having been diagnosed with POS for women with endometrial carcinoma versus controls.
   b What is the 95% CI for this association?
   c What can be concluded for these data?
   d Is there an association between POS and endometrial cancer based on these data?

References

1 Last JM. *A Dictionary of Epidemiology*, 3rd ed. (New York: Oxford University Press, 1995).

2 Greenberg RS et al. *Medical Epidemiology*, 4th ed. (New York: Lange Medical Book, 2005).

3 Savitz DA. *Interpreting Epidemiologic Evidence*. (New York: Oxford University Press, 2003).

4 Karatas AF, Miller EG, Holmes, L Jr. Cerebral palsy patients discovered dead during sleep: Experience from a comprehensive tertiary center. *J. Pediatr. Rehabil. Med.* 2013;6:225–231.

5 Mausner J, Kramer S. *Epidemiology—An Introductory Text*, 2nd ed. (Philadelphia, PA: Saunders).

6 Holmes L Jr, Kalle F et al. Health disparities in pediatric asthma: comprehensive tertiary care center experience. *JNMA*. 2015;107(3):1–7.

7 MacMahan B, Trichopoulos D. *Epidemiology, Principles & Methods*, 2nd ed. (Boston, MA: Little, Brown, 1996).

8 Rothman KJ. *Epidemiology, An Introduction*. (New York: Oxford University Press, 2002).

9 Holmes L Jr, Shutman E et al. Aberrant epigenomic modulation of glucocorticoid receptor gene (NR3C1) in early life stress and major depressive disorder correlation: Systematic review and quantitative evidence synthesis. *Int. J. Environ. Res. Public Health*. 2019;16(21):4280. doi: 10.3390/ijerph16214280.

10 Holmes L Jr et al. Lower regional pediatric in-hospital mortality albeit racial/ethnic disparities. *J. Natl. Med. Assoc.* 2018,110(6):583–590. doi: 10.1016/j.jnma.2018.03.007. Epub 2018 Apr 25.

11 Holmes L Jr et al. DNA methylation of candidate genes (ACE II, IFN-γ, AGTR 1, CKG, ADD1, SCNN1B and TLR2) in essential hypertension: A systematic review and quantitative evidence synthesis. *Int. J. Environ. Res. Public Health*. 2019;16(23):4829. doi: 10.3390/ijerph16234829.

12 Holmes L Jr. *Applied Epidemiologic Principles and Concepts*. (Boca Raton, FL: Taylor & Francis Publisher, 2018).

13 Epigenomic public access data source: Available at: https://epigenie.com/epigenetic-tools-and-databases/ - [Accessed 21 May 2023].

7
ECOLOGIC DESIGN

7.1   Introduction—Ecologic Design

The ecologic design simply reflects a group-level assessment rather than individual subject or patient data or information [1–4]. The examination of subpopulation data in comparing risk determinants in one subpopulation relative to the other facilitates individual subject risk and predisposing factors in morbidity and mortality. For example, if one population in a specific geographic locale is exposed to railroad air pollutants and the prevalence of bronchitis and/or chronic obstructive pulmonary disease (COPD) is higher in such a population compared to the unexposed population, this reflects an ecologic study. With such data, a need arises for individual subject studies such as cross-sectional design, thus marginalizing ecologic fallacy toward a causal inference.

7.1.1   Epigenomic Modulation and Group Assessment

Epigenomic modulation that is implicated in heritable alteration in gene expression is observed in impaired protein synthesis and cellular dysfunctionality (malignant neoplasm); however, this modification occurs without any alteration in DNA sequence. While DNA remains a statistic in the process of ontogeny, epigenetic code undergoes dramatic alteration during embryonic development, initiating differential patterns of gene expression within developing tissues. The observed epigenetic codes comprise chemical modifications to DNA as well as histones, which are proteins that are central to tightly coiling and packaging DNA into nucleosomes.

DNA methylation, as stated earlier, occurs within the CpG regions as CpG islands in the promoter or enhancer region of the gene which is linked to

DOI: 10.4324/9781003094487-9

transcriptional silencing. The epigenetic regulation of transcription as a transcriptome is driven by histone modification, namely acetylation, methylation, phosphorylation and ubiquitination, with histone acetylation remaining very essential and fundamental in histone transcriptional regulation. Specifically, histone acetylation implies the addition of the acetyl group to lysine residues on the amino-terminal tails of the histones, resulting in the neutralization of the positive charge and hence decreasing their affinity for the DNA. This process allows for increased accessibility of transcriptional regulatory proteins to chromatin templates, as well as being regulated and catalyzed by enzymes such as acetyltransferases and deacetylases. Basically, DNA methylation and histone modification may inter-correlate, collectively enhancing or influencing the accessibility of chromatin to RNA polymerase and transcription factors. Additionally, gene expression modulation is enhanced by non-coding RNA which regulates gene activities at transcriptional as well as posttranscriptional levels.

Epigenomic modulations have been implicated in nutritional imbalance. For example, obesity, T2D, CVDs, osteoporosis and cognitive impairment have been observed in nutritional imbalance as under-nutrition and over-nutrition, with significant variations in DNA methylation and histone modifications. The observed differentials signal a causal pathway in these health conditions with nutritional environment. Without individual data on DNA methylation or histone modification, group-level data, although not causal, could be utilized in the understanding of how nutritional imbalances predispose to these conditions, and thereafter individual-level data by a cross-sectional design.

7.2 Ecologic Design Concept and Application

Ecologic designs, also called group-level ecologic studies [2], correlational studies or aggregate studies, obtain data at the level of a group or community often by making use of routinely collected data. Second, when the population, rather than the individual, is the unit of study and analysis, such a study is correctly characterized as ecologic. This design involves the comparison of aggregate data on risk factors and disease prevalence from different population groups in order to identify associations. Because all data are aggregated at the group level, relationships at the individual level cannot be empirically determined but are rather inferred. Thus, because of the likelihood of an ecologic fallacy, this type of study provides weak empirical evidence.

Basically, the focus of ecologic studies is the comparison of groups, and not individuals, implying the missing of individual data on the joint distribution of variables within the group. This focus places the need for ecologic inference about effects on group levels. The question is: why conduct an ecologic study given the critique of this method among some epidemiologists? The rationale involves feasibility and data reliability and accuracy in generating testable hypothesis. Ecologic studies are conducted when there are no initial data on a health problem, no individual-level data are available, data are available at the group level and there are limited research resources and time (rapid conduct).

7.2.1   Ecologic Design: Advantage

The advantages of ecologic design include its ability to generate hypotheses for individual-level data design and analysis, being inexpensive, and requiring a short period of time to conduct. The required data for ecologic studies may be obtained from published literature or public access databases, rendering the conduct less time-consuming and inexpensive [1, 4–6]. While ecologic fallacies have been observed to be the main disadvantage of ecologic design, individual-level studies are not completely immune from them, implying careful ascertainment of exposure and disease variables in the conduct of ecologic studies.

Ecologic designs are used for geographical comparison of diseases, such as investigating the correlation between childhood brain cancer in certain regions of the United States, implicating clusters in some regions relative to the state. If, in the same region, there is a low consumption of extra virgin olive oil, hypotheses can be generated about the association between brain cancer and extra virgin olive oil. However, care must be exercised in the interpretation of such ecologic studies given the potential for confounding factors such as age, sex, Socio-economic status (SES), education and access to primary care. Ecologic studies are also useful in assessing time and secular trends in disease [5]. While rates of acute conditions such as bronchiolitis fluctuate over time, rates of chronic diseases tend to remain stable over time. Ecologic studies may be used to generate hypothesis if disease rates illustrate a correlation with environmental changes. For example, increasing rates of upper respiratory disorders in children during the summer may be due to carbon monoxide car emissions during the summer months.

Migrant studies remain a typical example of ecologic designs for hypothesis generation. These studies provide the opportunity to examine genetic, environmental and gene-environment association or determinant of disease. For example, if a migrant population in the United States (i.e., Asians) is observed to have a higher incidence of prostate cancer in the United States compared to Asians in Asia, the higher rate of Prostate cancer (CaP) among Asians in the United States may be due to environmental conditions in the United States. Also, the observed higher incidence of CaP among Asians in the United States may be due to selective emigration from Asia, implying those who were more susceptible to prostatic adenocarcinoma or hormonally related malignancies in general. Race/ethnicity, mortality, chronic obstructive pulmonary disease and occupation illustrate the correlation. African Americans have higher

Epigenome – Normal Modulation vs. Aberrant Modulation

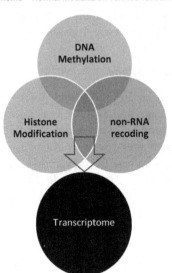

FIGURE 7.1 The epigenomic mechanistic processes: DNA methylation, histone modification and non-RNA recoding. These mechanistic processes influence the transcriptomes, resulting in protein synthesis and cellular functionality. If these processes become aberrant, they can lead to adverse gene expression, impaired protein synthesis, as well as abnormal cellular differentiation and proliferation.

age-adjusted mortality compared to whites, and are more likely to be employed in low-paying jobs, which correlates with higher mortality. On the basis of these correlations, hypotheses on the association between COPD incidence and low-paying jobs could be generated (Figure 7.1).

7.3 Conducting an Ecologic Study

To conduct an ecologic study, we need aggregate information on groups or subpopulations on the dependent or outcome variable of interest and the independent, explanatory or predictor variable [6–9]. For example, to determine the effect of alcohol consumption on stroke, we can obtain information on the prevalence of stroke in populations A, B and C and then determine alcohol consumption in these three populations. Finally, we correlate alcohol consumption and stroke prevalence in these three populations. If alcohol is a risk factor for the development of stroke, the population with the highest alcohol consumption will be associated with the highest prevalence of stroke. Alternately, if alcohol consumption per capita is protective, then the population with the highest alcohol consumption will be associated with the lowest prevalence of stroke.

7.3.1   *Importance of ecologic data*

One situation where ecologic data are particularly useful is when a powerful relationship that has been established at the individual level is assessed at the ecologic level in order to confirm its public health impact [4–6, 8–10]. If a risk factor is a major cause of a condition (in terms of population attributable fraction as well as the strength of association), then a lower presence of that factor in a population should presumably be linked to a lower rate of the associated outcome.

7.3.1.1   Examples of Ecologic Studies in Epidemiologic Evidence Discovery

A study on prostate cancer mortality and dietary practices and sunlight levels as environmental risk factors for geographic variability in the CaP rate was conducted using an ecologic design. The CaP mortality rate was compared in 71 countries. The per capita food consumption rate and sunlight levels were correlated with age-adjusted mortality rate in CaP. The study indicated an increase in CaP mortality rate with total animal fat calories, meat, animal fat, milk, sugar, alcoholic beverages and stimulant consumption, but an inverse correlation with increased sunlight level, soybeans, oilseeds, onions, cereal grains and rice [10]. Caution must be exercised in the application of these aggregate data in clinical decision-making regarding the recommendation of these food products and sunlight exposure. Like all aggregate or group-level data, the geographic variation in lifestyle and potential CaP confounders remain to be assessed. Additionally, countries may differ in the presence of effect measure modifiers which may explain part of the observed correlation in these data.

Hypothetical Study: Ecologic Study of the Association between Extra Virgin Breast Cancer Mortality (age-adjusted) Rate in Five Countries

7.3.2   *Statistical Analysis in Ecologic Design*

The estimate of the effect of exposure/s on disease or health-related events involves not just a correlation coefficient but a predictive parameter [1]. To estimate the effect or association, we have to regress the group-specific disease or outcome rates (Y) on the group-specific exposure prevalence (X). Therefore, the linear regression model remains useful in estimating the effect or association in ecologic studies. The prediction equation in this context is represented by $Y = \beta 0 + \beta 1 X 1$, where $\beta 0$ is the intercept on the Y-axis (coefficient without the effect of the exposure) and $\beta 1$ is the slope. The predicted outcome rate ($Yx = 1$) in a group with the exposure, or entirely or mostly exposed, is $\beta 0 + \beta 1(1) = \beta 0 + \beta 1$, and for the group that is less exposed or unexposed, the predicted rate for ($Yx = 0$) is $\beta 0 + \beta 1(0) = \beta 0$. Consequently, the estimated rate difference is $\beta 0 + \beta 1 - \beta 0 = \beta 1$, while the rate ratio is $(\beta 0 + \beta 1)/\beta 0 = 1 + \beta 1/\beta 0$.

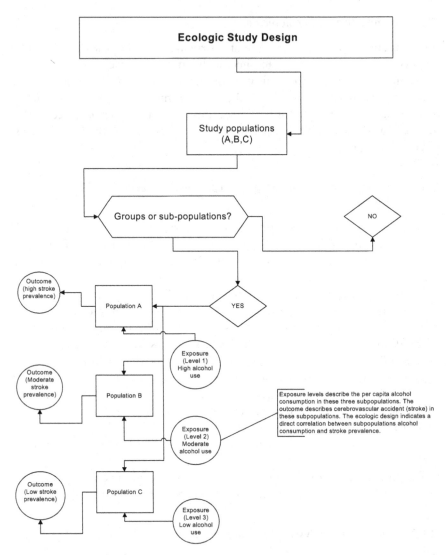

FIGURE 7.2 Ecologic study design structure. With respect to histone modifications such as histone acetylation and CDKN2A/CDKN2B in B-precursor ALL, the loss of these genotypes is observed in an estimated 40% of B-precursor ALL, adversely affecting cell cycle regulation in ALL. The assessment of the epigenomic modulations based on group data may facilitate the contributory effect of these genotypes in this malignant neoplasm, requiring individual case data for specific and individual adverse gene expression.

7.3.2.1 Ecologic Evidence: Association or Causation?

Data from ecologic design indicate association and not causation. However, etiologic studies are often based on initial ecologic investigations.

Biological Pathway: Association involves a possible biological mechanism. For example, extra virgin olive oil consumption (group level) and female breast cancer mortality rate among women in the five selected countries (hypothetical). The biologic pathway reflects the inhibition of abnormal cellular proliferation given extra virgin olive oil consumption. These data showed an inverse correlation between olive oil consumption and breast cancer mortality, implying that countries with high extra virgin olive oil consumption have a lower breast cancer mortality rate.

Group Level: Association is based on group-level exposure in the countries examined. For example, women who consume extra virgin olive oil may be exposed to more vegetable and fruit consumption, as well as physical activities, than women who do not, and breast cancer has been associated with vegetable and fruit consumption as well as physical activities.

Contextual: Association involves biological mechanism as well as ecologic or group-level exposures (Figure 7.2).

7.3.2.2 Limitations of Ecologic Study Design

Despite several practical advantages of ecologic studies, there are methodological issues that limit causal inference, including ecologic fallacies and cross-level bias, unmeasured confounding, within-group misclassification, a lack of adequate data, temporal ambiguity, collinearity and migration across groups [4, 5]. Ecologic fallacies typically represent the absence of association observed at one level of grouping to correlate to an effect measure at the group level of interest. Specifically, ecologic bias or fallacies refer to the absence of an association at the individual-level data despite the observed association at the group level [10–15]. Additionally, study limitations using this design reflect geographic variability in the ascertainment of exposure and disease, implying the need for uniformity of exposure and disease exposure across geography [11–13].

7.4 Summary

The ecologic design assesses the relationship between the exposure and outcome of interest at a group level and does not involve individual-level analysis as applicable to cohort, case-control and cross-sectional classic designs. These designs are feasible when group-level data are available and inference is required on such a level and not at individual-level risk. It is analytic since the measure of effect, the correlation coefficient, is an essential inference when provided with the coefficient of determination. Since individual data are not assessed in an ecologic design, an inference about individual risk from such a design remains invalid, leading to an ecologic fallacy.

The analysis of ecologic design involves different measures of effect and association and includes the correlation coefficient but mainly predictive parameters, namely the linear regression model. While the linear regression model is appropriate in the analysis of ecologic research data, temporality (cause-and-effect association) and confounding remain major issues in the interpretation and application of ecologic findings in public health policy formulation as well as in intervention mapping.

While epigenomic assessment based on causal inference of DNA methylation or histone modification is not adequate, the availability of existing data at the subpopulation level such as cyclin-dependent kinase inhibitor 2A (CD-KN2A) (9p21.3) and AT-rich interactive domain 5B (ARID5B) (10q21.2) may facilitate the understanding of these epigenotypes in ALL and the application of individual-level data in epidemiologic designs such as case-control studies and, most relevant in causal inference, prospective cohort design.

7.5   Questions for Review

1 A study is planned to investigate the benefits of agent X in drinking water (agent X is measured at group level) and the risk of developing dental caries in children.

   a Which design should be used if individual-level data is not available?

   b What are the advantages and disadvantages of ecologic design? Comment on ecologic fallacy.

   c What is the measure of effect or association in ecologic design, and how is it interpreted?

2 Suppose you are required to examine the effect of maternal education on learning abilities in Sweden, Norway, Finland, Austria, Australia, the United Kingdom and the United States, and there are no data on individual cases. How will you begin to conceptualize the study? What design will be most feasible to draw an inference on the association between maternal education and learning disabilities in children?

3 Consider a study to determine whether or not there is an association between extra virgin olive oil consumption and breast cancer. If data are obtained from several countries on extra virgin olive oil consumption and the incidence of breast cancer, what design could be feasible in assessing this relationship? Second, on the basis of these aggregate data, what sort of causal inference could be drawn, if any? Comment on the distinction between biologic and ecologic causality.

4 Suppose you are required to assess poverty among children and education attainment in adulthood and data are only available in different countries on poverty level and mathematical skills in children. What design should be feasible in this case? What will be the measure of effect? Comment on the association between education and poverty, and discuss the implications of this for the subsequent health status of children.

5 If a study observed ARID5B SNP rs10821936 allele frequency as an ALL predisposing factor based on control and ALL cases assessment as ALL susceptibility, as well as the association of this genotype among whites with European ancestry. How could an ecologic design be conducted to determine whether or not this genotype reflects epigenomic aberration by subpopulations, namely whites, blacks/AA and Hispanics?

References

1 Holmes L Jr. *Applied Epidemiologic Principles & Concepts.* (Boca Raton, FL: Taylor & Francis Publisher, 2018).

2 Rothman KJ. *Epidemiology, An Introduction.* (New York: Oxford University Press, 2002).

3 Morgensen H. Ecologic studies in epidemiology: Concepts, principles and Methods. *Annu. Rev. Public Health.* 1995;16:61–81.

4 Morgenstern H, Thomas D. Principles of study design in environmental epidemiology. *Environ. Health Perspect.* 1993;101(Suppl 4):23–28.

5 Holmes L Jr. *Basics of Public Health Core Competencies.* (Sudbury, MA: Jones and Bartlett, 2009).

6 Rothman KJ. *Modern Epidemiology,* 3rd ed. (Philadelphia, PA: Lippincott, Williams & Wilkins, 2008).

7 Hennekens CH, Buring JE. *Epidemiology in Medicine.* (Boston, MA: Little Brown & Company, 1987).

8 Greenland S. Epidemiologic measures and policy formulation: Lessons from potential outcomes. *Emerg. Themes Epidemiol.* 2005;2:1–4.

9 Gordis L. *Epidemiology,* 4th ed. (Philadelphia, PA: Elsevier Saunders, 2014).

10 Colli JL, Colli A. International comparison of prostate cancer mortality rates with dietary practices and sunlight levels. *Urol. Oncol. Semin. Orig. Investig.* 2006;24:184–194.

11 Elwood M. *Critical Appraisal of Epidemiological Studies in Clinical Trials,* 2nd ed. (New York: Oxford University Press, 2003).

12 Aschengrau A, Seage III GR. *Essentials of Epidemiology.* (Sudbury, MA: Jones & Bartlett, 2003).

13 Friis RH, Sellers TA. *Epidemiology for Public Health Practice.* (Frederick, MD: Aspen Publications, 1996).

14 Szklo M, Nieto J. *Epidemiology: Beyond the Basics.* (Sudbury, MA: Jones & Bartlett, 2003).

15 Greenberg RS. *Medical Epidemiology,* 4th ed. (New York: Lange, 2005).

8

CROSS-SECTIONAL STUDY DESIGN (NON-EXPERIMENTAL)

8.1   Introduction—Epigenomic Modulations and Design

A cross-sectional design (CSD) is a snapshot study, classified as an instant co-hort [1–3]. This design simultaneously examines exposure as a risk or predic-tor as well as the outcome. In this design, which may be indicative of reverse causal inference, the identification of a predictor or exposure variable, such as race, ethnicity, age and sex, prior to the outcome variable remains causal.

Epigenomic studies require the assessment of aberrant epigenomic modula-tions in health outcomes such as hypertension, cardio-metabolic disorders and neuropsychiatric disorders. For example, perinatal anxiety and stress, mater-nal deprivation and separation in early life, and disparities in maternal access and care utilization may reflect cognitive impairment, neuropsychiatric condi-tions, major depressive disorder as well as cardio-metabolic conditions. The application of genome-wide and candidate gene studies with respect to gene expression such as DNA methylation, histone modification as acetylation, methylation and phosphorylation, and non-coding RNAs facilitates the un-derstanding of early life stress as well as isolation and subordination in aberrant epigenomic modulations, hence poor health outcomes in a specific popula-tion. A CSD that allows for data collection on maternal separation during early postnatal time has been implicated in neuroendocrine regulation disruption, namely hippocampal glucocorticoid receptor upregulation as well as hypotha-lamic corticotropin-releasing factor (CRF) and increased corticosterone and adrenocorticotropic hormone, and is required in assessing DNA methylation as well as histone modification. This design approach enables the comparison of the methylation index (MI) with either correlation or mean in the process

DOI: 10.4324/9781003094487-10

of understanding aberrant epigenomic modulations by comparing maternal separation or deprivation with non-maternal separation or deprivation.

A CSD is a non-experimental epidemiologic design that is feasible and ethical when a randomized clinical trial cannot be conducted and other non-experimental designs are less feasible or inefficient. This design basically assesses the association between diseases or health-related events and other variables or factors of interest as potential risk factors in a defined population at a particular time [2–8]. Contrary to the sampling method involved in case-control design, cross-sectional studies obtain data on exposure and disease status at the same time, implying the prevalence measure and not disease incidence data.

While the outcome of CSDs is determined at the same time as the exposure or intervention, this design remains effective in quantifying the prevalence of disease or risk factors, especially in circumstances where resources are limited to apply other designs. Appropriate sampling is optimal for inference, and this applies to CSD as well [4]. In effect, the sampling frame used for the sample selection and the response rate in CSD determine the extent of its generalizability. Consequently, if epidemiologists select a random sample in the conduct of a cross-sectional study (CSS), then the sample will be representative, yielding a reliable inference. Additionally, the response rate should be reasonable to reflect sample representation. What should clinicians or those conducting CSS aim to accomplish in an attempt to address sampling representation? Clinicians could minimize a low response rate by: (a) using telephone and mail prompting, (b) sending second and third mailings of surveys, (c) offering reasonable incentives and (d) communicating clearly the importance of the study to potential participants. Clinicians should be cautious of biased responses which may be associated with recall bias in participants without the outcome of interest. For example, consider a CSS on passive smoking and asthma where a door-to-door survey is conducted during working hours. The groups more likely to be interviewed are women, girls, mothers, children and the elderly, and asthma is more likely to be higher in this group, biasing the outcome assessment in a given population.

CSS designs are conducted in situations where multiple exposures could be explored, implying the clinician's ability to gather lots of data without a threat of loss of follow-up as experienced in longitudinal or cohort studies. Additionally, CSS is recommended in clinical or public health settings for public health and healthcare planning, examining predisposing factors to disease, and generating hypotheses for multiple and complex disease etiologies.

CSDs are limited by: (a) lack of temporal sequence—disease and exposure sequence, (b) biased identification of cases—a high proportion of prevalent cases of long duration and a low proportion of prevalent cases with short duration, and (c) healthy worker survivor effect bias—those employed are healthier relative to those who remain unemployed [1, 2, 4–6].

Because non-experimental studies can yield valid epidemiologic evidence on the relationship between exposure and disease, a well-designed cross-sectional can address important clinical research questions regarding disease prevention, treatments and possible etiologies as implicated in aberrant epigenomic modulations in cardiovascular diseases, malignant neoplasms and T2D.

8.2 Rationale and Basis of a Cross-Sectional Study

Whereas cohort studies (prospective) are designed to measure the incidence (new events or changes) of a disease or an event of interest, cross-sectional studies assess the prevalence and hence focus on existing states [6–10]. Thus, no matter the frequency of data collection from a specified population, unless data are collected more than once from the same population, such a design cannot be termed longitudinal or concurrent. CSD remains a snapshot of exposure and outcome (response) [11–13].

CSDs can also be used for causal association because prevalence, as pointed out earlier, reflects both the incidence rate and the duration of the disease [1, 2, 14]. As a result, these studies yield associations that reflect both the determinants of survival with the disease and the disease etiology (Figure 8.1).

8.2.1 Feasibility of Cross-Sectional Design

A CSD is used to measure the prevalence of health outcomes, health determinants or both in a population at a point in time or over a short period of time. Such information can be used to explore disease risk factors. For example, a study was conducted to examine demographic and lifestyle predictors of the intention to use a condom in a defined population [15]. The prevalence of the intent to use a condom was the response or outcome, while demographic and lifestyle variables were the predictors, independent or explanatory variables, and were both measured at the same time from a survey instrument. Since exposure (demographics and lifestyle) and outcome (intent to use a condom) were measured simultaneously for each subject, the cross-sectional design used by these authors was qualified. In this study, the authors first identified the population of subjects and determined the presence or absence of the intent to use a condom, as well as the lifestyle and demographics for each subject. Using a 2 × 2 table, they compared the prevalence of lifestyle and demographic features in those with the intent to use a condom and compared it with those without the intent to use a condom: $(A/A+C) \div (B/B+D)$. A CSD represents a snapshot of the population at a certain point in time.

Because of the inability to establish the cause-and-effect relationship, any association in this design must be interpreted with caution. Second, bias may arise because of selection into or out of the study population. Due to the

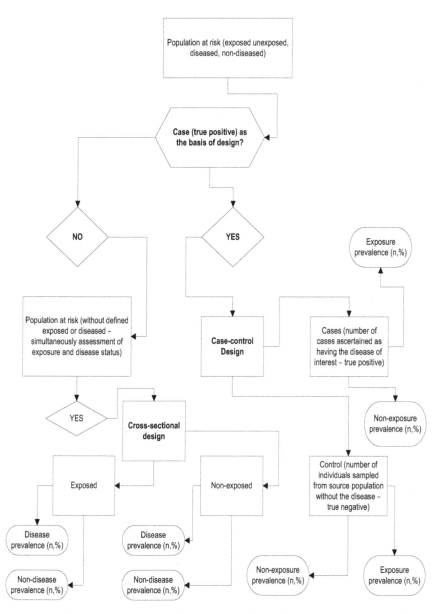

FIGURE 8.1   A cross-sectional design as a snapshot, implying an instant cohort study.

issues arising from a lack of temporality (cause-and-effect relationship), cross-sectional studies of causal association are best conducted to examine accurate disorders, clinical conditions with little disability, or presymptomatic phases of serious and chronic disorders.

8.3   Strengths and Limitations of Cross-Sectional Design

8.3.1   Strengths (Advantages)

Below are the strengths and advantages of conducting non-experimental epidemiologic studies based on the research questions, aims and the hypotheses, as well as the nature of the data, such as preexisting secondary data or current data collection:

- Generalizability, given that a sample is usually obtained from large population
- Relatively inexpensive
- Relatively easy to conduct
- Rapid in conduct and data acquisition
- Assessment of multiple outcomes and exposures or risk factors
- No loss to follow-up

8.3.2   Limitations (Disadvantages)

Below are the study limitations which are driven by preexisting data as well as the conceptualized study:

- Inability to assess the temporal sequence between exposure and disease or health-related events if exposure changes over time
- Preponderance of prevalent cases, indicative of survivorship
- Healthy worker survival effects, implying an association or prevalence odds/risk ratio reflecting survival after the health-related event rather than the risk of developing the event or disease [2, 4]

CSDs could also be used in planning health care. For example, a prostate cancer epidemiologist planning a chemoprevention intervention with micronutrient supplements to reduce the incidence rate of prostate cancer among African American men in Delaware State might wish to know the prevalence of prostate cancer in this subpopulation by age and other factors so that the epidemiologists could address the chemoprevention intervention accurately.

8.3.2.1   Cross-sectional Design and Case-Control Comparability

While the case-control study is not fully discussed in this chapter but was mentioned previously, there is a need to examine the CSD with case-control.

A Cross-Sectional Design

- Cross-sectional studies, also called surveys and prevalence studies, are designed to assess both the exposure and outcome simultaneously.

- However, since exposure and disease status are measured at the same point in time (snapshot), it is difficult, if not impossible, to distinguish whether the exposure preceded or followed the disease, and thus cause-and-effect relationships are not certain, lacking temporal sequence.
- No matter how frequent a CSS is conducted, it does not represent a longitudinal study since one is unable to ensure a repeated measure from the same sample from baseline.

B Case-Control Design

- A case-control design classifies subjects on the basis of outcome (disease and non-disease or comparison group) and retrospectively identifies the exposure of interest.
- This design could be prospective as well.
- In this design, the history or previous events for both cases and comparison groups are assessed in an attempt to identify the exposure or risk factors for the disease.
- If properly designed with a representative sample, both cross-sectional and case-control designs can generate valid and reliable results.

It is unlikely that any sample provided is representative and could be used to provide a generalizable result from both designs. For example, the fact that only older women with chronic kidney disease (CKD) are studied with respect to hypertension as a predisposing factor does not render the results unreliable, provided inference is drawn from older women. The problem is assuming that hypertension predisposes to CKD in young women and men who were not in the sample studied.

8.4 Atypical Cross-Sectional Design: Novel Design with "Big Data"

This design involves the application of preexisting data with a large sample size as "big data" in the assessment of the exposure effect of an outcome [2]. The rationale behind this design is to ensure adequate generalizability rather than relying on random error quantification such as the p-value since the p-value does not reflect the point estimate reliable difference as clinically or biologically meaningful difference, confounding or effect measure modifier but the sample size (sampling variability). While the assessment of preexisting data does not require sample size estimation, the process of accurate and reliable finding requires an approach that utilizes sampling from a sample, also termed "Bootstrapping."

The atypical CSD involves the utilization of the case or exposure and the non-case or none-exposed from the total sample. In such a dataset, the investigative team will identify the exposed as well as the unexposed and apply systematic random sampling in the process of identifying the non-exposed that will not be more than four times (4×) the exposed sample size within the large dataset in order to obtain a reliable, valid and accurate point estimate and inference in the risk estimation [2].

The benefit of this design is the application of a biologically and clinically meaningful difference comparing the non-case (non-exposed) with the case (exposed) rather than random error quantification as study generalizability. With this approach, caution must be implied in the interpretation of the random error quantification, p-value as well as the cautious interpretation of the point estimate comparing the case with the non-case.

VIGNETTE 8.1. Cross-Sectional Design

Consider a study that is interested in the possible association between low serum lycopene levels (exposure) and prostate cancer (disease). The population is surveyed and serum lycopene levels are determined for all subjects, while Prostate specific antugen (PSA) for prostate cancer is performed; both the exposure and the outcome are determined at the same time.

Could this constitute a CSD? Calculate the prevalence risk ratio if 20 of the 60 men with low serum lycopene levels had prostate cancer and 10 of the 80 men with high serum lycopene levels had prostate cancer.

Computation: Prevalence risk ratio: a/a+b/c/c + d. Substituting →
20/80/10/90 = 0.25/0.11 = 2.27.

A CSS was conducted using a health fair survey to examine the prevalence of chronic disease among participants who take part in at least 45 minutes of daily exercise versus those who do not during the past 12 months. The data obtained are summarized in the 2 × 2 table.

2 × 2 TABLE: Physical Activities and Chronic Disease (Hypothetical Data)

	Physical Activity (≥45 Minutes)	Physical Activity (<45 Minutes)	Total
Chronic Disease (+)	45 (A)	100 (B)	145
Chronic Disease (−)	155 (C)	35 (D)	190
Total	200 (A + C)	135 (B + D)	335

The prevalence odds ratio = odds in the exposed/odds in the unexposed = AD/BC = 45 * 35/100 * 155 = 1575/15,500 = 0.10. The crude estimate indicates a protective effect of physical activity >45 minutes per day for chronic disease. Thus, those who exercised, according to this hypothetical data, were

90% less likely to be told that they had any form of chronic disease. We can determine the statistical stability of these data by quantifying the random error (p-value) and precision (95% CI)

STATA Application: (command/syntax)

cci 45 100 155 35:

2 × 2 TABLE: Cross-Sectional Study Using Case-Control computation (Hypothetical Data)

Chronic Disease	Exposed (Physical Activities)	Unexposed (No Physical Activities)	Odds Ratio	95% CI
Control (–), WCD	*155*	*35*	*Referent*	*Referent*
Case (+), NCD	45	100	0.10	0.06–0.17

Notes and Abbreviations: WCD = with chronic disease; NCD = no chronic disease. The physical activities (≥45 minutes) were associated with low chronic disease prevalence compared to those with <45 minutes of physical activities. Compared with those with <45 minutes of physical activities, those with ≥45 minutes of physical activities were 90% less likely to develop chronic disease (OR = 0.10, 95% CI, 0.06–0.17, p < 0.001).

The STATA output indicates a statistically stable inference, p <0.001, 95% CI, 0.060–0.17 (precision). Since older individuals are more likely to have chronic disease and are less likely to exercise, age may be a confounding or effect measure modifier in the relationship between physical activity and chronic disease. Therefore, the observed inference may be misleading without assessing for confounding or the modifying effect of age.

VIGNETTE 8.2. Aberrant Epigenomic Modulation and Maternal Depressive Episode

The glucocorticoid response elements of FKBP5, an HPA-axis regulating gene, are observed in childhood trauma, with DNA demethylation associated with increased stress-dependent gene transcription as well as long-term dysregulation of the stress hormone and immune system.

1 Examine the stress-related methylation levels of the brain-derived neurotrophic factor (BDNF) gene and its key role in neural and behavioral plasticity, as well as this gene's expression in the prefrontal cortex.

2 Determine whether or not maternal depression during the gestational period reflects the decreased levels of methylation in the promoter region of the SLC6A4 gene, utilized in serotonin transporter encoding in maternal

peripheral leukocytes, and compare this effect with the BDNF gene in this maternal depressive mood.

8.5 Summary

Cross-sectional studies are used to examine the relationship between exposure and disease at the same point in time. These studies measure the prevalence of the exposure and disease or outcome of interest. One issue in this design is the difficulty in establishing temporal sequence as well as over- or underestimation of disease prevalence.

The feasibility of the research question or issues and the available resources determine which of these designs is to be used in evidence discovery. Therefore, if appropriately applied, these designs could generate standard and reliable results in addressing clinical and public health issues, thus improving and maintaining health.

There are obvious advantages to CSD, mainly that it is inexpensive, rapid and easy to conduct. Remarkably, this design could generate reliable and generalizable findings given the large and random samples. However, the lack of temporal sequence tends to limit its application to association and hypothesis generation for causal or etiologic studies. A clear ambiguity on the causal pathway is the association between milk and peptic ulcer. Does milk cause peptic ulcers or are those with peptic ulcers more likely to consume milk to reduce the hyperacidity seen in this condition? Despite the observed limitations, a well-conceptualized and performed CSS could benefit clinical medicine and public health in terms of health care and public health program planning respectively.

While causal inference is difficult to estimate in an a CSD, understanding exposure prior to outcome as a snapshot facilitates a causal inference evaluation. Remarkably, this design upon accurate findings allows for an evidence-based scientific discovery through a prospective cohort study design.

8.6 Questions for Review

1 Suppose you are a physician and have seen a few patients with prostate cancer, almost all of whom report that they have been exposed to milk and red meat. You and your colleagues hypothesized that the exposure to milk and red meat is related to the development of prostate cancer in these patients.

   a Which study design will be adequate in testing this hypothesis?
   b Do you need a control, and how will you select your control?
   c What would be the measure of association in your design?
   d What are the benefits and disadvantages of this design?

e Comment on the measure of the effect of the exposure on the disease as a direct measure of risk.

2 A "healthy worker survivor effect" bias has been identified as one of the limitations of cross-sectional design. Comment on this.

3 If you were expected to examine the association between obesity and TV watching, would you consider cross-sectional design? What are the anticipated problem with sampling and response rate? Comment on the causal association in this relationship.

4 Cross-sectional studies are often criticized for their lack of temporal sequence. Can this same criticism be applied to case-control design, and why?

5 Consider a hypothetical study performed in an outpatient clinic on the association between vaccination and developmental disorders, such as autistic spectrum disorder (ASD), in children. If data were gathered on mothers with and without children with autism as outcome and history of vaccination before the diagnosis of autism was gathered simultaneously (survey questionnaire) as exposure, what is the design used in this study? Is it difficult or simple to establish a causal relationship between exposure and outcome on the basis of this design? Suggest other alternative designs that may lead to causal association inference. Can we assess relative risk on the strength of this design? Finally, if among 300 of the children vaccinated, (ASD) was ascertained in 15, and among 400 unvaccinated children, there were 30 children with ASD, what are the odds and the odds ratio?

6 Suppose among 200 children with cerebral palsy, 125 had feeding difficulties, and among 180 controls, 75 had feeding difficulties. Test the hypothesis that feeding difficulties are associated with cerebral palsy.

a Compute the odds ratio relating cerebral palsy to feeding difficulties in children.

b Provide a 95% CI for the estimate.

c What can you conclude from these data?

7 In a population-based study of pediatric with SEER dataset, 2000–2018, African American children presented with higher or excess mortality compared by their white counterparts.

a Could the observed survival advantage of AA be explained by the ALL immunophenotype (T-ALL, B-ALL, T-ALL non-specified)?

b Does chromosomal translocations such as t(12,21) with ETV6-RUNX1, t(1,19) with TCF3, PBX1 fusion, t(9,22) with BCR-ABL1 fusion and MLL rearrangements at 11q23 explain this survival differential?

c Is it possible that TCF3-PBX1 is overexpressed among AA?

d Is it possible that PIP4K2A locus rs7688318 is associated with ALL risk differentials by race/ethnicity?

e Based on the GWAS (genome-wide association studies), is the IKAROS family zinc finger 1 (IKZF1) (7p12.2) associated with ALL susceptibility among whites and AA?

f With respect to ARID5B and PIP4K2A loci, what epigenomic mechanistic process could be utilized in the aberrant epigenomic modulation in the pediatric survival differentials explanation?

References

1 Levin KA. Study design III: Cross-sectional studies. *Evid. Based Dent.* 2006;7:24–25.

2 Holmes L Jr. *Applied Epidemiologic Principles & Concepts.* (Boca Raton, FL: Taylor & Francis Publisher, 2018).

3 Savitz A. *Interpreting Epidemiologic Evidence.* (New York: Oxford University Press, 2003).

4 Morgenstern H, Thomas D. Principles of study design in environmental epidemiology. *Environ. Health Perspect.* 1993;101(Suppl 4):23–28.

5 Holmes L Jr. *Basics of Public Health Core Competencies.* (Sudbury, MA: Jones and Bartlett, 2009).

6 Rothman KJ. *Modern Epidemiology*, 3rd ed. (Philadelphia, PA: Lippincott, Williams & Wilkins, 2008).

7 Hennekens H, Buring JE. *Epidemiology in Medicine.* (Boston, MA: Little Brown & Company, 1987).

8 Gordis L. *Epidemiology*, 4th ed. (Philadelphia, PA: Elsevier Saunders, 2014).

9 Rothman KJ. *Epidemiology, An Introduction.* (New York: Oxford University Press, 2002).

10 Elwood M. *Critical Appraisal of Epidemiological Studies in Clinical Trials*, 2nd ed. (New York: Oxford University Press, 2003).

11 Aschengrau A, Seage III GR. *Essentials of Epidemiology.* (Sudbury, MA: Jones & Bartlett, 2003).

12 Friis RH, Sellers TA. *Epidemiology for Public Health Practice.* (Frederick, MD: Aspen Publications, 1996).

13 Szklo M, Nieto J. *Epidemiology: Beyond the Basics.* (Sudbury, MA: Jones & Bartlett, 2003).

14 Greenberg RS. *Medical Epidemiology*, 4th ed. (New York: Lange, 2005).

15 Essien J, Holmes L Jr et al. Emerging sociodemographic and lifestyle predictors of intention to use condom in human immunodeficiency virus intervention among uniformed services personnel. *Mil. Med.* 2006;171:1027–1034.

9

CASE-CONTROL (COMPARISON/ NON-CASE) DESIGN

9.1   Introduction

Aberrant epigenomic modulations and epigenetic abnormalities have been identified in developmental syndromes and disorders, malignant neoplasm, and chronic diseases such as essential hypertension (eHTn) and psychiatric conditions. This aberration can affect individual genes, or globally, such as genome-wide DNA hypomethylation, loss of DNA methylation boundaries at CpG islands, as well as loss of balance between active and repressive histone modifications. There is a dysregulation of DNA methylation that is pervasive in disease, which may facilitate a case-control epidemiologic as well as non-experimental design in some pathologies, namely malignant neoplasms, T2D, eHTn, major depressive disorder (MDD), etc. Specifically, malignant cells exhibit both global DNA hypomethylation and focal hypermethylation. DNA hypomethylation often occurs in low-density CpG regions, repeats, satellite DNA and regions associated with nuclear envelope lamina as well. This DNA hypomethylation may spread over large blocks of DNA. Unlike DNA hypomethylation, locus-specific DNA hypermethylation occurs in CpG islands and lower-CpG-density CpG islands as well as CpG shores. The hypermethylation of CpG islands in promoter or enhancer regions results in gene silencing, as observed in tumor suppressors, p27 and p53. Similarly, promoter hypomethylation has been observed in oncogene activation as well as in loss of imprinting [1].

A genomic study as genetic that implies TCF3-PBX1 fusion in T-ALL, ETV6-RUNX1 translocation in ALL, as well as Down syndrome (trisomy 21) in ALL, requires a case-control study on the DNA methylation of these epigenomic markers for reliable and accurate therapeutics in ALL. With prenatal exposure to higher body fat, a higher BMI, obesity, a lipid profile, primary

DOI: 10.4324/9781003094487-11

insulin resistance, glycemic dysregulation and immune system dysfunction, this gestational environment (cases) may predispose to aberrant epigenomic modulations, leading to excess disease outcomes among those with these conditions compared with the control (non-cases).

Case-control studies are traditional to epidemiology and refer to a design that compares subjects or patients ascertained as diseased, with the specific outcome of interest, subclinical conditions or risk determinants, with comparable subjects or patients who do not have the disease or outcome of interest, and examines retrospectively (most cases) to determine the frequency of the exposure or risk factor in each group, with an attempt to assess the relationship between the exposure/risk factor and the disease/outcome [2–7]. As simple as it may appear in conceptual terms, implying the cases as the basis of design upon which controls are sampled. This sampling difficulty, which may create non-comparable controls, renders evidence from this design unreliable as controls may not reflect similar experiences or other exposures experienced by the cases (differences in related risk factors that may not be known—unknown confounding).

In the previous chapter, an ecologic epidemiologic design with a focus on multiple groups and group-level analysis was presented. In this chapter, an attempt is made to present an individual-level design with individual-level analysis [1–4]. While randomized placebo-controlled clinical trials (RCTs) are the gold standard of clinical research in determining therapeutic benefits, thus providing evidence to guide clinical or surgical practice, they are not always feasible or ethical. Randomization of study participants into treatment and control ensures the balance of baseline prognostic factors and implies that the differences between the groups compared result from the trial or intervention and are not confounded by baseline differences between them [2, 4, 5–8]. Despite the advantages of RCT, ethical issues remain potential obstacles to the application of this design in clinical research, requiring epidemiologists or investigators to use non-experimental designs that are feasible for addressing the research questions. In addition, non-experimental studies are efficient in clinical epidemiology, population science or medicine since they could be used in assessing a wider range of exposures relative to RCTs.

Case-control studies are classically retrospective designs in which investigators identify and enroll cases of the disease or outcome of interest and sample the source population (control or comparison group) that generated the cases [9–12]. Since case-comparison studies are relatively inexpensive and faster to conduct, the availability of cases, as in rare diseases, should suggest the application of this design. There are limitations to this design, but this should not discourage the use of a well-designed case-control study in examining the exposure status of those with and without the outcome or disease of interest, especially when exploring rare outcomes or when the induction or latent periods are long, as in malignancies. Therefore, investigators should prefer a case-control design when limited information is available on disease etiology or exposure. This approach allows investigators to generate information on the exposure distribution, thus indirectly comparing the rate of the disease or outcome in exposed and unexposed groups.

This chapter describes the notion, design process, measures of association or effect, and strengths and limitations of case-control design. First, case-control is presented along with the variants of this design. Second, the notion of case-control as a prospective design is mentioned, but not discussed in detail due to the scope of this book. For example, if all the cases did not occur at the time of study initiation and new cases were included as the study progressed, such a design represents prospective case-control. However, while this notion of prospective case-control is not widely used among epidemiologists, the inclusion of incident cases in ongoing case-control studies represents an "ambi-directional case-control" design. Next, the limitations of case-control are discussed with the intent of describing the inherent inadequacies of this design despite its widespread use in epidemiologic studies, especially in the context of rare diseases. Finally, the recommendations are made to reflect how to report the method and results in case-control designs (Figure 9.1).

9.2 Case-Control Design: Conceptualization and Application

9.2.1 Basis of Case-Control Design

A traditional case-control study represents non-experimental designs that begin with cases who have the disease or experience events of interest and the selection of the control subjects without the disease or events of interest from the source population. These controls are comparable with the cases except for the outcome of interest. In terms of directionality, this design uses outcome to determine the exposure and is mainly retrospective with respect to timing, rendering temporal sequence difficult to properly ascertain; sampling is based on the outcome [3, 5]. In a case-control study, patients who have developed a disease are identified and their past exposure to suspected etiological factors is compared with that of controls or referents who do not have the disease. This design allows the estimation of odds ratios (OR; but not attributable risks). For example, a case-control study was conducted to examine the association between intraoperative factors and the development of deep wound infection. The investigators retrospectively ascertained 22 cases over a period of ten years and sampled controls from the source population (patients with neuromuscular scoliosis who underwent spine fusion for curve deformity correction).

Case-control studies have been shown to be efficient in assessing many exposures, indicating their unique strength; however, caution must be exercised

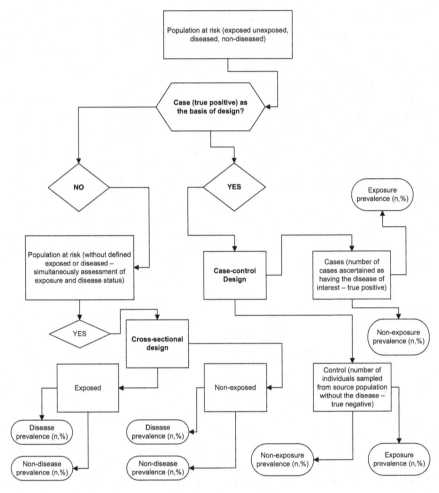

FIGURE 9.1 Case-control and cross-sectional designs. While these two designs are retrospective as traditional epidemiologic designs, case-control ignores the simultaneous assessment of the risk as exposure and the outcomes, which is implicated in cross-sectional design as a "snapshot." For example, if there are 88 ALL patients (cases) and 53 healthy blood donors (control) and the methylation index is required for TCFL5(20q13.33) and DSC3(18q12.10), the case-control design reflects an appropriate design.

in determining the association of the exposures with the disease. A study with 12,461 cases and 14,637 controls on obesity (body mass index [BMI], hip, waist, waist-to-hip ratio) and the risk of myocardial infarction indicated a graded and highly significant relationship with waist-to-hip ratio but not with BMI. This association persisted after adjustment for age, sex, region and smoking, indicative of the relevance of waist-to-hip ratio in the obesity and disease relationship [13].

Another example involved the association between neck circumference and childhood asthma severity, in which children with severe asthma (cases) were compared with those with low and moderate asthma (controls) with respect to neck circumference as exposure. Data were also collected on hips, waists and the calculated waist-to-hip ratio. Investigators utilized the electronic medical records to identify children diagnosed with asthma severity as cases (n = 11) and obtained controlled samples using stratified systematic sampling techniques to obtain age-matched controls (children with mild and moderate asthma, n = 44, 1:3 ratio). With the age-adjusted neck circumference, cases were compared with controls for differences in exposure experience (unpublished paper). This example reflects the use of hospital-based control by selecting control from the hospital which may not represent the source population where the cases were obtained. However, alternatives to hospital-based design, such as sampling the controls from the population where the hospital is located, may not provide a comparable control if the hospital has proven quality outcomes and low costs (value care), implying the referral of cases nationally and globally.

Case-control presents a unique issue in the ascertainment of exposure since the controls may not have similar or comparable exposure to the cases if the source population where the cases originated differs from the control, as in the example of a hospital-based or clinic-based case-control study on asthma severity and neck circumference. Epidemiologists are challenged with uniformity in the ascertainment of exposure and the balance between the exposure experiences of the controls if the controls differ from the cases.

9.2.2 Cases Ascertained in Case-Control Studies

9.2.2.1 Selection of Cases

The starting point of most case-control studies is the identification of cases. This requires a suitable case definition, as in the example above of a deep wound infection. In addition, care is needed so that bias does not arise from the way in which cases are selected. A study of a deep wound infection after posterior spine fusion in children with neuromuscular scoliosis might be misleading if cases were identified from hospital admissions and admission to the hospital was influenced not only by the presence and severity of neuromuscular scoliosis but also by other variables, such as medical or specific health insurance. In general, it is advantageous to use incident (deep wound infection) rather than prevalent cases since prevalence is influenced not only by the risk of developing the disease of interest but also by factors that determine the duration of illness. Please recall that the prevalence proportion = $I \times D$, where I is the incidence rate and D is the mean duration of illness. This formula is applicable when the prevalence of the disease is small—less than 10%.

It is adequate because with small prevalence, prevalence proportion will approximate the prevalence odds. Furthermore, if disease has been present for a long time, then premorbid exposure to risk factors may be harder to ascertain, especially if assessment depends on subjects' recall.

In the previous example, deep wound infection case ascertainment was based on the combination of signs and symptoms, physical and microbiologic examination, and results of these diagnostic tests. Investigators should apply existing standard criteria to define the cases with as much accuracy as possible to avoid selection and misclassification bias. With standard criteria for case ascertainment, the next step is to identify cases and enroll them in the study by gathering data on them. The sources of data in this case were the medical records. In typical case-control studies, other sources of data include patients' rosters, death certificates, birth certificates, MRI, CT, X-ray, PET, etc. It is important to recognize the role of accuracy and efficiency in the ascertainment of the cases. Depending on the research question, incident cases may be preferred to prevalent cases. Therefore, if the intent is to study risk factors, it is preferable to study incident cases since prevention cases reflect factors that affect the disease duration and not the factors that cause the disease itself. However, regardless of the cases used in case-control studies, investigators should apply caution in the interpretation of the results. Therefore, it is important to point out if the factors studied affect the disease etiology, its duration or a combination of the two. A 2 × 2 contingent table could be used to illustrate point estimate or association and effect in a case-control design (unmatched design). The odds of the exposure in the case relative to the control are provided by cross product exposed/case (a) and control/non-case (d), divided by the cross product exposed/non-case (false positive) and non-expose/case (false negative). Mathematically, the measure of effect or association in a case-control design is given by ad/bc [3, 10].

9.2.3   Selection of Controls in Case-Control Studies

Usually, it is not too difficult to obtain a suitable source of cases, but selecting controls tends to be more difficult, since the control must be comparable to the cases, except for the disease status or outcomes of interest. Controls are expected to come from the same source population as the cases and are expected to meet these two requirements:

1 Within the constraints of any matching criteria, their exposure to risk factors and confounders should be representative of that in the population "at risk" of becoming cases—that is, people who do not have the disease under investigation but who would be included in the study as cases if they did.
2 The exposure/s status of controls should be measurable with similar accuracy to those of the cases. Geographic variation and temporal factors

must be considered in the ascertainment of cases and control if different geographic locales are involved in cases and controls sampling. Specifically, the diagnostic criteria, implying disease ascertainment, may differ from one location to another.

9.2.4   Case-Control Design: Strengths and Limitations

Case-control or case-comparison design, while reliable and efficient, has some limitations and disadvantages. However, there are no scientific findings that are driven by absolute certainty, since *the p-value for random error quantification is* never 0.00, implying all scientific findings driven by "uncertainties."

Strengths (Advantages)

- Efficient for rare diseases (desirable design)
- Efficient for diseases with long induction and latent periods
- Adequate for evaluating multiple exposures in relation to a disease (desirable when little is known about exposure variables in a given disease).
- Rapid and inexpensive relative to prospective cohort design

Limitations (Disadvantages)

- Recall and selection bias due to the retrospective nature of design
- Difficult to assess temporal sequence between exposure and disease or health-related events if exposure changes over time
- Information bias and poor information on exposure (retrospective nature of design)
- Inefficient for rare exposure

9.3   Hybrids of Case-Control Studies

Nested Case-Control

- A case-control study conducted within a cohort study
- Involves an ongoing study with a defined cohort
- Random sampling of cases and controls is very feasible

Case-Cohort

- Applicable where the source population is a cohort and every individual in the cohort has an equal opportunity of being selected as a control
- Person-time contribution of the cohort is not relevant
- Efficient when the measure of effect of interest is the incidence proportion ratio or average risk

- Mathematically: Re (incidence proportion among exposed sub-cohort) = De/Ne, where De is the number of the diseased among the exposed and Ne is the total population of the exposed. Likewise, Ru (incidence proportion in the unexposed sub-cohort) = Du/Nu, where u is unexposed
- Incidence proportion ratio = Re/Ru
- To be reliable as design to measure the incidence proportion ratio, the ratio of the number of exposed controls (Re) to the number of the exposed sub-cohort (Ne) should be similar to the ratio of the number in the unexposed control (Ru) to the number of unexposed sub-cohort (Nu)

Density Case-Control

- Can be used to estimate risk ratio—if the ratio of person-time denominators Te/Tu is accurately estimated by the ratio of exposed to unexposed controls (De/Du)
- Involve the selection of controls such that the exposure distribution among them is the same as it is among the person-time in the source population—density sampling

9.3.1   Case-Cross Over: Conduct and Measure of Effect/Association

9.3.1.1   Sources of Controls

There are two commonly used sources of controls:

1 General or source population: Controls selected from the general or source population have the advantage that their exposures are likely to be representative of those at risk of becoming cases. However, assessment of their exposure may not be comparable with that of cases, especially if the assessment is achieved by the subject's recall; as cases are more likely to recall factors that may be related to their illness relative to healthy controls.

2 Hospital-based control: If controls are selected from a group of patients with a disease that is different from the disease of interest in the case-control study, then controls are more likely to recall the exposure. Therefore, measurements of exposure can be made more comparable by using patients with other diseases as controls, especially if subjects are not told the exact focus of the investigation. However, their exposures may be unrepresentative. For example, a case-control study of prostate cancer (CaP) and an agent used to enhance erectile function could give quite erroneous findings if controls were taken from the impotence clinic. If other patients are to be used as referents, it is safer to adopt a range of control diagnoses rather than a single disease group. In that way, if one of the control diseases happens to be related to a risk factor under study, the resultant bias is not too large.

When cases and controls are both freely available, then selecting equal numbers will make a study most efficient. However, the number of cases that can be studied is often limited by the rarity of the disease under investigation. In this circumstance, statistical confidence can be increased by taking more than one control per case. There is, however, a law of diminishing returns, and it is usually not worth going beyond a ratio of four or five controls to one case [9, 11, 12].

9.3.2   Ascertainment of Exposure

A wide variety of exposures are involved in disease causation or association and include but are not limited to lifestyle, environment, job, occupation, heredity or genes, diet, alcohol and drugs. In any of these exposure circumstances, information is required on the source, nature, exposure frequency and duration of exposure. Many case-control studies ascertain exposure from personal recall, using either a self-administered questionnaire or an interview. The validity of such information will depend in part on the subject matter. People may be able to remember quite well where they lived in the past or what jobs they did. However, long-term recall of dietary habits is probably less reliable. For example, in a study of the relation between intraoperative factors and deep wound infection, the information for the cases and controls was ascertained by searching their medical records. Provided that records are reasonably complete, this method will usually be more accurate than one that depends on memory. Occasionally, long-term biological markers of exposure can be exploited. Biological markers are only useful, however, when they are not altered by the subsequent disease process. For example, serum cholesterol concentrations measured after a myocardial infarction may not accurately reflect levels before the onset of infarction [13].

9.4   Case-Control Analysis—Measure of Effect or Association

The statistical techniques for analyzing case-control studies are discussed in previous chapters. The odds of exposure, given the disease (cases), and the odds of exposure, given non-disease (control), are computed as follows:

The odds of case exposure = exposed cases/all cases ÷ unexposed cases/all cases.

Mathematically, this appears as follows:

Odds (of exposure) Ratio (or) = AD/BC, also termed Relative Odds (RO)
$(A/A{+}B) \div (B/A + B) = A/B$

where AD and BC represent the cross products from the 2 × 2 contingency table.

The odds of control exposure, implying odds of exposure in the control group = C/D,

Odds Ratio (OR)/(RO) = odds of case exposure/odds of control exposure =
(A/B) ÷ (C/D) = A*D/B*C.

Because the two groups are sampled separately, rates of disease, disability or injury in the exposed or unexposed groups cannot be calculated, nor can relative risk be measured directly. However, the OR can be computed; it is the primary measure of association in a case-control design. Because of the sampling used, the total number exposed is not a + b, and the risk in exposed subjects is not a/(a + b).

It is important to note that the attempt at event (exposure or outcome) estimate is not to directly derive disease incidence in the exposed and unexposed groups, but to estimate the odds of exposure in the cases and in the controls. Additionally, if the controls are sampled from all subjects initially at risk, then this design can directly estimate the risk ratio, but if controls are sampled from those who are still disease-free at the time where all cases are obtained (end of follow-up, no more new cases), then it is possible to estimate the OR for the disease (odds of disease ratio). Finally, if the controls are sampled (time matching of controls with the case ascertained) from those still at risk at the time that each case is ascertained, then it is possible to estimate the rate ratio.

9.4.1 Variance of Case-Control Design

Nested case-control is advantageous to the classic case-control in that it minimizes and eliminates recall bias; it ensures or reduces the uncertainty with the temporal sequence, thus making it easy to determine whether the exposure preceded the disease; and it is relatively inexpensive and rapid, compared to prospective cohort design. Nested case control is limited in that the non-diseased may not be fully representative of the original cohort because of loss to follow-up or death. The OR is a good estimate of relative risk, except when the outcome is very frequent (high prevalence).

9.4.2 Case-Cohort Design

Density case-control studies require that the control series represent the person-time distribution of exposure in the source population. Epidemiologists establish this representativeness by sampling controls in such a way that the probability that any person in the source population is selected as a control is proportional to his or her person-time contribution to the incidence rates in the source population. Regarding case-cohort study:

- It is a case-control study in which an individual selected as a control may also be a case.
- Every person in the source population has the same chance of being included as a control regardless of how much time that individual has contributed to the person-time experience of the cohort.
- Each control participant represents a fraction of the total number of individuals in the source population, rather than a fraction of the total person-time.
- The point estimate is similar to that of the density case-control study, but the estimated odds represent the risk ratio, while the odds estimated in the density case-control study is a measure of the rate ratio.

9.4.3   Odds Ratio in Case-Control and Cohort Designs

The odds and probability (case-control versus cohort design): Odds differs from probability (P) but is related by the following equation.

Odds $= P \div (1 - P)$.

For example, if the **probability** of the diseased individuals being exposed is 80% (0.8), the **odds** of the diseased individuals being exposed are 4.0, which is 80/20 ($P/1 - P$), where P = probability and $1 - P$ = "non-probability" of the disease.

In a cohort design, the probability that the exposed will develop a disease is a/a + b and the odds that a disease will develop in the exposed is a/b ($P/1 - P$). The probability that the disease will develop in the unexposed is c/c + d; similarly, the odds of the disease developing in the unexposed is c/d ($P/1 - P$). The OR (incidence rate ratio) in cohort design is presented mathematically as follows:

Incidence Rate Ratio (IRR) $= A/B \div C/D = A*D/B*C$.

These are the odds that an exposed person develops a disease divided by the odds that a non-exposed person develops the disease.

9.4.4   Measure of Disease Effect or Association Obtained in Matched Case-Control

The OR from a matched case-control study using a 2×2 contingency table is assessed by Table 9.1.

TABLE 9.1 Matched Case-Control 2 × 2 Table

	Control Exposed	*Control Unexposed*	*Total*
Case exposed	A	B	A+B
Case unexposed	C	D	C+D
Total	A+C	B+D	A+B+C+D

Notes: A = both case and control are exposed; B = case exposed but control unexposed; C = case unexposed but control exposed and D = case unexposed and control unexposed. A and D are concordant pairs.

Assuming 1:1 matching, the OR is given by the following equation:

Odds Ratio (1:1) Matched Pair = B/C (Discordant Pairs)

where B (case exposed and control unexposed) and C (case unexposed and control exposed) are the discordant pairs, implying exposed case divided by unexposed case.

9.4.5 *Interpretation of Odds Ratio (OR) or Relative Odds (RO) in Case-Control Study*

Suppose a case-control study was conducted to examine the association between postnatal steroid use and cerebral palsy, and investigators obtained an OR of 3.6. What does this mean? Simply, the odds of the use of postnatal steroid for children with cerebral palsy is over three times greater than the odds for the use of postnatal steroid among the control (children without cerebral palsy) in the study.

Consider another example of a case-control study on the association between measles-mumps-rubella (MMR) vaccination and autism. With 96 cases, investigators sampled 192 matched controls (year of birth, sex and general practitioners). Investigators used a conditional logistic regression model to assess the association between MMR vaccination and autism. The adjusted OR for MMR (vaccinated versus non-vaccinated) after adjusting for mother's age, medication during pregnancy, gestation time, perinatal injury and Apgar score was 0.17, 95% CI, 0.06–0.52 [14]. What is the basic interpretation of this result? First the odds of developing autism was 83% lower among children vaccinated with MMR compared to unvaccinated children. In addition, the 95% CI (unadjusted type I error level tolerance for multiple comparison/multivariable logistic regression) does not include "1," implying a statistically precise point estimate.

While the interpretation of associations in non-experimental epidemiologic studies may be straightforward, that is not the case in case-control designs. Specifically, the observed point estimate or association or no association may be due to: (a) selection bias, (b) information bias (exposure) and (c) confounding (assessment and adjustment).

9.4.6   Scientific Reporting in Case-Control Studies: Methods and Results

The scientific statement on the reporting of observational (non-experimental) studies, termed Strengthening the Reporting of Observational Studies in Epidemiology (STROBE), recommends the result section include participants (numbers potentially eligible, study sample, actually analyzed participants, flow diagram to reflect eligibility and actual sample), descriptive statistics mainly on participant characteristics (demographic, clinical, social) as well as missing data on all variables examined. Additionally, the numbers in each exposure category or summary measures of effect (OR) should be reported as outcome data. Further, the main result should include unadjusted or crude (raw), and, where applicable, the adjusted estimate and their precisions (95% CI), including the confounders included in the adjusted model and the rationale for their inclusion. Other reports such as subgroups, interaction, propensity and sensitivity analysis should be presented in the result section.

STROBE recommended the method section to report on the design used in conducting the study, study setting (location or site), participants (eligibility criteria, data source, sampling method), variables, data sources and measurement, sample size and power estimation, and statistical analysis. The statistical analysis should include a description of all methods used (summary statistics, crude and adjusted), methods for subgroup and interaction analysis as well as an explanation for missing data, if applicable [15, 16].

VIGNETTE 9.1: Case-Control (Hypothetical)

A study was conducted to examine the role of selenium in the development of CaP. There were 15 cases of older men with localized incident CaP and 15 controls (older men without prostate or any other malignancy). The proportion of cases and controls who ingested selenium as a daily supplement was estimated from the data. Among cases of CaP, three reported of having had selenium supplement daily during the past five years, while 13 did so among the controls. On the basis of these data, is there an association between routine selenium intake and the development of CaP?

Using STATA statistical software, we are able to obtain the frequency of the cases of CaP and controls who took selenium. The syntax "tab exposure (0,1) disease (0,1)" generates the frequency distribution of the exposure within the disease status (case/control) (Tables 9.2 and 9.3).

tab exposurestatus_seleniumuse disease_caP (STATA command)

To examine the association between selenium intake and CaP, we can use the software again by entering the appropriate syntax: cc outcome (var) exposure (var) (Table 9.4):

TABLE 9.2 2 × 2 Tabulation on Association between Selenium and Prostate Cancer

Exposure	Disease		Total
	Non-Disease (0)	Disease (CaP (1))	
Non-selenium (0)	2	13	15
Selenium use (1)	12	3	15
Total	**14**	**16**	**30**

Notes: Selenium is an anti-oxidant, implying normal cellular proliferation and stenosis inhibition. The table reflects hypothetical relationship between anti-oxidant selenium and CaP (cancer of the prostate gland).

TABLE 9.3 Hypothetical Data on Selenium Use and Prostate Cancer Incidence

ID	Age	Race	Exposure (Selenium)	Disease (CaP)
001	50	1	1	1
002	45	2	0	1
003	60	3	0	1
004	70	1	0	1
005	66	2	0	1
006	65	1	1	0
007	48	1	1	0
008	50	2	1	0
009	55	1	0	0
010	63	2	0	1
011	43	1	0	1
012	67	2	0	1
013	75	3	0	1
014	64	3	0	1
015	65	1	1	0
016	48	2	1	0
017	50	4	0	1
018	55	1	1	1
019	63	1	1	1
020	43	1	0	1
021	67	1	0	1
022	65	1	1	0
023	48	2	1	0
024	50	1	1	0
025	55	2	1	0
026	63	2	1	0
027	43	2	0	0
028	67	2	1	0
029	59	1	1	0
030	61	2	0	1

Data code: Age is in years, race/ethnicity; Caucasian = 1; African American = 2; Hispanic = 3; Asian = 4, 0 = absence of exposure or outcome, and 1 = presence of exposure or outcome. R = Race, Ex = exposure to selenium.

TABLE 9.4 2 × 2 Table on Exposure Effect in Case-control Design

Disease	Exposed	Unexpored	Total	Proportion
Cases (CaP)	1	13	16	0.19
Control	12	2	14	0.86
Total	15	15	30	0.50

Notes: Selenium = exposed while unexposed are those without selenium. This table requires the application of odds ratio in the association between selenium and CaP development.

TABLE 9.5 Exposure Effect of Selenium in Prostate Cancer Incidence

Disease	Exposed	Unexposed	Total	Proportion
Cases (CaP)	3	12	15	0.2000
Controls	13	2	15	0.8667
Total	16	14	30	0.5333

Notes: Selenium = exposed while unexposed are those without selenium. This table requires the application of odds ratio in the association between selenium and CaP incidence.

cc diseasecap exposurestatusseleniumuse (STATA command)

The above syntax generates the OR, 95% confidence interval (CI) and the p-value. According to these data, the odds of developing CaP are significantly lowered by selenium intake. Selenium is associated with a 99.6% decrease in CaP development, OR = 0.04, 95% CI, 0.003–0.35, $p < 0.001$ (Table 9.5).

cci 3 12 13 2 (STATA command)

The odds of exposure among the cases and controls can be determined by using the frequency (aggregate data) without the entire data. The STATA syntax cci three (selenium intake and developed CaP), twelve (do not take selenium and develop CaP), two (do not take selenium, and do not develop CaP) and thirteen (do take selenium and do not develop CaP) allows us to perform this computation.

9.5 Summary

Epidemiologic studies are essentially non-experimental (observational), experimental and ecologic. Non-experimental studies are conducted when RCTs, "the gold standard" of clinical research, are not feasible or are unethical. The choice of non-experimental designs depends on several factors, some of which are research design and hypothesis to be tested, financial constraints, time, disease frequency and exposure frequency.

Case-control studies are warranted when the disease is rare, as when the induction and latent periods of the disease are long, as observed in malignancies. Though these designs do not estimate the risk directly, if well designed, they could approximate the risk of the disease by comparing the exposure risk or odds in the diseased (case) and the non-diseased (control).

Hybrids or variances of case-control studies include case-cohort, nested case control, density case control, cumulative case control, case only, case cross-over and case specific, also termed hypothetical case-control. The choice of a particular hybrid design depends on the research question and the manner in which the cases occurred, as well as other conditions that characterize the case. For example, the attempt to examine risk factors implying incident cases reflects the need to consider nested-case control.

The major limitation in case-control design is selection bias since the controls are sampled from the source population and should be comparable to the cases except for the outcome of interest or the disease. The efficiency of this design depends on the careful selection of controls, as well as the accuracy in the measurement of the exposure. In addition, because the controls are healthy subjects in most circumstances, these subjects are less likely to recall their exposure experience, and recall bias minimization is required for a valid epidemiologic inference from case-control designs.

9.6   Questions for Review

1 Read the study by Yusuf S, Hawken S, Ounpuu S, et al. Obesity and the risk of myocardial infarction in 27,000 participants from 52 countries: a case-control study, Lancet 2005:1640–1649 [13]. (a) Comment on the eligibility criteria and the analysis used in determining the implication of waist-to-hip ratio in myocardial infarction risk. (b) Is the analysis used by the authors to determine the graded association between waits-to-hip ratio and MI appropriate? (c) Do you consider the appropriate design for this study to be ecologic? Why and why not?

2 Consider a hypothetical study performed to assess the association or relation between education and cervical cancer. A total of 780 samples (case and control) were studied. Among cases (400), 119 had cervical cancer and were never educated (never attended school), while among controls (380), 64 had cervical cancer and were never educated (never attended school). Using the 2 × 2 table, calculate the OR and the 95% CI. Also use chi-square to determine whether or not the relationship is statistically significant at 5% type I error tolerance.

3 Suppose you conducted a case-control study on the association between artificial sweeteners, namely saccharin, and bladder cancer. The data showed that of the 600 total samples, 500 were diagnosed with bladder cancer and 450 were exposed to saccharin, while among controls, 60 were exposed to saccharin. (a) On the basis of these data, is it possible to create a 2 × 2 table? (b) Is there any association between the exposure and the diseases? (c) What may possibly explain the lack association if data point to that

direction? (d) Do you consider sampling insufficiencies to account for this crude result?

4 Suppose among 200 children with cerebral palsy, 125 had feeding difficulties, and among 180 controls, 75 had feeding difficulties. Test the hypothesis that feeding difficulties are associated with cerebral palsy. (a) Compute the OR relating cerebral palsy to feeding difficulties in children. (b) Provide a 95% CI for the estimate. (c) What can you conclude from these data?

5 Examine the association between depression and the 5-hydroxytryptamine transporter (5HTT) gene and the SLC6A4 gene. (a) Explain the DNA methylation of the promoter regions of these genes. (b) Does hypermethylation or hypomethylation predispose to depression? (c) Explain the mechanistic process that results in the alteration of the methylation and its impact on depression. (d) Perform a hypothetical study on 5HTT methylation among depressed patients and healthy volunteers using a case-control design.

6 Explain the genetic implication in asthma. (a) What are the environmental determinants of asthma? (b) Is the 17q12-21 locus a widely replicated genetic locus for asthmatic conditions? (c) Observe the effect of SNPs in this locus (17q12-2), given higher levels of methylation, on asthma risk reduction or increased risk. (d) Does the IL-4R gene variant (rs3024685) associate with asthma predisposition or risk as a genetic variant? Explain how polymorphisms in this context affect the epigenomic modulation of this gene, IL-4R, in asthma risk and predisposition.

References

1 Holmes L Jr et al. DNA Methylation of candidate genes (ACE II, IFN-γ, AGTR 1, CKG, ADD1, SCNN1B and TLR2) in essential hypertension: A systematic review and quantitative evidence synthesis. *Int. J. Environ. Res. Public Health.* 2019;16(23):4829. doi: 10.3390/ijerph16234829.

2 Gordis L. *Epidemiology*, 3rd ed. (Philadelphia, PA: Elsevier Saunders, 2004).

3 Rothman KJ. *Epidemiology, An Introduction.* (New York: Oxford University Press, 2002).

4 Holmes L Jr. *Applied Epidemiologic Principles and Concepts.* (Boca Raton, FL: Taylor & Francis Publisher, 2018).

5 Hennekens CH, Buring JE. *Epidemiology in Medicine.* (Boston, MA: Little Brown & Company, 1987).

6 Elwood M. *Critical Appraisal of Epidemiological Studies in Clinical Trials,* 2nd ed. (New York: Oxford University Press, 2003).

7 Aschengrau A, Seage III GR. *Essentials of Epidemiology.* (Sudbury, MA: Jones & Bartlett, 2003).

8 Friis RH, Sellers TA. *Epidemiology for Public Health Practice.* (Frederick, MD: Aspen Publications, 1996).

9 Szklo M, Nieto J. *Epidemiology: Beyond the Basics.* (Sudbury, MA: Jones & Bartlett, 2003).

10 Schlesselman JJ. *Case-Control Studies: Design, Conduct, Analysis.* (New York: Oxford University Press, 1982).

11 Holmes L Jr. *Basics of Public Health Core Competencies.* (Sudbury, MA: Jones and Bartlett, 2009).

12 Greenberg RS. *Medical Epidemiology*, 4th ed. (New York: Lange, 2005).

13 Yusuf S, Hawken S, Ounpuu S et al. Obesity and the risk of myocardial infarction in 27,000 participants from 52 countries: A case-control study. *Lancet.* 2005;366:1640–1649.

14 Mrozek-Budzyn D, Majewska R. Lack of association between measles–mumps–rubella vaccination and autism in children: A case-control study. *Pediatr. Infect. Dis. J.* 2010;29:397–400.

15 Colli JL, Colli A. International comparison of prostate cancer mortality rates with dietary practices and sunlight levels. *Urol. Oncol. Semin. Orig. Investig.* 2006;24:184–194.

16 Vandenbroucke JP, von Elm E, Altman DG et al. Strengthening the reporting of observational studies in epidemiology (STROBE): Explanation and elaboration. *PLoS Med.* 2007;4:e297. [PMC free article] [PubMed].

10

COHORT DESIGNS

Prospective, Retrospective, Ambi-Directional

10.1 Introduction

While epidemiologic studies do not primarily aim to establish causality but rather association, prospective cohort studies (also termed longitudinal, concurrent, follow-up and incidence studies) are more likely to demonstrate cause and effect or temporal sequence relative to other non-experimental or observational designs [1–4]. A cohort design in epidemiology simply refers to a non-experimental study that involves follow-up of subjects with common characteristics, namely exposed (toxic waste, air pollutants, chemicals, fatty nutrients, etc. in the environment) and unexposed (in an adequate healthy environment). This design may involve an open or dynamic cohort, a fixed cohort and a closed cohort. In these examples, loss to follow-up is not uncommon, except in the closed cohort, where no losses occur. Whereas the measure of effect or association in the open and closed cohort designs is the relative risk or rate, the measure of effect in the closed cohort is the cumulative incidence or average risk since no losses occur because of the short observation or follow-up period.

To illustrate a cohort study, let us consider a hypothetical study to determine the effect of DNA methylation (mDNA) among adolescents on the development of chronic myeloid leukemia (CML). This study will involve: (a) a well-defined cohort of children by age, sex, geographic locale, air quality, socio-economic status, etc.; (b) a well-defined cohort of high school girls who do not have CML; (c) ascertainment of outcome, specifically mDNA as the inverse mean correlation of gene expression, at the onset and after 12 months during the study duration; (d) gathering of information on potential confounders from the two groups, which will allow the investigators to balance

DOI: 10.4324/9781003094487-12

baseline differences (assuming factors such as weight, nutritional status, other sports involvement, time spent in an environment that induces aberrant epigenomic modulations) during the analysis phase of the study; (e) a defined follow-up period for mDNA—ETV6/RUNX1, t(12;21)(p13;q22), TCF3/PBX1, t(1;19)(q23;p13.3) as part of outcome ascertainment; and (f) determination of whether or not mDNA (ETV6/RUNX1, t(12;21)(p13;q22), TCF3/PBX1, t(1;19)(q23;p13.3)), as aberrant epigenomic modulation, is associated with CML.

Epigenomic modulation that implies mDNA in predicting acute lymphoblastic leukemia (ALL) subtypes could be applied using a prospective cohort design. This approach allows for risk stratification improvement and the application of these findings to the accurate allocation of ALL subtypes of patients to accurate and reliable therapeutics. The application of mDNA remains an anticipated direction in facilitating the current ALL diagnostic strategies.

Childhood ALL genetic subtypes are characterized by large-scale chromosomal aberrations, such as aneuploidies and translocations. The Karyotyping, fluorescent in situ hybridization (FISH), reverse transcriptase polymerase chain reaction (RT-PCR) and array-based methods for copy number analysis are routinely used to detect high hyperdiploidy (HeH, 51–67 chromosomes), the translocations BCR/ABL1, t(9;22)(q34;q11), ETV6/RUNX1, t(12;21) (p13;q22), TCF3/PBX1, t(1;19)(q23;p13.3), 11q23/MLL-rearrangement, dic(9;20)(p13.2;q11.2), and intra-chromosomal amplification of chromosome 21 iAMP21 (RUNX1 X >3), are observed to be recurrent in patients with ALL. The accuracy of detecting chromosomal abnormalities by karyotyping, FISH and PCR is generally high; however, mDNA allows detection of all the aberrations caused by gene and environment interactions in gene expression. This approach may benefit ALL therapeutics, but requires accurate laboratory techniques, data acquisition, design, analysis and interpretation.

Specifically, with respect to epigenomic modulations discussed earlier, the methylation of cytosine (5mC) residues in CpG dinucleotides is an epigenomic modulation that plays a significant role in the establishment of cellular identity by influencing gene expression. There are approximately 28 million CpG sites in the human genome that are targets for mDNA. The pathogenesis and phenotypic characteristics of leukemic cells are in part explained by specific and genome-wide alterations in mDNA.

By way of recapitulation, non-experimental studies are designs in which investigators do not assign study subjects to the study groups but passively observe events and determine the measures of association or effect. The goal is generally to draw inferences about a possible causal relationship between exposure and some health outcome, condition or disease. These studies (cohort) are broadly characterized as analytic. The analytic designs are traditionally identified as cross-sectional, case-control and cohort, as well as the several hybrids of these designs (nest case-control, case-cohort, case-crossover, etc.), but such characterization remains inappropriate since every analytic study has a descriptive component [1, 3–6].

10.2 Prospective Cohort Design

Prospective cohort studies (where the investigator collects information about the exposed and unexposed at the commencement of the study and follows both groups for the occurrence of the outcome/s) relative to other non-experimental epidemiologic studies can be relatively expensive and time-consuming. However, these designs can provide information on a wide range of outcomes and can be used appropriately to assess the time sequence of events. In a retrospective cohort, the investigator collects information on exposure (for example, operative and non-operative patients) and outcomes (for example, nosocomial infection) that were recorded at some time in the past and then determines whether or not the outcome (nosocomial infection) occurs more or less frequently in the operative (index) or non-operative (referent) group. A retrospective cohort is less expensive and less time-consuming, but it is difficult to establish a clear temporal sequence and it can introduce measurement (selection and information) bias into the results of the study [7–9] (Figure 10.1).

As indicated in previous chapters, cohort study is one of the most commonly employed non-experimental epidemiologic designs, as it is most efficient in studying a rare exposure and reliable in establishing the temporal sequence (cause-and-effect relationship) and in assessing multiple disease/outcome/health-related event incidences. Therefore, cohort studies examine a single exposure in order to determine the outcome/s. Typically, study subjects are defined by exposure status and followed over a well-defined period of time to determine the occurrence or incidence of the outcome, disease or health-related event. This chapter describes the types of cohort designs, namely prospective, retrospective and ambi-directional cohort designs. A detailed discussion is provided on the design, conduct and analysis of prospective and retrospective cohort studies. Finally, the advantages and limitations of the two main designs are presented [1, 2, 9–13].

10.2.1 Cohort Designs

Cohort studies are non-experimental designs that commence with the identification of the exposure status of each subject and involve following the groups over time to determine the outcome for both the exposed and unexposed subjects. And like most epidemiologic studies, cohort designs are intended to allow inferences about whether exposure influences the occurrence of disease. Whereas sampling (selection of study subjects) in case-control is based on the disease or health outcome, in cohort designs, sampling is performed without

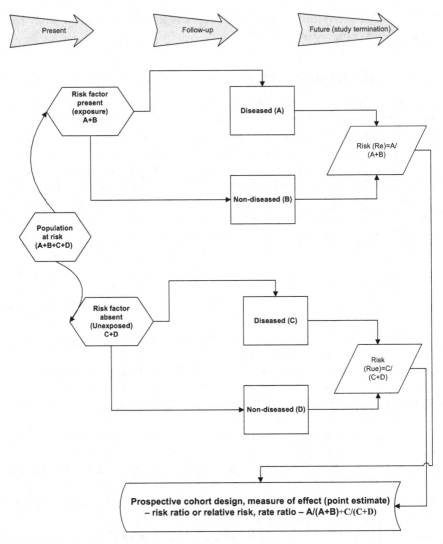

FIGURE 10.1 Prospective cohort design. Exposure to an environment such as nutritional imbalance in colorectal cancer may implicate KRAS (co-dons,12, 13), BRAF (codon 600) and p53 (exons 5-8), APC/β, RASSF1A, SFRP1 mutation. The observed colorectal and control hypermethylation of these genes in this malignant neoplasm from baseline to the follow-up period reflects a prospective cohort design with reliable findings if the confoundings are reliable addressed.

regard to the disease or health outcome but only exposure status. In contrast to a cohort study, a cross-sectional design, which is an "instant cohort," involves sampling without regard to exposure or disease status.

Cohort design is basically classified into prospective cohorts and retrospective cohorts. Basically, prospective (concurrent events) and retrospective (historical events or non-concurrent events) denote the timing of the events under investigation in relation to the time the study begins or ends. While this distinction is theoretically and conceptually useful, caution must be applied in the use of this dichotomy to describe designs, as it is not uncommon to have prospective cohort designs with a retrospective measurement of some variables and vice versa [1, 11, 14].

10.2.2 Prospective Cohort Design

A prospective cohort design is one in which exposure and the subsequent outcome status of each participant are determined after the initiation or onset of the study. This design involves selection of a sample from the population, measurement of the exposure or predictor variable (for example, exposed and unexposed gestational X-ray status or absence or presence of obesity) and measurement of the outcome that developed during the follow-up period (for example, a higher proportion of leukemia in offspring of mothers exposed to X-ray or a higher incidence of type II diabetes mellitus in the overweight and obese group).

10.2.3 Retrospective Cohort Design

A retrospective cohort design, like a prospective design, is defined by exposure status and involves historical information on exposure and the subsequent outcome. This design involves: (a) identification of a cohort that has been assembled in the past, such as through historical records or past medical records; (b) collection of data on the predictor or exposure variable—for example, a retrospective cohort was designed to study the risk of postoperative pancreatitis after spinal fusion in patients with neuromuscular scoliosis [1–4, 15–17]. The investigators used the medical records of all patients who underwent posterior spine fusion and ascertained gastro-esophageal reflux, reactive airway disease and seizures as potential exposure variables to the outcome (postoperative pancreatitis); and (c) collected data on the outcome, which was measured in the past according to the same medical records—for example, the outcome in the above retrospective design was postoperative pancreatitis. This measure occurred prior to the onset of the study.

10.2.4 Measure of Disease Frequency and Association

The measure of association, in cohort studies, is the risk ratio (RR), or relative risk, which is quantified as the risk among the exposed divided by the risk among the unexposed. A RR greater than 1.0 is indicative that the exposure increases the risk of the disease; a RR of 1.0 implies that there is no association between the exposure and the disease, while a RR less than 1.0 implies that the exposure is protective of the disease. Later in this chapter, the computation of relative risk will be discussed, which differs from the assessment of the odds ratio from the probability of the exposure given the case and comparison experience. However, it is important to note that the variability in sampling schemes between case-control and cohort studies influences the assessment of the relationship between exposure and outcome [1, 5, 6, 18–20].

10.2.5 Cohort Risk Assessment

A/A + B (risk in exposed) divided by C/C + D (risk in unexposed).

Other measures used in cohort designs include the attributable risk (AR) percentage, the number needed to harm, the number needed to treat, etc. AR refers to the proportion of exposed cases who would not have contracted the disease if they had not been exposed. For example, if investigators conducted a prospective cohort study to determine the incidence of oral cavity neoplasm associated with smokeless tobacco, the AR would be the proportion of those with oral cavity neoplasm who would not have developed the disease (oral cavity neoplasm) if they had not been exposed to smokeless tobacco. AR is computed by subtracting the rate of disease in a population that does not have a risk factor from the rate of disease in a population with a risk factor. Also related to AR is AR fraction (ARF), which is a proportion of the rate among the exposed; it is attributable to the exposure [1, 21–23]. ARF is mathematically given as follows:

Attributable Risk Fraction (ARF) = Re – Ru/Re

where Re and Ru are the risks in the exposed and unexposed subjects respectively. The AR percentage refers to the measure of the proportion of the total risk among the exposed subjects that is related to the exposure, if the exposure is associated with the disease or outcome.

10.2.6 Prospective Cohort (Longitudinal/Concurrent) Study

Design: Cohort designs represent a non-experimental study method for determining the incidence and natural history of a condition and may be prospective or retrospective; sometimes two cohorts are compared. In a prospective design, a group of subjects is chosen who do not have the outcome of interest (for example, diabetes mellitus). The investigator then measures a variety of variables that might be relevant to the development of Diabetes mellitus (DM). Over a period of time, the subjects in the sample are observed to see whether they will develop the outcome of interest, DM. In a single-cohort study, the participants who do not develop the outcome of interest are used as internal controls. Where two cohorts are used, one group has been exposed—for example, through obesity/being overweight or being treated with an antidiabetic/antihyperglycemic agent of interest like insulin—while the other doesn't, thereby acting as a control (unexposed).

10.2.7   Longitudinal (Cohort) Studies

While a cohort study is classified as longitudinal, a retrospective cohort design is not very appropriately characterized as longitudinal. Below are the basic characterizations of cohort (group) design.

- Cohort studies are based on exposure status for sampling controls.
- These studies could be retrospective, prospective or ambi-directional but must utilize >1 data point for assessment of effect, unlike a cross-sectional design (baseline and follow-up measures).
- The type of design depends on the temporal relationship between the initiation of the study and the occurrence of outcome.
- A design is considered a retrospective, also termed historical or non-concurrent, if the exposure and outcomes of interest have already occurred prior to the initiation of the study.
- In a prospective design, the exposure which defines the cohort has occurred in this exposed group prior to the initiation of the study but the outcome of interest has not occurred.
- Both groups (exposed and unexposed or controls) are followed to assess the incidence rate of the outcome or event of interest.
- Both retrospective and prospective designs compare the exposed group to the unexposed group in order to determine the measure of the effect of the exposure.

10.2.8   Prospective Cohort Study Conduct

The first step in conducting a prospective study is defining the specific cohort or group based on the exposure status and not on the outcome of interest or the disease [1, 3, 6]. If the specific group definition is based on disease or outcome, then the design constitutes a case-control or case-comparison study. In a cohort investigation, each subject must have the potential to develop the outcome of interest (that is, both males and females should be included in a cohort designed to study, for example, the association between being overweight/obese and DM). Additionally, if a study is designed to examine the risk of cancer of the prostate (CaP) given exposure to fruits, vegetables, serum lipids and red meat, all subjects recruited (men older than 40 years of age) must have the potential to develop prostate cancer (CaP). Furthermore, the sampled cohort or population must be representative of the general population if the study is primarily designed to determine the incidence and natural history of the disease. However, as in the previous example with DM, a representative sample may involve studying females of a certain age only. In addition, if the investigators' aim is to examine the association between predictor variables and outcomes (analytical), then the sample should contain as many subjects or patients likely to develop the outcome (DM) as possible; otherwise, much time and money will be spent collecting information of little value (inability to detect the significant association because of the small study size).

10.2.9 Feasibility of Prospective Cohort Design

While the randomized controlled clinical trial remains the gold standard among clinical research designs, its conduct may not be feasible because of ethical concerns on allocations of subjects to potential risk factors [1, 6, 8]. For example, one cannot deliberately allocate or expose pregnant subjects to X-rays in order to determine the risk of ionizing radiation for childhood thyroid cancer or leukemia. A prospective cohort becomes a feasible alternative design in determining such associations. As cohort studies measure potential etiology prior to the outcome, this design can demonstrate that these "causes" preceded the outcome, thereby avoiding the issue of temporal sequence—cause-and-effect nexus.

In addition, cohort designs have an advantage of allowing the examination of various outcome variables. For example, cohort studies of obesity as an exposure can simultaneously look at deaths from cancer and cardiovascular and cerebrovascular disease as end-points or outcomes. A prospective cohort design allows the computation of the effect of each variable on the probability of developing the outcome of interest, measured by relative risk. However, since the design of the prospective cohort study is based on exposure, if the outcome is rare, this design is rendered inefficient. For example, a design to study the natural history of benign unicameral bone cysts with osteosarcoma as an outcome of interest may be inefficient because of the rare occurrence of osteosarcoma. The efficiency of a prospective cohort study increases as the incidence of any particular outcome increases. Therefore, a study of union after cervical spine fusion in patients with cervical instability of C1 through C2 will be efficiently investigated with a prospective cohort design if most patients who receive surgery experience union. Another problem with prospective cohort studies is the loss of some subjects to follow-up, which can significantly affect the outcome, thus resulting in biased estimate of effect [1, 3–6].

10.2.10 Measure of Effect/Association

The measure of association or effect in cohort studies is the RR, or relative risk, which is quantified as the risk among the exposed divided by the risk among the unexposed. Primarily, this design describes incidence or natural history, analyzes predictors or risk factors or variables thereby enabling calculation of relative risk, and measures events in temporal sequence thereby distinguishing causes from effects. Mathematically, relative risk is computed by using a 2 × 2 table:

Relative Risk (or Risk Ratio) = $(a/(a + b))/(c/(c + d))$.

VIGNETTE 10.1: Incidence Rate

A prospective study conducted by Boice and Monson on the exposure to X-ray fluoroscopy and breast cancer reported 41 cases among the exposed with a 28,010 person-time (year) observation and 15 cases among the unexposed with a 19,017 person-time observation. What is the incidence rate (Table 10.1)?

STATA syntax (command): iri 41 15 28010 19108
  .iri 41 15 28010 19108
  Using the 2 × 2 table, a = 41, b = 15, c = 28,010 (person-years for the exposed) and d = 19,108 (person-years for the unexposed). The 95% CIs for the measures of disease association support the rejection of the null hypothesis of no association between X-ray fluoroscopy and the development of breast cancer. The incidence rate ratio of 1.85 (95% CI, 1.00–3.61) indicates a significant (85%) increased incidence of breast cancer among those exposed to fluoroscopy.

VIGNETTE 10.2: Risk Ratio Estimation

Glass et al. (1983) conducted a prospective cohort with a ten-day follow-up among 30 breast-fed infants colonized with vibrio cholera, as measured by anti-lipopolysaccharide antibody titers in the mother's breast milk. The high antibody was found in seven children with diarrhea out of 19 children with diarrhea; nine children without diarrhea out of 11 without diarrhea had high antibody. Construct a 2 × 2 table of this cumulative incidence study and calculate the RR.

A 2 × 2 Table of Association between Diarrhea and Antibody Level

Disease	Exposure–Antibody Level		Total
	High Antibody (Exposed)	Low Antibody (Unexposed)	
Diarrhea	7 (a)	12 (b)	19 (a+b)
Non-Diarrhea	9 (c)	2 (d)	11 (c+d)
Total	16	14	30

Using STATA syntax (command): csi 7 12 9 2

A 2 × 2 Table of Association between Diarrhea and Antibody Level: Risk Estimation

Disease	Exposed	Unexposed	Total
Cases	7	12	19
Non-cases	5	2	11
Risk	0.44	0.86	0.63
Risk Ratio	----	---	0.51

Abbreviations and Notes: The exposure is high anti-lipopolysaccharide antibody titters (ALAT) in breast milk, while the unexposed is low ALAT. Case = childhood diarrhea.

The STATA output indicates the protective effect of high anti-lipopolysaccharide antibody titers in the mother's breast milk with respect to childhood diarrhea (RR, 0.51, 95% CI, –0.028–0.93, p = 0.02).

TABLE 10.1 The Exposure Effect of X-Ray Fluoroscopy on Breast Cancer

	Exposed	Unexposed	Total
Cases	41	15	56
Person-time	28010	19108	47118
Incidence rate	.0015	0.0010	0.0012
	Point Estimate		**95% CI**
Inc. rate diff.	0.001		0.0001–0.0013
Inc. rate ratio	01.86		1.01–3.63 (exact)
Attr. Frac. Ex.	0.46		0.01–0.72 (exact)
Attr. Frac. pop	0.34		

Notes: iri above in stata syntax represents incidence rate command when data is aggregate. (summary data), CI = confidence interval, Inc. rate diff. = incidence rate difference; Attr. Frac. Ex. = attributable fraction exposed, Attr. Frac. Pop = attributable fraction of the population.

VIGNETTE 10.3. Population Attributable Fraction

L. Fleiss et al. (2003) reported infant mortality by birth weight for 72,730 live births among whites in 1974 in New York. There were 1,040 deaths during this period, and 618 deaths were reported among low birth weights (≤2,500 g), while 422 deaths were reported among those with normal birth weights (>2,500 g). Of the 71,690 who were alive, 5,215 were born with prematurity. Construct a 2 × 2 table, and estimate the population attributable fraction (PAF) and the attributable fraction for the exposed.

Table of the Association between Diarrhea and Birth Weight

Disease	Exposure–Birth weight		Total
	≤2,500 g (Exposed)	>2,500 g (Unexposed)	
Diarrhea	618 (a)	422 (b)	1,040 (a+b)
Non-Diarrhea	4,597 (c)	67,093 (d)	71,690 (c+d)
Total	5,215 (a + c)	67,515 (b + d)	72,730

With this syntax, *csi 618 422 4597 67093* the risk is estimated, as risk ratio (RR) = 19.0, 95% CI, 16.8–21.4, p < 0.001. The attributable fraction of the exposed is 0.94, 95% CI, 0.94–0.95. The attributable fraction of the population is 0.56.

Examples of cohort studies include the following:

a Lerner, D.J., and W. B. Kannel. "Patterns of Coronary Heart Disease Morbidity and Mortality in the Sexes: A 26 Year Follow-Up of the Framingham Population." *Am Heart J* 111 (1986):383–390.
b Doll, R., and H. Peto. "Mortality in Relation to Smoking: 40 Years Observation on Female British Doctors." *BMJ* 208 (1989):967–973.
c Smith, George Davey, Carole Hart, David Blane, and David Hole. "Adverse Socioeconomic Conditions in childhood and Cause Specific Adult Mortality: Prospective Observational Study." *BMJ* 316 (1998):631–635.

10.2.11 Comparison of Prospective Cohort Study with Case-Control

Cohort studies, as compared to case-control studies, have outcome/s that are measured after exposure, yield accurate incidence rates and relative risks, may uncover unanticipated associations with outcome, are best for common outcomes, are expensive, require large numbers, take a long time to complete, are prone to attrition bias (which can be compensated for by using person-time methods) and are prone to the bias of change in methods over time. Unlike previously thought, case-control could be prospective, implying the ascertainment of the cases during the process of conducting the study [1, 3–6, 14].

10.2.11.1 Other Measures of Effect in Prospective Cohort Designs

10.2.11.1.1 Attributable Population Fraction and Attributable Fraction in the Exposed

STATA syntax (command): csi 618 422 4597 67093

The csi command is used to estimate RR, attributable population fraction and attributable fraction in the exposed in a cumulative incidence data.

Interpretation: prematurity, which is the exposure, characterized by birth weight less than or equal to 2,500 g, accounts for 94.7% of the deaths among the premature children. This result represents the attributable population fraction. An estimated 56.3% of the mortality in this population could be prevented if prematurity (low birth weight) were eliminated (attributable exposure fraction).

10.2.12 Risk Ratio in Cumulative Incidence Data

STATA syntax (command): csi 7 12 9 2. The csi command is used to estimate the RR in cumulative incidence data.

Using STATA syntax (command): csi 7 12 9 2, exact

Disease	Exposed	Unexposed	Total
Cases	7	12	19
Non-cases	5	2	11
Risk	0.44	0.86	0.63
Risk ratio	–	–	0.51

Notes: The exposure is high anti-lipopolysaccharide antibody titters (ALAT) in breast milk, while the unexposed is low ALAT. Case = childhood diarrhea. Fisher's exact, p = 0.02.

The RR of 0.51 indicates a significant (49%) decreased risk of diarrhea among children with high antibody compared to those with low antibody, RR = 0.51, 95% CI, 0.28–0.93, p = 0.02.

10.2.13   *Basic Distinctions of Epidemiologic Study Design (Prospective versus Retrospective)*

- A design that begins with exposure/s of interest and disease-free subjects and aims to assess the outcome in the future by following the subjects represents a prospective cohort study.
- The time relation in a prospective cohort study is present and future (continuing).
- A case-crossover design uses the previous experience of the cases as a substitute for a control series to estimate the person-time distribution in the source population.
- Ambi-directional cohort is a design that is both retrospective and prospective in its observation of the outcome.
- Retrospective cohort (historical cohort study) is a design in which the cohorts are identified from recorded information and the time during which they are at risk for disease occurred before the beginning of the study.

  - Simply, a retrospective study is conducted by defining the cohort and collecting information which applies to past time.

- Case-control is a design in which the groups of individuals are defined in terms of whether they have or have not already experienced the outcome under consideration and the exposure is then measured.

10.3   Retrospective (Historical/Non-concurrent) Cohort Study

A retrospective cohort design involves the use of data already collected for other purposes. The methodology is the same, but the study is performed historically or as post hoc and the cohort is "followed up" retrospectively. The study period may be many years, but the time to complete the study is only as long as it takes to collect and analyze the data. Depending on the time when the cohort study is initiated relative to the occurrence of the disease(s) to be studied, a distinction could be made between historical (retrospective) and current (prospective) cohort studies. In a current cohort study, as described above, the data concerning exposure are assembled prior to the occurrence of disease. In a historical cohort study, data on exposure and occurrence of disease are collected after the events have taken place, implying that the cohorts of exposed and non-exposed subjects are assembled from existing records or medical or healthcare registries. The methodological principle of historical cohort studies is, however, the same as those of prospective studies [1, 3–6].

10.3.1   *Retrospective Design*

An observational or non-experimental design in which the medical records/registries of groups of individuals who are alike in many ways but differ by a certain characteristic (for example, androgen-deprivation therapy (ADT) and non-ADT) are compared for a particular outcome (such as locoregional CaP survival). This design is also termed historical cohort study.

10.3.2 Retrospective Study Conduct

This design is essentially the same as that of prospective, but it involves the investigator collecting data from past records and does not involve prospective follow-up of subjects/patients [12–18]. The starting point of this study is the same as for all cohort studies, with the first objective being to establish two groups—exposed versus non-exposed. The groups are then followed up in the ensuing time period (past). Compared to a concurrent cohort design, this design is relatively less expensive and less time-consuming. For example, to assess the effectiveness of ADT in the prolongation of survival of older males with locoregional CaP, the investigator utilized the NCI, SEER data for a period of time, retrospectively followed these men (ADT and non-ADT) and captured the mortality events in the two cohorts (an outcome that had occurred prior to the onset of the study). We illustrate the design and conduct of a retrospective cohort study of the association between radiation exposure and TC in Figure 10.2.

10.3.3 Feasibility of Retrospective Cohort Study

The term "retrospective" in a clinical research environment often portrays an inherently less reliable design and lower level of evidence compared to a prospective cohort. But this is an incorrect claim. However, a retrospective cohort study could be as reliable as a prospective one if the methods of variable measurement preclude the possibility that exposure information could have been influenced by the disease. Therefore, high-standard and valid results could be obtained from retrospective designs if selection and information biases are substantially minimized [1, 3, 13–15].

Where data are available (preexisting information on exposure and disease/outcomes), such as with medical records and disease registry, a retrospective design is a feasible epidemiologic design. However, the preexisting data may affect study validity if selection bias and missing-data bias significantly influence this historical ascertainment.

10.3.4 Measure of Effect or Association in a Retrospective Cohort Design

The measure of effect or association in this design is similar to that of prospective, but since temporality is questionable in some instances, care is required in using risk and rate ratio in the interpretation of retrospective cohort data.

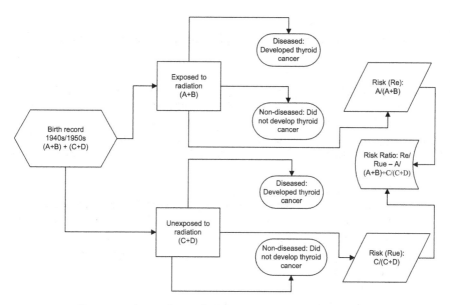

FIGURE 10.2   Retrospective cohort design. Epigenomic study in this direction requires the identification of thyroid cancer genomes as well as epigenomes.

Notes: Thyroid cancer (TC) had occurred prior to the initiation of the study; both the exposed and unexposed are screened for thyroid cancer and compared with respect to the risk of thyroid cancer in the exposed (radiation) versus the non-exposed for the outcome (TC). The mDNA data as pre-exiting and the utilization of these data on thyroid cancer versus non-malignant subjects allow for the implication of DNA hypermethylation of such genes in thyroid carcinogenesis and malignant neoplasm.

Mathematically, the rate ratio (data are based on the rate of the outcome—disease or event) is given as follows:

Rate Ratio (RR) = Rate of outcome among the exposed/Rate of outcome among the unexposed

where rate is described as the number of the outcome (disease/event) divided by the person-time. With this, the RR = A/PT (exposed)/B/PT (unexposed), where A is the number or count of the exposed subject with the outcome of interest and B is the number or count of the unexposed subject with the outcome of interest (2 × 2 table).

The RR is often used as an appropriate measure of effect or association in a retrospective cohort study. Mathematically, the RR is given as follows:

RR = Risk (exposed)/Risk (unexposed)

where risk in the exposed is measured by A/A+C and risk in the unexposed is measured by B/B + D (2 × 2 table). For example, in the retrospective study conducted to examine how developmental motor delay, sex of patients and age at walking were related to Thoracolumbar kyphosis (TLK) progression, the RR was used as the measure of effect or association. To illustrate the use of this measure, the investigators used the binomial regression model to present the RR as the measure of the association between sex and TLK progression. Using the data from this study, a (male with TLK progression) = 11, b (male without TLK progression) = 10, c (female with TLK progression) = 9 and d (female without TLK progression) = 18. The RR is 11/(11 + 9)/10/ (10 + 18) = (11/20)/(10/28) = 0.55/0.36 = 1.53. This means that males were 53% more likely to have TLK progression. However, this association may be due to factual association, chance, confounding or bias. To assess the possibility of chance in this effect measure or point estimate, STATA statistical software was used (as shown here) to compute the RR, significance and the 95% confidence interval.

STATA syntax (command): csi 11 10 9 18

Using STATA syntax (command): csi 11 10 9 18

Disease	Exposed	Unexposed	Total
Cases	11	10	21
Non-cases	5	18	11
Risk	0.55	0.36	0.63
Risk Ratio	–	–	1.54

Notes: The risk ratio as point estimate (RR = 1.54, 95% CI, 0.81–2.91, p = 0.18).

The STATA syntax csi is used to fit the estimate for aggregate data that simultaneously assesses the association between exposure and outcome (preexisting data) or a cross-sectional design.

Using binomial regression to assess the RR associated with sex and TLK progression: the STATA syntax binreg is used to estimate risk in binomial regression involving failure and success (outcome) given the exposure such as sex.

STATA syntax (command): binreg varlist (dependent/response) varlist (independent); binreg TLK sex, rr

The RR computation and tabulation on the implication of sex in TLK progression are indicative of the protective effect of female sex or gender in TLK progression.

SEX	Risk Ratio	Standard Error	Z	p	95% CI
Male	1.0	Reference	Reference	Reference	Reference
Female	0.64	0.22	–1.32	0.19	0.33–1.25

Notes and abbreviation: CI= confidence interval.

This result (using a regression model, binomial) indicates that girls were 36% less likely to have TLK progression: RR = 0.64, 95% CI = 0.33–1.25. However, this finding is not statistically significant, implying that one should fail to reject the null hypothesis of no association between TLK progression and sex in children with achondroplasia, but not that there is no clinical relationship between sex and TLK progression, given the magnitude of the protective effect of sex on TLK progression.

10.3.5 Retrospective Cohort Study Example: Pediatric ALL

With respect to pediatric ALL, environmental risk has been observed, mainly infections, ionizing radiation, alkylating chemotherapy, topoisomerase-II inhibitors as well as urbanicity and socio-economic status. ALL is the most commonly diagnosed childhood malignancy, with leukemia in general accounting for an estimated 34% of all childhood malignancies. While childhood ALL incidence continues to increase in the United States, survival has substantially improved, albeit with subpopulation variances in morbidity and mortality, with black/African Americans (AA) and males relative to whites and females being disproportionately affected. ALL cytogenetics remain a viable pathway to B-ALL predictive prognostic value, but such is yet to be achieved in T-ALL, the most biologically aggressive ALL with increased relapses and survival disadvantage. The understanding of T-ALL immunophenotype in pediatric ALL prognosis and survival may provide additional translational guidelines for intervention mapping in risk reduction and racial/ethnic disparities gap narrowing in survival. We aimed to assess ALL survival by race, and to determine the exposure function of T-ALL immunophenotype in the survival disadvantage of blacks/AA.

The Surveillance, Epidemiology and End Result (SEER) data on children with ALL, 1973–2015, were examined with retrospective cohort design modeling. The National Cancer Institute (NCI) SEER is a representative sample of pediatric cancer cases in the United States. We assessed time as a function of survival, median survival time, ALL tumor prognostic factors, social determinants of health and sociodemographics. Survival was assessed using the Kaplan-Meier and log-rank tests for subpopulation variability as well as the predictive margin plots, while the Cox proportional hazard model was utilized for the predictors of survival and multilevel modeling.

Of the 18,720 cases of pediatric ALL diagnosed during this period, ALL cumulative incidence was highest among B-ALL, 11,669 (62.5%); intermediate among ALL-unspecified, 5,437 (29%); and lowest among T-ALL, 614 (8.6%). Racial and sex variabilities were substantially observed in ALL mortality and survival. Compared to whites, blacks with ALL were 42% more likely to die, hazard ratio (HR) = 1.42, 95% CI = 1.27–1.59. Survival varied by ALL immunophenotype, with T-ALL and ALL-unspecified indicating survival disadvantages relative to B-ALL. There was a significant 54% increased risk of dying among children with T-ALL relative to B-ALL (HR = 1.54, 95% CI = 1.37–1.74). Similarly, children with ALL-unspecified were 81% more likely to die relative to B-ALL (HR= 1.81, 95% CI = 1.68–1.94). After controlling for confoundings, blacks compared to whites with T-ALL were 61% more likely to die, adjusted HR (aHR) = 1.61, 99% CI = 1.10–2.39, while blacks with B-ALL relative to their white counterparts were 31% more likely to die, aHR = 1.31, 99% CI = 1.03–1.66.

The T-cell immunophenotype predicts the survival disadvantage of blacks with pediatric ALL relative to their White counterparts. These findings are suggestive of subpopulation epigenomic investigation of T-ALL, given the observed aberrant epigenomic modulation and excess genomic instability in this malignancy relative to B-ALL.

10.4 Cohort Studies: Confounding—Assessment and Application

There are several factors as environmental such as stress, isolation, discrimination, racism and Socio-economic status (SES) that tend to influence any disease outcome. Assessing these factors as confounding factors allows for accurate and reliable evidence discovery. Mainly, controlling for confoundings allows for: (a) baseline comparability between the subgroups of interest in any study, (b) unbiased assignment, and (C) a reliable and accurate point estimate.

10.4.1 Confounding as an Aspect of Internal Validity of a Study

- Confounding is derived from the Latin word "confondere" meaning "to pour together" and indicates the confusion of two supposedly causal variables so that part or all of the estimated effect of one variable (exposure) is actually due to the other (confounder).

- A confounding variable is considered an extraneous variable since it competes with the independent variable (exposure of interest) in explaining the outcome.
- In a study conducted to assess whether exposure (A) causes disease (B), C is a confounder if:

  1 C (smoking) is associated with A (coffee drinking) in the population that produced the cases of B (pancreatic cancer).
  2 C is an independent cause or predictor of B.
  3 C is not an intermediate step in the causal pathway between A and B.

Since confounding distorts the measure of effect or association, implying causal inference, this needs to be addressed in any evidence discovery in intervention mapping and therapeutics. Similar to other non-experimental studies, confounding affects the internal validity of the study and should be assessed and controlled for prior to the interpretation of the results of an epidemiologic investigation. It is worth observing that confounding, while not a bias, can lead to a biased estimate of effect unless adjusted for in the association. There are ways to determine if a variable is a confounder or not. One approach is to examine the association between the suspected confounding variable and both the exposure and outcome. The first step is to examine the association between the confounder and the outcome among the exposed and unexposed. If there is an association, then the variable may be a confounder (suspect possible confounding effect of the variable). The next step is to examine the association between the confounder and the exposure. Therefore, if there is an association, then the variable is a confounder.

10.5   Controlling for Confounding

A confounding effect may be addressed at the analysis phase of the study through stratified analysis and multivariable analysis. At the design phase, matching is recommended in a non-experimental design while the randomization process is required in an experimental design. The primary intent of these two strategies is to balance the baseline factors, thus achieving group comparability prior to exposure to treatment or placebo in an experimental design or follow-up in non-experimental cohort and case-control designs.

Specifically, we can examine whether or not there is a distortion in the anticipated association, given a potential confounding as the third external variable. First, the estimated measure of the association (odds ratio) will be compared before (crude) and after adjustment for the potential confounder (stratified) with Cochran-Mantel-Haenszel Stratification Analysis. Second, if the difference between the crude and adjusted odds ratio is 10% or more, then the potential confounder is an actual confounder. Mathematically, the magnitude of confounder is determined by: Crude Odds Ratio – Adjusted Odds Ratio/ Adjusted Odds Ratio. Third, if age is clinically related to second thyroid cancer, regardless of statistical significance (p > 0.05), then age will be considered a confounder. Finally, if age is the only confounder, the stratum-specific odds ratios will be similar to one another but will differ from the crude OR estimate by 10% or more. In effect, then age will be adjusted for in the multivariable model.

In a hypothetical retrospective cohort study to determine the effect of extra virgin olive oil on the risk of female breast cancer, investigators assessed the potential confounding effect of family history of female breast cancer on the association. Using a stratified analysis, family history of female breast cancer was assessed. Examine these outputs to determine whether or not family history of female breast cancer is a confounder.

STATA syntax (command): cc fbc evoo, by (fh)

Family History as Potential Confounding in Nexus between Female Breast Cancer and Extra virgin Olive Oil (Hypothetical Data)

Exposure	OR	95% CI	M-H Weight
Family History			
No	1.70	0.18–15.1	0.9
Yes	3.50	0.24–196.5	0.4
Crude	1.40	0.35–5.45	
M-H-adjusted	2.20	0.54–9.20	

Notes and abbreviations: FH = Family history of breast cancer, OR = odds ratio, fbc = female breast cancer, evoo = extra virgin oil. This stratified analysis allows for the assessment of the crude estimate as well as the adjusted estimate of female breast cancer, given family history (fh) as confounding. Test of homogeneity (M-H) chi2(1) = 0.23 p = 0.6284; test that combined OR = 1: Mantel-Haenszel chi2(1) = 1.20, p = 0.2740.

Also, the M-H stratification analysis could be used after examining the crude odds ratio.

STATA syntax (command): tabodds fbc evoo, or

Association between Extra Virgin Olive Oil and Female Breast Cancer (Hypothetical Data)

EVOO	Odds Ratio	Chi2	p-value	95% CI
YES	1.00	Referent	Referent	Referent
NO	1.40	0.29	0.59	0.41–4.76

Notes and abbreviations: EVOO = extra virgin olive oil, CI = confidence interval, Chi2 = chi-square. The homogeneity test (chi-square (chi2) = 0.29, p = 0.59) as well as the score test for the trends of odds (chi2 = 0.29, p=0.59).

10.5.1   Confounding Control

The M-H analysis utilized in controlling for family history as a confounding factor in the association between female breast cancer and extra virgin olive oil is provided below:

STATA syntax (command): mhodds fbc evoo, by(fh)

Maximum likelihood estimate of the odds ratio, comparing evoo==1 versus evoo==0 by fh

Association between Extra Virgin Olive Oil and Female Breast Cancer Controlling for Family History (Hypothetical Data)

FH	Odds Ratio	Chi2	p-value	95% CI
Yes	3.50	1.06	0.30	0.27–44.8
No	1.67	0.30	0.59	0.26–10.51

Notes and abbreviations: FH = family history, CI = confidence interval, Chi2 = chi-square. The homogeneity test (chi-square (chi2) = 0.29, p = 0.59) as well as the score test for the trends of odds (chi-square (chi2) = 0.29, p = 0.59). While controlling for family history, the risk associated with female breast cancer and non-consumption of extra virgin olive oil decreases (RR = 2.20, 95% CI, 0.51–9.76).

10.5.2   Further Examples of Cohort Designs

Meirik, O., and R. Bergstrom. "Outcome of Delivery Subsequent to Vacuum Aspiration Abortion in Nulliparous Women." *Acta Obstet. Gynecol. Scand.* 62 (1983):499–509.

This study of the outcome of delivery subsequent to induced abortion provides an example of a historical cohort study. This study aimed to examine if an induced abortion increases the risk of preterm birth or low birth weight in pregnancies following the abortion. From 1970 to 1975, the investigators assembled information on the date and type of abortion and the personal identification number of women who had an induced abortion in one hospital in Sweden. Sources of information were a computerized hospital discharge registries and ledgers kept in the surgical unit of the department of obstetrics and gynecology of the hospital. Information was obtained on 95% of the 5,292 induced abortions performed during the period studied. The computerized data on women who had a previous abortion were linked by means of the personal identification number to a national medical birth registry, which contains information on the outcome of all births in Sweden, including gestational duration and infant birth weight. Through this procedure, the investigators could identify women who gave birth after having had an induced abortion and were provided with information on the outcome from the medical birth registry. A control group was selected from the medical birth registry. The abortion history of women in the control group was checked from their antenatal care records. In this cohort study, the data collection was carried out from 1978 through 1981, whereas the abortions (exposure) had taken place from 1970 to 1975 and the deliveries (outcomes) from 1970 to 1978.

Coffey, Carolyn, Friederike Veit, Rory Wolfe, Eileen Cini, and George C. Patton. "Mortality in Young Offenders: Retrospective Cohort Study." *BMJ* 2003;326:1064. doi: 10.1136/bmj.326.7398.1064 (available at http://www.bmj.com/cgi/reprint/326/7398/1064.

10.6 Hybrids of Cohort Designs

10.6.1 Ambi-Directional Cohort Design

In clinical research, we sometimes need to collect data on certain measures after the studies have begun. This leads to a design that combines prospective measurement of some variables with retrospective measurement of some variables. A study that involves a mixture of prospective and retrospective measurements is sometimes called an ambi-directional cohort design [1, 3]. If presented with a mixed design, some epidemiologists have suggested the description of the study as prospective if the exposure measurement could not be influenced by the disease and retrospective if influenced by the disease. In addition, the measured variables could be described differently for different analyses. A different analysis is required since a study with retrospective data is subject to concern that disease occurrence, diagnosis or treatment outcomes (following medication or surgery) affect exposure evaluation (observers, information, misclassification, selection biases), thus influencing the internal validity of the study and making generalization questionable (external validity).

10.6.2 Rate Ratio Estimation in Cohort Study (Retrospective)

The rate ratio may be estimated by rate in the exposed (Re)/rate in the unexposed (Ru). The Re is estimated by A/Person-time [PT] (exposed), while Ru is expressed by B/PT (unexposed). Rate ratio: A/PT(exposed)/B/PT (unexposed).

Rate Ratio Estimation in Cohort Study (Person-Time Denominator)

	Exposed	*Unexposed*	*Total*
Number of outcomes	A	B	A + B
Person-time	PT (exposed)	PT (unexposed)	PT (total)

Abbreviation and notes: PT = person-time that involves the estimated time of all the subjects involved in the study.

VIGNETTE 10.4. Rate Ratio Estimation

A CaP study on the effect of selenium and vitamin D in reducing the risk of CaP was conducted (hypothetical). The study involved 12,000 older men on selenium and vitamin D and 8,000 controls, who were enrolled between 2000 and 2002 and followed for ten years. At the end of the study, 136 men developed CaP among those on selenium and vitamin D, while 66 developed CaP among the unexposed (no selenium/vitamin D). Is selenium associated with decreased risk of CaP (Figure 10.3)?

Rate Ratio Estimation Using the 2 × 2 Table

	Selenium/VitD	Non-selenium/VitD	Total
Number of outcomes	136(a)	66(b)	202
Person-time	118,640(c)	79,340(d)	197,980

Rate ratio = 136/118,640 ÷ 66/79,340. The obtained rate ratio indicates no benefit of selenium/vitamin D in reducing the risk of CaP.

10.7 Summary

Cohort studies are non-experimental epidemiologic designs that are feasible for examining the outcomes or effects of an exposure, implying risk as exposure function of the outcome. In terms of timing, this design could be prospective, retrospective or ambi-directional. These studies, namely prospective cohort, can provide valid and reliable scientific evidence in support of the effectiveness of surgical, medical, public health and behavioral intervention. Additionally, these studies have the potential to generate incidence and, hence, temporality in terms of cause and effect. Prospective cohort design, also termed incidence, longitudinal and follow-up, involves:

(a) ascertainment of exposure, (b) identification or selection of the exposed group, (c) selection of the comparable group or groups, and (d) follow-up of the cohort (exposed and unexposed) for the occurrence or incidence of the outcome (disease or health-related event). Practical considerations in the design of cohort studies are the definition of the research question and hypothesis, selection of an appropriate comparison group, confirmation of outcome-free status, determining the method of measuring the outcome, reducing the effect of confounders and limiting the attrition rate or loss to follow-up.

The advantages of prospective cohort designs are: (a) reliable data on incidence, (b) efficiency in the examination of the effect of rare exposure on

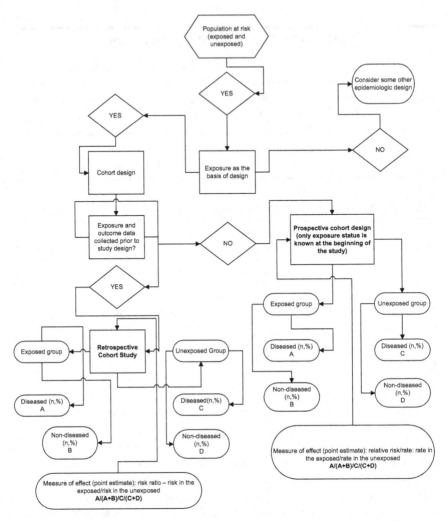

FIGURE 10.3 Prospective and retrospective cohort study design. While the point estimate is comparable in terms of assessment method, retrospective cohort design involves preexisting and secondary data.

outcome, (c) less prone to bias and (d) ability to establish a clear temporal sequence on the effect of exposure on the outcome.

The limitations or weaknesses of prospective cohort designs are: (a) inefficiency in studying rare outcomes or diseases (case-control remains a preferable design in this context) and (b) inefficiency in studying a disease with a long induction and latent period.

Retrospective cohort studies could be conducted if there are preexisting data, and if exposure status information does not suffer from misclassification bias, which may influence the result of the study toward the null. With this design, the advantage of prospective studies can be used without the need for the length of time required for prospective follow-up. The advantages of this design include the following: (a) efficiency for rare exposure, (b) capability of assessing multiple effects of an exposure and (c) efficiency for diseases with long induction and latent periods.

The disadvantages of this design include the following: (a) more vulnerable to bias relative to prospective cohort design or clinical trials, (b) inefficiency for rare outcomes and (c) more prone to bias relative to prospective and RCTs.

10.8   Questions for Review

1 Historical and concurrent groups remain the two common types of comparison groups in classical cohort design.

   a Suppose you are conducting a cohort study in which you are expected to use a historical comparison group; explain how data will be collected for this comparison.
   b What are the possible sources of data for the historical comparison group?
   c What are the limitations of using a historical control group? Can changes in clinical factors, such as nursing practices, rehabilitation protocols or adjunct medications, compromise the use of historical comparison?

2 Read the paper by L. Holmes, Jr., et al. (2007), and discuss the design and the analysis used to determine the effectiveness of androgen-deprivation therapy in prolonging the survival of older men treated for prostate cancer. What are the potential biases in this design?

3 Suppose you are conducting a retrospective cohort study on the effect of spinal fusion on deep wound infection among children with neuromuscular scoliosis, where you look back in time and examine exposure and outcomes that have already occurred by that time.

   a What are the advantages and disadvantages of this design?
   b Discuss the measure of effect or association.

4 Discuss how you will conduct a prospective cohort study to determine the incidence rate of prostate cancer among men who are on a vitamin E supplement.

   a What would the expected limitations of this design be, and will they be addressed?
   b Comment on the consequence of non-differential loss of participants due to follow-up.

5 Consider a study on epigenomic mechanistic process of prostate cancer with whole-genome bisulfite sequencing (WGBS) in the quantifying the methylation status of each cytosine in both CpG and non-CpG.

   a Is this approach reliable and appropriate in methylation profiling?
   b Are 70–80% of the WGBS reads are informative with respect to CpG methylation?
   c Is the Reduced Representation Bisulfite Sequencing (RRBS) more appropriate in selectively targeting the CpG sites?
   d In RRBS genomic DNA, digested with a methylation-insensitive restriction enzyme, does this process enhance the enrichment of the genomic regions containing CpG?
   e If the RRBS allows for rapid screening of many patients with bronchial or prostate carcinoma, which epidemiologic study design could be applied in this context?

References

1 Holmes L Jr. *Applied Epidemiologic Principles & Concept.* (Boca Raton, FL: Taylor & Francis Publisher, 2018).
2 Savitz DA. *Interpreting Epidemiologic Evidence.* (New York: Oxford University Press, 2003).
3 Morgenstern H, Thomas D. Principles of study design in environmental epidemiology. *Environ. Health Perspect.* 1993;101(Suppl 4):23–28.
4 Holmes L Jr. *Basics of Public Health Core Competencies.* (Sudbury, MA: Jones and Bartlett, 2009).
5 Rothman KJ. *Modern Epidemiology*, 3rd ed. (Philadelphia, PA: Lippincott, Williams & Wilkins, 2008).
6 Holmes L Jr. *Applied Biostatistical Epidemiologic Principles & Concept.* (Boca Raton, FL: Taylor & Francis Publisher, 2018).
7 Hennekens CH, Buring JE. *Epidemiology in Medicine.* (Boston, MA: Little, Brown, and Company, 1987).
8 Elwood M. *Critical Appraisal of Epidemiological Studies in Clinical Trials*, 2nd ed. (New York: Oxford University Press, 2003).
9 Aschengrau A, Seage III GR. *Essentials of Epidemiology.* (Sudbury, MA: Jones & Bartlett, 2003).
10 Friis RH, Sellers TA. *Epidemiology for Public Health Practice.* (Frederick, MD: Aspen Publications, 1996).
11 Szklo M, Nieto J. *Epidemiology: Beyond the Basics.* (Sudbury, MA: Jones & Bartlett, 2003).
12 Dawson-Saunders B, Trap RG. *Basic and Clinical Biostatistics*, 2nd ed. (Norwalk, CT: Appleton & Lange, 1994).
13 MacMahan B, Trichopoulos D. *Epidemiology, Principles and Methods*, 2nd ed. (Boston, MA: Little, Brown, 1996).
14 Boise JD, Monson RR. Breast cancer in women after repeated examinations of the chest. *J. Natl. Cancer Inst.* 1977;59:823–832.

15 Glass RI et al. Protection against cholera in breast-fed children by antibiotics in breast milk. *N. Engl. J. Med.* 1983;308:1389–1392.

16 Lerner DJ, Kannel WB. Patterns of coronary heart disease morbidity and mortality in the sexes: A 26 year follow-up of the Framingham population. *Am. Heart J.* 1986;111:383–390.

17 Doll R, Peto H. Mortality in relation to smoking: 40 years observation on female british doctors. *BMJ.* 1989;208:967–973.

18 Smith GD, Hart C, Blane D, Hole D. Adverse socioeconomic conditions in childhood and cause specific adult mortality: Prospective observational study.

19 Holmes L Jr, Chan W, Jiang Z, Du XL. Effectiveness of androgen deprivation therapy in prolonging survival of older men treated for locoregional prostate cancer. *Prostate Cancer Prostatic Dis.* 2007;10(4):388–395.

20 Meirik O, Bergstrom R. Outcome of delivery subsequent to vacuum aspiration abortion in nulliparous women. *Acta Obstet. Gynecol. Scand.* 1983;62:499–509.

21 Coffey C, Veit F, Wolfe R, Cini E, Patton GC. Mortality in young offenders: Retrospective cohort study. *BMJ.* 2003;326:1064.

22 Kelsey JL, Whittermore AS, Evans AS, Thompson WD. *Methods in Observational Epidemiology*, 2nd ed. (New York: Oxford University Press, 1996); Prospective Cohort Studies: Planning and Execution, 86–112.

23 Jackowski D, and Guyatt G. A guide to health measurement. *Clin. Ortho Relat. Res.* 2003;413:80–89.

11
HUMAN EXPERIMENTAL DESIGN— CLINICAL TRIALS

11.1 Introduction

Clinical trials (CTs) translate the results of basic scientific research into better ways to prevent, screen, diagnose or treat diseases/clinical conditions. A CT thus refers to a designed experiment involving human subjects in which investigators assign participants to treatment or control groups (randomized treatment allocation in a comparative CT) [1–6]. CTs differ from non-experimental or observational designs since active manipulation of the treatment by the investigator remains the basis of this design. Because this design involves a controlled environment that resembles a laboratory setting (chance assignment or unbiased treatment assignment, same physical environment), if conducted as designed and appropriately, a more scientifically rigorous result could be obtained compared with observational epidemiologic designs. Randomized clinical trials (RCTs) in comparative CTs balance the baseline prognostic factors and hence allow investigators to efficiently determine the effect of the treatment per se [1, 2, 5, 6]. However, despite the advantage of RCTs (more scientifically valid results due to minimized bias and confounding) over observational epidemiologic designs, there are ethical issues that will restrict this conduct in human research until prospective cohort design becomes feasible.

A randomized trial is considered the ideal design for assessing the effectiveness and side effects of new forms of intervention (treatment, procedure, behavior change or modification). The description and differentials between CTs and non-experimental epidemiologic studies, types of CTs, phases of CTs, designing and conducting RCTs, and analysis and interpretation of CTs. The measure of association in RCTs as well as the advantages and limitations of

DOI: 10.4324/9781003094487-13

CTs is presented. Though not partitioned as one could have wanted them to be, given the introductory nature of this chapter, the goal was to present three landscapes in the performance of CTs: conceptualization, design process and statistical inference [1, 2, 6] (Table 11.1).

11.1.1   Clinical Trial: Basic Notion—Human Experimental Design

- A biomedical, biomechanical or behavioral research study involves human subjects designed to answer specific questions about biomedical, clinical or behavioral interventions (drugs, treatments, devices or new ways of using known drugs, treatments or medical devices such as pulse oximeter and epigenomic devices for gene expression in the future).
- CTs are used to determine whether new biomedical, clinical, medical or behavioral interventions are safe (Phase II), efficacious (Phase III) and effective (Phase IV).
- CTs of an experimental drug, treatment, device or intervention may proceed through four phases (I, II, III, IV).

TABLE 11.1 Clinical Trial versus Cohort Studies Characterization

Design Perspective	Clinical Trials	Cohort Studies
Comparison group	Two or more exposure groups	Two or more exposure groups
Follow-up	Participants followed for the development of the outcome/s	Participants followed for the development of the outcome/s—prospective/ambi-directional
Outcome and outcome measure	Determines more than one outcome using incidence rates as the measure of effect	Determines more than one outcome, using incidence rates as the measure of effect
Subjects selection	Selection with randomization, thus balancing baseline prognostic factors	Selection to obtain comparability and efficiency without randomization (exposure versus non-exposure)
Subject allocation	Investigator allocates exposure to the treatment group or placebo	No active manipulation of exposure by investigators
Placebo assignment	Yes	No
Timing of study	Prospective	Prospective and retrospective

Notes: The objective of clinical practice is to modify the natural history of a disease so as to prevent or delay death or disability and to improve the patient's health and quality of life, and clinical trials provide the pathway for such assessment.

11.1.2 Goals of Clinical Trial

The art of designing trials is to provide a degree of error reduction that is efficient for the purpose of clinical objectives and the application of this perspective in treatment and survival [1, 2, 6, 7–10].

- Controls the effect of random error—sampling error due to small sample size reflecting variability and non-representative sample.
- Controls the effect of bias (nonrandom error), including systematic error which may occur as a result of measurement error and inaccuracy.
- Selection bias, observation bias, information bias and misclassification bias.
- Confounding (not bias but may lead to a biased estimate of effect)—the mixing effect of the third variable on the relationship between, for example, the disease and the treatment drug.

11.2 Clinical Trial as Experimental Design

The core of the experimental design is the subject allocation. It denotes the assignment of individuals or subjects/participants by the investigator and may involve randomization [1, 2, 11–14]. The distinguishing feature from non-experimental or observational designs is that the investigator controls the assignment of the exposure or treatment, but otherwise the symmetry of potential unknown confounders is maintained through randomization. Properly executed, experimental studies provide the strongest empirical evidence. The randomization of subjects to treatment, control or control arms also provides a better perspective for statistical procedures than non-experimental studies.

A randomized clinical control trial (RCCT) is a prospective, analytical, experimental study using primary data generated in the clinical environment to draw statistical inferences on the efficacy of a treatment, device or procedure. Subjects similar at the baseline are randomly allocated to two or more treatment groups, and the outcomes from the groups are compared after a follow-up period [1, 2, 15–19]. This design, designated the gold standard, is the most valid and reliable evidence of the clinical efficacy of preventive and therapeutic procedures in the clinical setting. However, it may not always be feasible since subject allocation and misclassification bias may be implicated in this design. The randomized cross-over CT represents a prospective, analytical, experimental design using primary data generated in the clinical environment to assess efficacy as in an RCT. In this design, for example, subjects with a chronic condition, such as low back pain, are randomly allocated to one of two treatment groups, and after a sufficient treatment period and often a washout period, they are switched to the other treatment for the same period. This design is susceptible to bias if carried-over effects from the first treatment occur (sort of contamination).

11.2.1 Clinical Trial Purpose and Reliability

A randomized trial is considered a reliable and accurate design for assessing the efficacy, effectiveness and the side effects of new forms of intervention (treatment, procedure, behavior change, modification, normal epigenomic modulations as gene expression by demethylase agent) [1, 2, 6, 18, 19].

A reliable CT must employ a rigorous design and disciplined outcome ascertainment, involving:

- Complete and accurate specification of the study population at baseline
- Rigorous treatment ascertainment
- Bias as systematic error control
- Active ascertainment of end-points
- Confounding control due to randomization and comparable baseline data between active and control or placebo groups

11.2.2 Basics of Clinical Trial Design

- Experimental design, if feasible, is considered the gold standard compared with non-experimental or "observational" studies.
- The active manipulation or assignment of the treatment by the investigator is the hallmark that differentiates experimental designs from non-experiment studies.
- Whereas not all experimental designs utilize blindness to minimize bias, blindness is not a feature of non-experimental designs.
- Neither in observational nor experimental designs are investigators required to manipulate the outcome.
  - Outcomes are observed as they occur. Hence, both designs apply observations and hence observational.
- Experimental designs, like non-experimental designs, are conducted in human as well as animal populations (Figure 11.1).

11.3 Phases of Clinical Trials

What are the phases of a CT? There are four stages that are commonly identified in CTs. These phases are as follows:

Phase I (Pharmacokinetics/Pharmacodynamics): Testing in a small group of people (e.g., 20–80) to determine efficacy and evaluate safety (e.g., determine a safe dosage range and identify side effects). For example, in phase 1 cancer trials, small groups of people with cancer are treated with a certain dose of a new agent that has already been extensively studied in the laboratory. The dose is usually increased group by group in order to find the highest dose

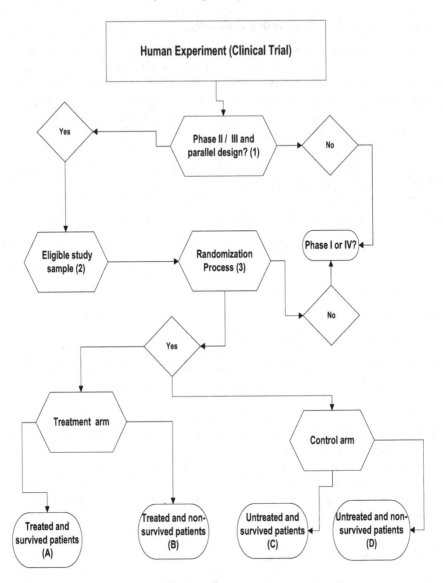

FIGURE 11.1 Clinical trial design structure and model. This illustration depicts the randomization process in phases II and III into treatment and control arms, as well as the application of a 2 × 2 table for estimating results, such as AD/BC as an effect (benefit) odds ratio and (A/AB)/(C/CD) as an effect risk (benefit) ratio.

that does not cause significant side effects. This process determines a safe and appropriate dose to use in a phase II trial [1, 2] (Figure 11.2).

Phase II (Drug Safety): This is a study in a larger group of people (several hundred) to determine efficacy and further evaluate safety. For example, people with cancer who take part in phase II trials have been treated with chemotherapy, surgery or radiation, but the treatment has not been effective.

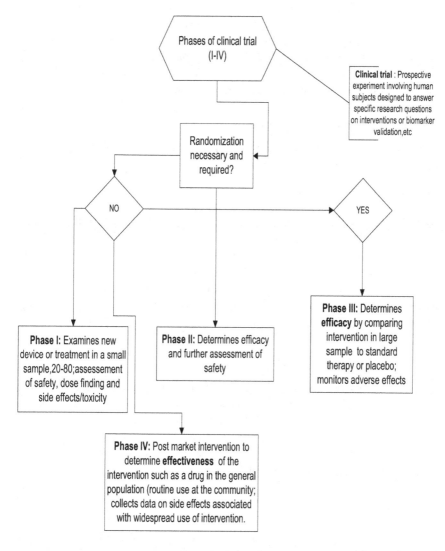

FIGURE 11.2   The Phases of Clinical Trial. The Phase I is kinetics and dynamics with respect to pharmacologic agent, while Phase II is the safety and Phase III is efficacy (benefit and side effects balance). The phase IV is the real world or community-based response and side effects.

Participation in these trials is often restricted based on the previous treatment received. Phase II cancer trials usually have less than 100 participants.

Phase III (Drug Efficacy): The phase III CT is conducted to determine efficacy in large groups of people (from several hundred to several thousand) by comparing the intervention to other standard or experimental interventions to monitor adverse effects and to collect information to allow safe use. The definition includes pharmacologic, non-pharmacologic and behavioral interventions given for disease prevention, prophylaxis, diagnosis or therapy. Community trials and other population-based intervention trials are also included.

Phase IV (Community-Based Drug Efficiency): This refers to studies conducted after the intervention has been marketed. These studies are designed to monitor the effectiveness of the approved intervention in the general population and to collect information about any adverse effects associated with widespread (routine real-world use).

11.3.1 Basic Design in a Clinical Trial

A sound scientific CT almost always demands that a control group be used against which new interventions can be compared. The process of randomization is the preferred way of assigning subjects to a control or treatment group. Here are the basic designs of CT:

(a) randomized, (b) non-randomized concurrent—assignment without randomization process, (c) historical—compares a group of participants on a new therapy or intervention with a previous group on a standard or control therapy, (d) cross-over—each participant is used twice, (e) factorial, (f) group allocation and (g) sequential—involves interim analysis [1, 2, 5, 6, 18, 19].

11.3.1.1 Feasible Clinical Trial Design

A good CT requires the following ingredients: it is randomized and controlled, able to ask a good question (testable research question), well designed and conducted, adequately powered (appropriate sample size), free from bias (measurement, selection, information) and generalizable to the target population; it has independent data collection and analysis; and it has unbiased reporting of findings (report and publication).

11.3.1.2 Blinding in Clinical Trial

Blinding is ensuring that patients, healthcare providers and researchers do not know to which group specific patients are assigned. Trials are said to be single, double or triple blinded, depending on how many of the relevant participants in the trial are unaware of patient assignment. The purpose of blinding is to minimize patients receiving different care or having their data interpreted differently based on the intervention they are assigned [1, 2, 18].

An open-label trial or open trial is a type of CT in which both the researchers and participants know which treatment is being administered. This contrasts with single-blinded and double-blinded experimental designs, in which participants are not aware of what treatment they are receiving (researchers are also unaware in a double-blinded trial). Open-label trials may be appropriate for comparing two very similar treatments to determine which is more effective. An open-label trial may be unavoidable under some circumstances, such as comparing the effectiveness of a medication to intensive physical therapy sessions. An open-label trial may still be randomized. Open-label trials may also be uncontrolled, with all participants receiving the same treatment.

11.3.2 Elements of a Randomized Clinical Trial

1 Comparative—two, three or more arms, for example, a comparison of the standard versus a new treatment for asthma among children.
2 Minimizes bias—selection bias due to baseline study characteristics is balanced, making the control as similar as possible to the treatment arm.
3 Randomization—assigns patients to treatment arms by chance, avoiding any systematic imbalance in characteristics between patients who will receive the experimental versus the control intervention. Usually, patients are assigned equally to all arms, although this need not be the case. With a simple two-arm trial (one experimental and one control), randomization can be accomplished with the flip of a coin. When there are more than two arms or unequal numbers of patients are to be assigned to different arms, computer algorithms can be used to ensure random assignment.

11.3.3 Types of Clinical Trial Designs and Statistical Inference

11.3.3.1 Parallel Design

This is a design in which subjects in each group simultaneously receive one study treatment. For example, if a study is conducted to determine the efficacy of drug A among men with advanced prostate cancer, a parallel design will involve men in the treatment group receiving drug A and men in the control arm receiving the standard drug (drug B) over the same calendar period. Elements of parallel designs are: (a) efficiency—if a randomized and controlled parallel design is considered effective; (b) treatment—each subject receives one treatment; (c) comparison—between patients comparison and average difference between the treatment groups should be much larger than differences between subjects; and (d) analysis—two groups, two independent sample t-tests as a parametric test and the nonparametric alternative, which is the Mann-Whitney, also termed the two-sample Ranksum test, and if more than two groups are involved, the appropriate test is the one-way ANOVA or its nonparametric alternative, the Kruskal-Wallis.

11.3.3.2 Series Design

Comparison within subjects or patients: Differences between subjects or patients do not affect the treatments. Comparison within subjects reduces variability, giving a more precise comparison.

1 **Statistical analysis**: The analysis involving two groups utilizes a paired t-test and Wilcoxon signed-rank test for parametric and nonparametric data respectively, while for groups greater than two, a two-way analysis of variance (ANOVA) and Friedman's test are appropriate test statistics for parametric and nonparametric data respectively.
2 **Disadvantages**: It is not suitable for acute conditions where treatment is curative but is adequate for chronic conditions, and it is prone to analysis issues with loss of follow-up/withdrawals.
3 **Design and conduct**: Series design involves assessing the results after a few subjects and deciding that one treatment is superior, and then the trial stops or more subjects need to be tested. This design can detect large differences quickly.
4 **Conduct:** Conducting this type of study requires grouping subjects or patients; it is suitable for the evaluation of rapid outcomes and minimizes numbers of subjects when there are clear differences between subjects.

11.3.3.3 Cross-over Design

Different groups have treatments in different orders. Basically, in this trial, all participants receive all of the treatments; what differs is the order of the treatments. Unlike parallel treatment trials, the groups usually switch treatments at the same time, and a washout period is normally expected. A washout period is the interval between the end of one treatment and the start of another treatment.

11.3.3.4 Factorial Design

In factorial design, subjects receive a combination of treatments—for example, placebo, drug X, drug Y, drug X plus drug Y. This design involves the consideration of interactions. No interaction occurs if drug X increases the response in the same amount regardless of whether or not the subject takes drug Y.

11.4   Elements of a Clinical Trial

CTs involve a huge amount of organization and coordination. Simply, the elements include the consideration of: (a) study subjects—CTs involve human subjects, (b) design direction—prospective in design, (c) comparison group—new treatment versus placebo/standard care, (d) intervention measures—primary outcome (death, recovery, progression, reduction in SE, etc.), (e) effects of medication and surgery—relating to outcome, and (f) timing of CT—conducted early in the development of therapies.

Conducting the trial, which is the design and implementation, distinct from conceptualization, requires the investigators to perform the following tasks: (1) review existing scientific data and build on that knowledge, (2) formulate testable hypotheses and the techniques to test these hypotheses, (3) consider ethics, (4) determine the scientific merits of the study through statistical inference, and (5) mitigate validity issues—biases and confounding [1, 2, 6].

11.4.1   The Conceptualization and Conduct of a Clinical Trial

Key to the conceptualization of CTs are the following factors:

a Primary question and response variable: The question must be carefully selected, clearly defined and stated in advance [1, 2, 9, 14]. The primary research question is the one that the investigator is most interested in answering and one that is capable of being adequately answered. This could be framed in a form of hypothesis testing, for example, "The outcome in the treatment will be different from the outcome in the control."

11.4.1.1   Clinical Trial Conduct: Research Question

The research question reflects PEICO, implying population (P), exposure (E), intervention (I), control group (C) and outcome (O). The research question conceptualization is indicative of the following:

- The concept development process assimilates observations from a variety of sources and frames a formal research question and testable hypothesis.
- In clinical research, this process often results in a trial concept document.
- The "what" and "why" questions raised in the previous section are particularly relevant to this process.
- Statement of research question.
- Translation of research question to testable hypothesis.

b Outcome: The outcome in a CT could be survival prolongation, ameliorating an illness, reducing symptoms, improving quality of life, or modification of intermediate or surrogate characteristics (for example, blood glucose, blood pressure). For example, a trial could be designed to determine whether or not drug X compared with nitroglycerin prolongs survival in patients with angina pectoris.

c Secondary objective: This is related to the primary question and/or the subgroup hypothesis.

d Secondary question: Survival differs by the ethnic/racial group of patients with angina pectoris treated with drug X.

e Subgroup hypothesis: This hypothesis is proposed to examine effects by sex, race, age, etc. In subgroup hypothesis testing, statistical power (SP) remains an issue. However, it is essential to conduct such an analysis even if it was not proposed at the beginning of the study, for example, in a factorial design trial of aspirin and streptokinase on vascular and total mortality in patients with MI (subgroup—astrological birth signs, Gemini or Libra, showed the worst outcome).

11.4.1.2 Design and Statistical Inference

The CT specific design is dependent on the conceptualized research question.

- Study design is critical for inference—good trial design and conduct is considerably more important than analysis.
- No matter how sophisticated an analysis is, it cannot reliably fix selection and observer biases.
- Systematic errors, such as selection bias, must be minimized during the design and implementation phases of the study.
- Imprecision in the estimate of the treatment effect must be taken into consideration in the interpretation of the results.

In addition, adverse effects could be used to answer some questions in a trial. However, primary and secondary questions should be scientifically and medically relevant or have public health significance.

11.4.1.3 What Is the Study Population in Clinical Trial?

The study population is the subset of the population with the condition or characteristics of interest defined by the eligibility criteria. This must be defined in advance, stating very clearly the inclusion and exclusion criteria (study eligibility). The selection of the study will involve the population at large, the population with the condition, entry criteria met, the study population, enrollment and a study sample. The participants with potential to benefit from the intervention are great candidates for enrollment if they met the inclusion criteria.

Adequate selection of study subjects requires that investigators select the subjects in whom the intervention may work, subjects in whom there is a likelihood of detecting the difference (hypothesized result of the intervention). There must be a reasonable number of participants, and it must be driven by a finite amount of funding, the effect size and the scale of measurement of the response or outcome variable, such as continuous (fewer subjects) versus binary (increased number of subjects).

11.4.1.4 Study Sample Size

To address this question, the investigators need to set the SP of the study, which is the ability of a study to show a difference should one truly be present. Beta, SP = 1 − β (tolerable type II error of 0.2). SP = 1 − 0.2 = 0.8 (80% minimum SP to detect the difference if one really existed). They must determine effect size—difference in mean, considering the standard deviation (SD) or proportion between the treatment and controls, and the alpha or type I error (tolerable significance level of 0.05) and test statistic—proportion, mean and survival estimate (Hazard ratio). With these assumptions, the size of the study, which is always an estimation, is obtained [1, 2, 14–17].

Clinical Trial: Example

Title: Randomized Trial of Estrogen Plus Progestin for Secondary Prevention of Coronary Heart Disease in Postmenopausal Women [18]

Authors: Hulley, S, et al. Heart and Estrogen/Progestin Replacement Study (HERS) Research Group

Background/Purpose: This is the women's health initative (WHI) randomized placebo-controlled trial of 16,608 healthy postmenopausal women assessing the effects of estrogen and progestin. Investigators assumed that the HRT trial would find that hormone replacement therapy (HRT) reduces coronary heart disease (CHD) and provides overall benefits to recipients (Stampfer & Colditz 1991, Grady et al., 1992). After 5.2 years of average follow-up, the trial revealed an increase in breast cancer, CHD and pulmonary embolism due to HT that more than offset reductions in colorectal cancer and hip fracture. The trial ended early because of these findings.

Context. Observational studies have found lower rates of CHD in postmenopausal women who take estrogen than in women who do not, but this potential benefit has not been confirmed in CTs.

Objective. To determine if estrogen plus progestin therapy alters the risk for CHD events in postmenopausal women with established coronary disease.

Design. Randomized, blinded, placebo-controlled secondary prevention trial.

Setting. Outpatient and community settings at 20 US clinical centers.

Participants. A total of 2,763 women with coronary disease, younger than 80 years, and postmenopausal with an intact uterus. The mean age was 66.7 years.

Intervention. Either 0.625 mg of conjugated equine estrogens plus 2.5 mg of medroxyprogesterone acetate in one tablet daily (n = 1,380) or a placebo of identical appearance (n = 1,383). Follow-up averaged 4.1 years; 82% of those assigned to hormone treatment were taking it at the end of one year and 75% at the end of three years.

Main Outcome Measures. The primary outcome was the occurrence of nonfatal myocardial infarction (MI) or CHD death. Secondary cardiovascular outcomes included coronary revascularization, unstable angina, congestive heart failure, resuscitated cardiac arrest, stroke or transient ischemic attack, and peripheral arterial disease. All-cause mortality was also considered.

Results. Overall, there were no significant differences between groups in the primary outcome or in any of the secondary cardiovascular outcomes: 172 women in the hormone group and 176 women in the placebo group had MI or CHD death (relative hazard [RH], 0.99; 95% confidence interval [CI], 0.80–1.22). The lack of an overall effect occurred despite a net 11% lower low-density lipoprotein cholesterol level and a 10% higher high-density lipoprotein cholesterol level in the hormone group compared with the placebo group (each P, 0.001). Within the overall null effect, there was a statistically significant time trend, with more CHD events in the hormone group than in the placebo group in year one and fewer in years four and five. More women in the hormone group than in the placebo group experienced venous thromboembolic events (34 versus 12; RH, 2.89; 95% CI, 1.50–5.58) and gallbladder disease (84 versus 62; RH, 1.38; 95% CI, 1.00–1.92). There were no significant differences in several other end-points for which power was limited, including fracture, cancer and total mortality (131 versus 123 deaths; RH, 1.08; 95% CI, 0.84–1.38).

Conclusions. During an average follow-up of 4.1 years, treatment with oral conjugated equine estrogen plus medroxyprogesterone acetate did not reduce the overall rate of CHD events in postmenopausal women with established coronary disease. The treatment did increase the rate of thromboembolic events and gallbladder disease. Based on the finding of no overall cardiovascular benefit and a pattern of early increase in risk of CHD events, we do not recommend starting this treatment for the purpose of secondary prevention of CHD. However, given the favorable pattern of CHD events after several years of therapy, it could be appropriate for women already receiving this treatment to continue.

11.4.1.5 Experimental Designs: Description, Measure of Association, Strengths and Limitations

A reliable and accurate evidence discovery in any CT requires a clear study description, measures of association as causal, evidence strength and advantages, as well as study limitations [1, 2, 6].

11.4.1.6   Description

- Experimental and involves the random assignment of subjects to treatment and control groups.
- Best design of studying new interventions on individual or community basis.
- Prospective in time relationship.
- Gold standard of epidemiologic investigation when feasible; allows randomized double-blinded placebo-controlled assessment.

11.4.1.7   Measure of Association

- Same as prospective cohort study (relative risk, odds ratio, hazard ratio).
- Unlike prospective cohort, the analysis to yield the point estimate could be intent-to-treat analysis (data on the effectiveness of treatment under everyday practice condition; all randomized subjects whether or not there is an assurance on treatment compliance) and efficacy analysis (data on treatment effects under ideal conditions).

11.4.1.8   Strengths and Advantages

- Randomization—most appropriate way to control confounding.
- Double-blinded—most appropriate way to control bias.
- Provision of a direct measure of association for benefits or risk (relative risk, risk ratio, hazard ratio).

11.4.1.9   Study Limitations

- Loss to follow-up (prospective), especially in long-term trials involving many years of follow-up.
- Generalizability—efficacy treatment may not necessarily translate to effectiveness in real-world situations (community settings).
- Ethical consideration—patients cannot be assigned to exposures with known adverse effects, such as tobacco ingestion.

11.4.1.10   Blinding and Placebo-Controlled Designs

CTs can be single-blinded trials, in which the participants are not aware of which study arms they are being assigned to; double-blinded trials, in which neither the experimental nor the study subjects have knowledge of the intervention assignment; or triple-blinded trials, in which neither the study staff (investigators), nor study subjects, nor the committee monitoring the response or outcome have knowledge of the intervention assignment [1, 2].

Placebo control refers to a design in which the control group is given an inactive treatment (water pill/nondrug), which resembles the intervention drug.

VIGNETTE 11.1

Consider a CT of 2,000 subjects (close cohort) with angina pectoris (AP), of whom half (1,000, intervention/treatment) received nitroglycerin-G2 (new drug) and the other half (1,000, control) received the standard therapy (nitroglycerin). After five years of follow-up, 200 deaths were reported in the intervention group and 350 in the control. If we assume non-differential loss to follow-up or no loss in the two arms, what is the relative mortality associated with the new drug? What is your interpretation of the result?

Computation: Mortality rate in the intervention = Number of deaths/Population at risk. Substituting: 200/1,000 = 0.2 (20%). Mortality rate in the control = Number of deaths (control group)/Population at risk (control group). Substituting: 350/1,000 = 0.35 (35%). Relative mortality associated with the new drug = Rate in the intervention group/Rate in the control group. Substituting → 0.2/0.35 = 0.57.

Interpretation: Relative risk less than 1.0 is indicative of the protective effect of the new drug with respect to mortality in the intervention population compared to the control.

VIGNETTE 11.2

Consider a CT of a Bacillus Calmette-Guerin (BCG) vaccination in which 556 children were vaccinated and eight died and 528 were not (control) and eight died. Assuming this was a randomized CT, what is the relative risk of dying? Is the vaccine protective against dying compared with the placebo (control)?

Computation: Mortality rate in the vaccinated = Number of death in the vaccinated group/Population at risk (vaccinated children). Substituting → 8/556 = 0.014 (1.44%). Mortality rate in the control group = Number of deaths in the control group/Population at risk (control). Substituting → 8/528 = 0.015 (1.51%). Relative risk = Rate in the vaccinated children/rate in the control. Substituting → 1.44/1.51 = 0.95.

Interpretation: The relative risk less than 1.0 (null—no association) is indicative of the benefit of the vaccine in decreasing mortality in the vaccinated group compared with the control.

VIGNETTES 10.3

Regarding histone enzymes, histone acetyltransferases (HATs) and histone methyltransferases (HMTs) are associated with the addition of acetyl or methyl groups, respectively, while histone deacetylases (HDACs) and histone demethylases (HDMs) are related to the removal of either acetyl or methyl groups. Consider H3K9me3, H3K27me3, H4K20me1 and H4K20me3 in transcriptional silencing, as implicated in malignant cells. In addition, variations in methylation patterns of H3K9 and H3K27 are related to anomalous gene silencing in different types of malignant neoplasm. Further, several studies have observed various HMTs involved in abnormal silencing of tumor suppressor genes (TSGs) such as p53, EZH2 and p27. Conduct an experimental study on the overexpression of EZH2 (an H3K27 HMT) in breast and prostatic adenocarcinoma, as well as in hepatic carcinoma.

a   How is this aberrant epigenomic mechanistic process conceptualized?
b   What is the research question?
c   What are the laboratory assays and how could this be measured?
d   What is the statistical or bioinformatics approach in this quantification?

11.5   Summary

Often considered the father of physiology, Claude Bernard (1813–1878) observed that the first requirement in practicing experimental medicine is to be an observing physician and to start from pure and simple observations of patients made as completely as possible. The decision to provide a certain treatment to a patient may come from past experience, diagnosis, opinion and natural observation, none which is scientifically valid in determining the effect of treatment. The evaluation of therapeutic benefits or efficacy of treatment depends largely on CTs, especially randomized controlled CTs. These designs are ethically suitable and necessary in several circumstances of medical and public health uncertainties.

CTs are designed experiments on human subjects that involve, as a hallmark, the allocation of participants to treatment and control group/s. Unlike observational epidemiologic studies, the exposure status in CTs is assigned by the investigator. However, like prospective cohort studies, it presents the opportunity to study more than one outcome. And because of its potential for minimizing systematic errors (bias) and balancing baseline prognostic factors through randomization (allocation of study subjects by chance), it is considered the gold standard of epidemiologic designs. However, like other designs, care must be taken in the performance of RCTs by considering the impact of

(a) the size of the trial, (b) the design and (c) the analyses in the determination of treatment effect.

There are four phases in clinical trials:

Phase I (20–25 subjects) is usually conducted to assess drug distribution and elimination (pharmacokinetics). The intent is to quantify the kinetic parameters, such as drug elimination rate and half-life. The result from this phase is used to provide information on dosing, without evidence on efficacy.

Phase II (25–50 subjects) focuses on side effects, thus assessing treatment feasibility and toxicity and, if feasible, providing simple estimates of clinical efficacy as success and failure rates. This phase estimates the success and failure rates based on the predetermined criteria (based on the hypothesis t-tested).

Phase III (formal sample size and power estimations depending on the hypothesis to be tested) determines the relative effects of treatment. The measure of effect may be the mean difference, ratio (risk, rate) or other measures of effect. This phase may involve information on repeated measurements, such as when all patients undergo surgery, when outcomes are correlated with one another or when predictor variables change over time (time-dependent covariate).

Phase IV (large sample) is a non-randomized widespread assessment of treatment effectiveness and adverse effect in the general population. This phase is termed post-marketing and is conducted after the drug's efficacy has been established.

There are several designs and design concepts involved in RCTs: parallel, series design, cross-over, factorial, non-inferiority or equivalence design, superiority design, treatment masking or blinding, blocking, stratification, randomization, nesting and replication. While the understanding of these concepts is necessary in the gaining of knowledge on the design of RCTs, some were not covered in detail in this chapter. However, detailed discussions on these design perspectives are covered in well-written texts on CTs and include some of the ones referenced in this chapter.

The analysis of CTs data may involve simple analysis without statistical models. These techniques are covered in volume II (*Biostatistics*) of this presentation. Statistical techniques commonly used for time-to-event data analysis, such as Kaplan-Meier's survival estimates, are useful to know, as are the log-rank test used to examine the survival equality while comparing the treatment groups, Cox regression for the effects of covariates, ANOVA, logistic regression, etc.

11.6 Questions for Review

1 Suppose you are interested in determining the effect of vitamin C on the common cold, and your control group is to receive a placebo.

a What design would be adequate if all subjects are to receive the treatment but at different times? Discuss the advantages and how to address the potential limitations in the design that you select.

b How will the efficacy of vitamin C be measured?

c Would a repeated measure design be efficient in this context?

2 Discuss the advantages and limitations, if any, of the following design concepts in RCTs:

a randomization,

b stratified randomization,

c double and triple blinding,

d drop-in non-adherence and sample size,

e noninferiority design and

f difference in response rate to be detected and sample size.

3 Suppose you are to plan a safety and activity (SA) or phase II CT to study the efficacy and side effects of a new drug against hormonally refractory prostate cancer and the toxicity is likely to be low while the potential treatment effect is expected to be high based on animal studies. There is a constraint to complete the study as quickly as possible, because of cost and scientific priorities. Which design would you consider feasible in this study? Please discuss.

4 One could use a prospective cohort study or an RCT to study the effect of selenium on prostate cancer progression. Discuss the strengths and weaknesses of each, and recommend which design to use in yielding more scientific evidence.

References

1 Piantadosi S. *Clinical Trials*, 2nd ed. (Hoboken, NJ: Wiley-Interscience, 2005).

2 Holmes L Jr. *Applied Epidemiologic Principles and Concepts.* (Boca Raton, FL: Taylor & Francis Publisher, 2018).

3 Fleiss JL. *The Design of Clinical Experiments.* (New York: Wiley, 1986).

4 Friedman LM et al. *Fundamentals of Clinical Trials*, 3rd ed. (New York: Springer-Verlag, 1998).

5 Yusuf S et al. Why do we need some large, simple randomized trials? *Stat Med.* 3 (1984):409–420.

6 Holmes L Jr. *Applied Biostatistical Principles and Concepts*, (Boca Raton, FL: Taylor & Francis, 2018).

7 Gordis L. *Epidemiology*, 3rd ed. (Philadelphia, PA: Elsevier Saunders, 2004).

8 Brown BW. The cross-over experiment for clinical trials. *Biometrics.* 1980;36:69–79.

9 Everitt BS. *The Cambridge Dictionary of Statistics in the Medical Sciences.* (Cambridge: Cambridge University Press, 1995).

10 Greenberg RS. *Medical Epidemiology*, 4th ed. (New York: Lange, 2005).

11 Howard J et al. How blind was the patient blind in AMIS? *Clin. Pharmacol. Ther.* 1982;32:543–553.

12 Hansson L et al. Prospective randomized open-blind end-point (PROBE) study: A novel design for intervention trials. *Blood Pressure.* 1992;1:113–119.

13 Moscucci M et al. Blinding, unblinding, and the placebo effect: An analysis of patients' guesses of treatment assignment in a double-blind clinical trial. *Clin. Pharmacol. Ther.* 1987;41:256–265.

14 Donner A. Approaches to sample size estimation in the design of clinical trials—a review. *Stat. Med.* 1984;3:199–214.

15 Lachin JM. Introduction to sample size determination and power analysis for clinical trials. *Cont. Clin. Trials.* 1981;2:93–113.

16 Dawson JD, Lagakos SW. Size and power of two-sample tests of repeated measures data. *Biometrics.* 1993;49:1022–1032.

17 Shih WJ. Sample size re-estimation in clinical trials. In: Peace KE, ed. *BioPharmaceutical Sequential Statistical Applications.* (New York: Mercel Dekker, 1992).

18 Hulley S et al. Randomized trial of estrogen plus progestin for secondary prevention of coronary heart disease in postmenopausal women. *JAMA.* 1998;280(7):605–613.

19 Aschengrau A, Seage III GR. *Essentials of Epidemiology.* (Sudbury, MA: Jones & Bartlett, 2003).

12

EPIDEMIOLOGIC CAUSAL INFERENCE

Causality Web, Meta-Analysis, Quantitative Evidence Synthesis (QES)

12.1 Introduction

Causal inference reflects the application of the causal determinant of an effect, where the cause results in an effect as an outcome (morbidity, treatment, prognosis, survival, mortality). Specifically, if the cause such as a risk determinant, namely tetrahydrocannobinal (THC) consumption, results in bronchial carcinoma, and THC (cause) remains the exposure function of bronchial carcinoma (effect). Simply, if the predictor remains a cause of any disease outcome, this predictor is indicative of a causal inference as cause and effect. However, it is quite challenging to observe whether or not a single predictor or cause results in disease development, and if not, what else acts as an additional causative agent or phenomenon, resulting in an effect (disease). Additionally, if hypermethylation of the ACE II enzyme gene predisposes to essential hypertension in a specific population, what else besides this gene and environment interaction as aberrant epigenomic modulation results in increased stroke volume, cardiac rate and peripheral resistance, thus essential or primary hypertension. Subsequently, the DNA methylation of the ACE II inhibitor reflects the exposure function of hypertension in a specific population. Further, the DNA methylation of the enhancer or prompter region of the gene has been implicated in gene expression. Holmes et al. observed a quantitative correlation between the methylation level of CpG sites in the promoter or enhancer region of the gene and bidirectional allele-specific silencing, implying reduced gene expression involving gene subsets with variability or differences in the levels of DNA methylation [1]. Notwithstanding the inverse gene expression due to DNA methylation, varieties of other epigenomic modulation mechanistic processes

DOI: 10.4324/9781003094487-14

are also implicated in gene expression, namely non-coding RNA as well as histone protein chemical modification within the enhancer region of the gene. Epidemiologic evidence (non-experimental and experimental) requires that investigations be carefully designed to minimize measurement errors and bias and control for the effect of confounders on the association between exposure and disease/outcome, as well as account for effect measure modifiers [2–6]. The inability of studies to address these issues at the design phase (measurement errors/bias/confounding) or at the analysis phase (stratified and multivariable analysis to control for the effect of confounders) signals threats to the internal validity of the study. Since internal validity cannot be ensured given these methodological issues, the findings from such flawed studies cannot be generalized, hence the threat to external validity as well. However, despite the need to increase both the internal and external validity of studies, it is not feasible to use a single study to establish a causal inference in terms of epidemiologic evidence. Therefore, established epidemiologic evidence must come from mechanisms that involve the consideration of methods used to claim a cause-and-effect relationship as well as the quantitative combination of valid and reliable individual studies. Applied Meta-Analysis or quantitative evidence synthesis (QES), which is the combination of results or scientific evidence on a specific relationship or effect of treatment after a heterogeneity of studies has been assessed, remains one of the methods of assessing epidemiologic evidence and determining causality [1, 3, 4–9].

12.2 Causality and Causal Inference

Causal association involves the assessment of a given study for evidence of causation (causal inference). Arriving at causality is a complex process, which involves a causal and non-causal explanation of the association based on the evidence from the study. A balanced assessment of these explanations then presents the likelihood that the association is explained by causal factors and not by non-causal factors, such as confounding, bias and error.

The search for causal evidence involves the examination of evidence description, internal validity, external validity and comparison of results with other evidence. In assessing the description of evidence, the investigator or researcher is expected to determine or assess the exposure or intervention, outcome, study design, study population and study sample, and the main result. The internal validity of the study involves the consideration of both non-causal and causal, or positive, features of association. With respect to non-causal explanations of the association, the study should be assessed for observation bias, confounding and chance variation. The positive features of causation involve the assessment of temporality, which is the timing of the study on cause and effect; the strength or magnitude of an association; the dose-response relationship; consistency with other studies; and specificity within the study.

External validity is the generalization of the results of the present study to the target population or populations beyond the target population [2–5, 7–11]. External validity or generalizability is possible if the study result can be appropriately applied to the eligible, source or other relevant population. In terms of the comparison of the results with other evidence, it is essential to assess consistency with other studies, specificity, biologic plausibility and coherency (exposure and outcome distribution).

12.2.1   *Measurement and Observation Error Minimization*

Measurement and observation errors require minimization for accuracy and reliability of findings. The inability to address this reflects inaccurate point estimates and unreliable inference.

How are measurement and recording errors minimized?

- Precision, reliability and practicability must be combined.
- Study must be conducted by carefully planning and monitoring the phases or stages of the study.
- Methods used must be applied in the same way and with the same care to all the subjects in the study regardless of the groups compared.

Association in clinical research may be due to observation bias, confounding, chance or facts. The variation between the true value of a factor being assessed and the value of the variable chosen to represent that factor in the study simplifies error and its possible source. Consider a study to examine the association between electrocautery and deep wound infection after posterior spine fusion in children with neuromuscular scoliosis. How could electrocautery be best assessed? If a questionnaire was developed and used to extract information from medical records on whether a particular surgeon used electrocautery on each study subject, electrocautery as measured shows a considerable departure from the physio-electrical or biologic measure of this variable. Measurement of this sort does not appropriately reflect the causal hypothesis intended by the study. Therefore, a study designed to assess such an association must consider acceptability, reproducibility and the relevance of the measures of electrocautery to the outcome: deep wound infection.

The appraisal of evidence depends on the design used in the study. Let us consider randomized clinical trials (RCTs) using a hypothetical study.

12.2.2 Observation Error Classification

Observation errors, if not properly addressed in scientific evidence discovery, render the findings unreliable and inappropriate. What are the types and sources of errors in observations?

- Within-subject variation—random variation and biological variation, such as circadian or seasonal rhythms
- Measurement and recording methods—results from measurement techniques, the recording of the data (manually or electronically) and data transformation

12.2.3 Critique of Randomized Clinical Trials

The critical appraisal of RCTs involves a brief summary of the study in an abstract form, introduction, materials and methods, patient recruitment and assessment, end-point assessment, randomization processes and statistical analysis. The causal association follows the steps outlined earlier. Using a hypothetical RCT study on the efficacy of androgen deprivation therapy (ADT) in reducing prostate specific antigen (PSA) levels (biochemical end-point) in men with locoregional prostate cancer, the appraisal of RCTs is illustrated below.

12.2.4 Evidence Description

a Identification of exposure or intervention (treatment): What was the treatment or intervention? ADT.
b Identification of outcome: What was the outcome? PSA level (biochemical end-point) assessed with an intention-to-treat analysis.
c Identification of the study design: What was the specific study design? Randomized controlled parallel design.
d Identification of the study population: What was the study population? Eligible older men diagnosed with localized and regional prostate cancer and who were Medicare recipients.
e Identification of the main result: What was the main result of the study? Describe the summary of the results indicating which results were statistically significant and which ones were not.

12.2.5 Internal Validity of RCTs

Assess the study for non-causal explanations of the result. This assessment involves the following questions:

a Were the results of the study likely to be affected by observation bias? Assessing level of PSA may be influenced by observation bias, but if the end-point was assessing survival (dead or alive), this could be highly unlikely.

b   Were the results likely to be affected by confounding? Randomization might have balanced the differences in the baseline prognostic factors between the treatment group (ADT) and the non-ADT group (control). Assess the study for multivariable analysis and stratification, which are both useful in controlling for confounding during the analysis stage of the study. Also, the intent-to-treat analysis may protect against confounding. Therefore, randomization as a measure of balancing the difference in the baseline prognostic factor or confounding is realized or effective if the intention-to-treat analysis is appropriately utilized in the analysis of clinical trials data.

c   Were the results likely to be affected by chance variation? Assess whether appropriate statistical tests were used, such as the log-rank test for equality of survival, which is a chi-square with n − 1 degree of freedom. It is also essential to assess multiple testing. Below is the STATA syntax that graphically examines the equality of survival by race.

12.2.5.1   STATA Syntax (Command): sts Graph, by (Sex)

Additionally, Figure 12.1 shows a test of the effect of race on ependymoma survival. The STATA syntax is used to test the equality of survival by race, which simply determines the statistical stability of the observed racial differences in survival.

12.2.5.2   STATA Syntax (Command): sts Test Race

The log-rank test output above gives a chi-square value with three degrees of freedom of 7.23 (3) and a probability value, $p = 0.06$. So a difference as large as or larger than that observed would be expected to occur in 6.0% of trials if the true situation were that the four races/ethnicities had the same mortality or survival. By applying this statistical test, the researcher is attempting to answer the question of how likely it is that the observed racial difference in survival occurred by chance. More technically, the log-rank test estimates the probability of having obtained results as extreme or more divergent from the null as those observed, under the assumption that the null hypothesis is true (p-value interpretation). Formally or traditionally, the significance level or p-value is pre-established at 0.05; thus, when the observed p-value is below 0.05, we declare that the results are unlikely to have arisen by chance only if the null hypothesis is true. In contrast, the log-rank test of the equality of survival by race showed p = 0.06; therefore, we failed to reject the null hypothesis and declare that the results are likely to have arisen by chance alone, implying no statistically significant racial difference (Table 12.1).

12.2.5.3   STATA Syntax: sts Test Treat

The log-rank test for equality of survivor functions by treatment. Table 12.2 illustrates the observed and expected cell counts of the events of interest.

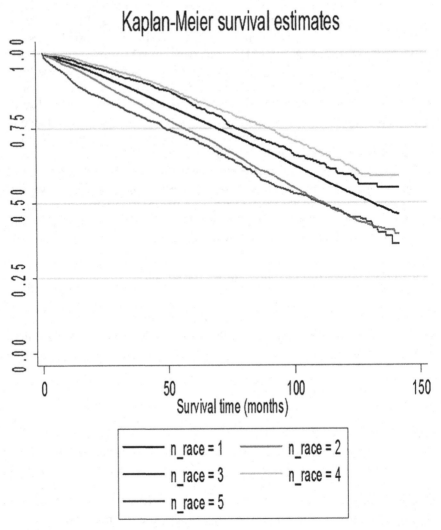

FIGURE 12.1 Kaplan-Meier survival estimates. This estimate illustrates the sex differentials in ependymoma survival.

Notes: This malignancy reflects abnormal ependymal cell proliferation within the brain and spinal cord. The survival time is by years, with females having a better survival rate in this malignancy compared with their male counterparts.

The log-rank test output above gives a chi-square value with three degrees of freedom of 326.34 and a p-value of <0.0001. So a difference as large as or larger than that observed would be expected to occur in <0.01% of trials if the true situation were that the four treatment groups had the same survival. Therefore, we reject the null hypothesis and declare that the results are unlikely to have arisen by chance alone, implying a statistically significant treatment difference in survival.

TABLE 12.1 Log-Rank Test for Equality of Survivor Functions

Race	Observed Cell Count	Expected Cell Count
White	657	632.6
Black/AA	157	154.1
Asian	26	39.0
Other	95	109.4
Total	935	935.0

Abbreviations and Notes: AA = African Americans. The chi-square value = 7.23, with three degree of freedom and the random error quantification, p-value = 0.06.

TABLE 12.2 Log-Rank Test for Equality of Survivor Functions

Treatment	Observed Cell Count	Expected Cell Count
0	94	44.42
1	591	381.41
2	109	144.99
3	141	364.18
Total	935	935.0

Abbreviations and Notes: AA = African Americans. The chi-square value = 326.3, with three degree of freedom (df) and the random error quantification, p-value < 0.001.

12.2.6 Clinical Trial Assessment and Evaluation: Scientific Evidence Discovery

The critical appraisal of clinical trials requires the understanding of study conceptualization, research questions, hypotheses, analysis, interpretation and discussion as current findings with supported scientific research in a comparable subject and direction [3, 8–15]. Below are the basic perspectives on these appraisals:

- Determine the null hypothesis—what was it?
- Groups tested—arms of study
- Study/sample size—adequate, estimated a priori
- Experimental and control arms selection—how was the selection made?
- Treatment regimens—were these adequately described?
- Blindness—was it single-, double- or triple-blinded?
- Analysis and Results—type of analysis, confidence interval (CI) used, power assessed, inference drawn from data; were the findings biologically plausible, and were they consistent with previous studies (Table 12.3)?

The above output indicates a dose-response risk of dying, given the tumor stage at diagnosis. The hazard ratio (HR) increases with the advancing stage of the tumor at diagnosis. While the Cox proportional hazard model will be discussed in detail, it is good to note that this model assumes that the effects of a covariate do not change with time. This model is expressed by h (t | x) = ho (t) exp (xβx) and is inherent to the linear predictor (xβx), which is the logarithm of the relative hazard exp (xβx). The linear predictor is the log relative hazard (LRH), xβx = xβx1, + xβx2, + xβx3, for k covariate.

12.2.6.1 STATA Syntax: xi:stcox i.treat

The above STATA output shows the results of treatment expressed here as HRs and indicates a significant (27%) decreased risk of dying comparing treatment 1 (referent group) to treatment 2 (HR = 0.73, 95% CI, 0.59–0.91); there was a 66% decreased risk of dying among patients who received treatment 2 compared to treatment 0 (HR = 0.34, 95% CI, 0.26–0.45), and an 82% decreased risk of dying among patients who received treatment 3 relative to treatment 0 (HR = 0.18, 95% CI, 0.13–0.23) (Table 12.4).

TABLE 12.3 Tumor Stage and Survival

Tumor Stage	HR	Z Score	p	95% CI
1	1.00	–	–	–
2	2.09	7.22	< 0.01	1.71–2.55
3	2.98	10.81	<0.01	2.44–3.63
4	4.88	15.61	<0.01	3.99–5.96
5	8.31	19.59	<0.01	6.72–10.63

Notes and abbreviations. HR=hazard ratio, z = z score or z-statistics, CI = confidence interval, p = random error quantity, p-value. *STATA syntax (command): xi:stcox i.stage.*

TABLE 12.4 Tumor Treatment and Survival

Treatment	HR	Z Score	p	95% CI	SE
1	1.00	–	–	–	
2	0.73	–2.78	<0.01	0.59–0.91	0.08
3	0.34	–7.54	<0.01	0.26–0.46	0.05
4	0.17	–12.98	<0.01	0.14–0.23	0.02

Notes and abbreviations: HR = hazard ratio, z = z score or z-statistics, CI = confidence interval, p = random error quantity, p-value, SE = standard error. *STATA syntax (command): xi:stcox i.stage.*

12.2.7 Internal Validity—Accuracy

Non-confounding and factual attributes of RCTs—assess for temporality (cause-and-effect relationship), magnitude of association, dose-response relationship, consistency and specificity [2, 3, 10, 13–16].

a **Temporality**: Was there a correct time relationship? Assess whether or not the outcome follows randomization. Was there a clear timing between the cause (intervention or treatment) and the effect (outcome)?

b **Magnitude of association**: Was the association strong? Assess whether the observed association is strong enough to be clinically important if the results are valid.

c **Dose-response relationship**: Was there a dose-response association? Assess whether the benefits are relative to the dose if a higher dose versus lower dose of the same agent was compared in the trial.

d **Consistency:** Are the results of the current RCTs consistent within the study? Assess whether or not the treatment produces improvement in some groups of patients. This is feasible if the trial was designed to answer questions about subgroups of patients. The use of posthoc analysis to examine subgroup effects may be affected by multiple comparison issues as well as comparisons between non-randomized groups. However, when feasible, subgroup analysis (though unplanned) is recommended since this could add more information to the study.

e **Specificity:** Was there any specificity within the study? Assess whether or not the drug expected to reduce mortality in cervical cancer, for example, is related to cervical cancer death reduction and not other cancers or other conditions in the study population.

If internal validity from causal explanation is possible as in well-designed large RCTs, we can claim that it is very unlikely that the observed results are due to confounding or observation bias and errors. However, given the significance level and p-value, chance variation may be a possible explanation if the p-value is greater than 0.05 (assuming that this was the set significance level for the hypothesis testing).

12.2.8 Study Accuracy: Validity—Systematic Error (Bias) and Random Error Quantification

The objective of a study, which is an exercise in measurement, is to obtain a valid and precise estimate of the effect size or measure of disease occurrence [14–18].

- Value of parameter is estimated with little error.
- This is related to the handling of systematic errors or biases and random errors.

- It involves the generalization of findings from the study to a relevant target or source population.
- It comprises validity and precision.

  - Validity refers to an estimate or effect size that has little systematic error (biases).
  - There are two components of validity: internal and external.

- **Internal validity** refers to the accuracy of the effect measure of the inferences drawn in relation to the source population.

  - Inference of the source population
  - A prerequisite for external validity

  - Measures of internal validity are: (a) confounding, (b) selection bias and (c) information bias (measurement error)

- **External validity** refers to the accuracy of the effect measure of the inferences in relation to individuals outside the source population.

  - Involves representation of the study population to the general population
  - Do factors that differentiate the larger or general population from the study population modify the effect or the measure of the effect in the study?
  - Involves combination of epidemiologic and other sources, for example, pathophysiology
  - Related to criteria for causal inference

- Precision refers to estimates or measures of effect or disease occurrence with little random error.

12.2.9 External Validity—Generalizing Study Results

- **Eligible population application**: Can the study results be applied to the eligible population? Assess what percentage of the subjects who met the inclusion criteria was randomized. Assess whether losses occurred after randomization. Assess whether the end-point PSA level was confirmed for every subject at the completion of the study, thus implying that the end-point data applied to all of the eligible population.
- **Source population application:** Can the result of the study be applied to the source population? The source population in this example is all older women with cervical cancer who were Medicare recipients in the cancer registries utilized for eligibility assessment. Assess whether the results could be applied to the source population based on the specific eligibility and exclusion criteria of the study population. For example, in the cervical

cancer hypothetical study, the external validity excludes younger women and women who are not recipients of Medicare.

- **Relevant population application**: Can the study results be applied to other relevant populations or beyond the target population? Assess whether the diagnostic procedure or treatment used in this study is consistent with those used in normal clinical practice. If the results of the study show a causal relationship with the treatment or intervention, it is likely that these results could be applied beyond the target population, for example, outside the cancer registries that the study populations represented in the hypothetical cervical cancer RCT. The application of the result to the relevant population should assess the difference in the natural history of the disease; for example, older women with cancer from other sites or concomitant disease affecting the cell or inflammatory disease may have a different natural history of cervical cancer. Further, since the natural history of the disease may vary by sex and age, care must be taken on the application of RCTs beyond the source or target population. This is an important consideration involving subgroup analysis, the absence of which does not necessarily imply that the results will be substantially different. Therefore, in the absence of a subgroup analysis, when the overall result is presented and is indicated to be efficacious, it is reasonable to expect no difference in treatment efficacy by sex or age group. Also consider the most generalizable measure of effect, which is relative risk, risk ratio or HR. In the example with cervical cancer and the risk of dying, compared with women who received drug 0, those who received drug 1 had a significant (27%) decreased risk of dying, with HR of 0.73, which corresponds to a risk difference of treatment 1 – treatment 0. That is the absolute benefit, and 1/absolute benefit = number of older women offered treatment 1 for one death prevented (number needed to treat [NNT]).

12.2.10 Comparison of Results with Other Evidence: Causal Relationship

a **Consistency of evidence:** Were the results consistent with other evidence? Assess whether or not the results of the RCTs are consistent with other evidence, especially evidence from studies of similar or more powerful design, such as randomized clinical trial Meta-Analysis or QES.

b **Specificity:** Does the evidence suggest specificity? Assess whether or not the end-point is specific to the treatment. For example, if the end-point was reduction in prostate cancer mortality, are there similar reductions shown equally with other diseases, such as cardiovascular diseases?

c **Biologic plausibility**: Are the results of the RCTs plausible in terms of the biologic mechanism? Assess the biologic, pathophysiologic and clinico-pathologic mechanism of the treatment.

d **Coherency**: If there is a large or major effect, is it coherent with the distribution of the exposure and outcome? Assess whether the result shown is of clinical importance, including assessing the NNT, side effects and cost effectiveness. Assess the result of the current study with results obtained from alternative methods.

The appraisal of other designs follows a similar approach. Therefore, regardless of the design, the basic approach is:

a Evidence description, which involves the identification of exposure or intervention, outcome, study design, study population and main result
b Non-causal explanations, which involve other possible explanations beyond factual for the observed results, such as bias and error, confounding and chance
c Factual attributes or positive features of studies: temporality, magnitude or strength of association, dose-response, consistency and specificity
d Generalizability as external validity: application of study findings to eligible, source and other relevant populations
e Comparison of results with other evidence: consistency, specificity, plausibility and coherence.

12.2.11 Number Needed to Treat (NNT)

- Number of patients needed to be treated or exposed to a procedure in order to prevent or cure one individual.
- Probability of a particular beneficial effect before, on average, one individual experiences the beneficial effect.
- The reciprocal of the absolute risk reduction (ARR): 1/ARR.
- ARR= Post-intervention absolute risk – pre-intervention absolute risk.
- Absolute risk decreases in the rate of specific adverse events associated with intervention.

12.2.12 Number Needed to Harm (NNH)

- Number of patients needed to be treated or exposed to a procedure in order to prevent or cure one individual.
- Probability of a particular beneficial effect before, on average, one individual experiences the adverse effect.
- The reciprocal of the ARR: 1/ARI.
- ARI = pre-intervention absolute risk – post-intervention absolute risk.
- Absolute risk increase is the rate of specific adverse events associated with intervention.

12.2.13 Special Consideration: Critical Appraisal of Public Health/ Epidemiologic Research

The appraisal of public health research utilizes a similar process as that discussed earlier. This section details the practical application of the outlines indicated here. Specific critical appraisals of observational studies include prospective cohort studies, retrospective cohort studies, case-control and matched case-control studies, and cross-sectional studies and large population-based studies.

Study Designs: Determine the study design to address the research questions: experimental (clinical trial, therapeutic, parallel, preventive, community, individual, etc.) and non-experimental (cross-sectional, case-control, cohort, etc.).

12.2.14 Scale of Measurement and Distribution

The scale of measurement and the shape of the data are essential in the selection of the test statistic. This aspect was covered in Part 1 of this book but needs to be reemphasized:

1 Determine the scale of measurement of the variables (nominal, categorical, discrete, ratio, interval) for the dependent and independent variables.
2 Determine if the data presented are assumed to follow normal distribution or not, parametric or nonparametric.
3 If data are assumed to be normally distributed, are the descriptive statistics appropriate (mean, standard deviation, standard error, etc.)?
4 If data are assumed to be nonparametric, are the descriptive statistics presented in terms of proportions or percentages?

Internal validity (random error, bias and confounding) refers to the accurate measurement of study effects without bias—bias presents threats to the internal validity of the study [2]. The precision and accuracy of measurement are essential to studying validity. Whereas precision refers to the degree to which a variable has nearly the same value when measured several times, accuracy pertains to the degree to which a variable actually represents what it is supposed to represent or measure. Precision may be enhanced by repetition, refinement, observer's training and performance verification, standardization and automation, which minimizes variability due to observers. Accuracy may be improved by specific markers and better instruments, unobtrusive measurement, blinding and instrument calibration.

12.2.15 Non-statistically Significant Result Interpretation

- A test based on a null hypothesis may suffer from random error, rendering the observed result smaller than the true result as well as losing statistical significance.

- To what extent can it be accepted that there is no true difference between the groups being compared?
- A type II or beta error is committed if the result is non-significant when there is a true difference (truth in the universe).
- Relying on the significance level in interpreting such a result is not encouraged and requires the computation of the confidence limits (for example, 95% CI), which will show the range of values of the association with which the results are compatible.
- If the non-significant result is due to a small sample size or study, the CI will be wide.
- A wide CI is indicative that one cannot conclude that there is no appreciable difference between the groups being compared.

  - It is uncommon to find two studies with inconsistent findings, which raises the question of type II errors.

Random Error Quantification: Assuming a random sample was taken from the population studied, is this sample representative of the population? Is the observed result influenced by sampling variability? Is there a recognizable source of error, such as quality of questions and faulty instruments? Is the error due to chance, given that there is no connection to a recognizable source of error? Random error can be minimized by improving design, enlarging sample size and increasing precision, as well as by using good quality control during study implementation. It is important to note here that the sample studied is a random sample and that it is meaningless to apply statistical significance to the results of designs that do not utilize random samples.

Null Hypothesis and Types of Errors: The null hypothesis states that there is no association between the exposure and the disease variables, which in most instances translates to the statement that the ratio measure of association is 1.0 (null), with the alternate hypothesis stated to contradict the null (one-tail or two-tail)—that the measure of association is not equal to 1.0. The null hypothesis implies that the statistics (mean, odds ratio [OR], relative risk [RR]) being compared are the results of random sampling from the same population and that any difference in OR, RR, relative odds (RO) or the mean between them is due to chance. There are two types of errors that are associated with hypothesis testing: type I (rejecting the null hypothesis when it is in fact true) and type II (failing to reject the null hypothesis when it is in fact false).

Significance Level (Alpha): The test statistics that depend on the design as well as the measure of the outcome and independent variables yield a p-value. The significance level or alpha (α) is traditionally set at 5% (0.05), which means that if the null hypothesis is true, we are willing to limit type

I error to this set value. The p-value (significance level) is the probability of obtaining the observed result and more extreme results by chance alone, given that the null hypothesis is true. The significance level is arbitrarily cutoff at 5% (0.05). A p-value less than 0.05 is considered statistically significant, implying that the null hypothesis of no association should be rejected in favor of the alternate hypothesis. Simply, this is indicative of the fact that random error is an unlikely explanation of the observed result or point estimate (which is statistically significant). With p greater than 0.05, the null hypothesis should not be rejected, which implies that the observed result may be explained by random error or sampling variability (which is statistically insignificant).

VIGNETTE 12.1: Study Interpretation

Consider a study to examine the association between physical inactivity and body mass index (BMI) among school-age children. Assume that the investigators observed that the risk of obesity (BMI > 30 kg/ m^2) was four times as likely among children with low levels of physical activity, and the p-value associated with the relative risk is 0.03. What is the possible explanation of this result, and is this result statistically significant?

Solution: This simply means that if the null hypothesis is true, there is a 3% probability of obtaining the observed result or one more extreme (RR = 4.0 or greater) by chance alone. Because p is < 0.05, the observed result is statistically significant.

12.2.16 Types of Errors in Hypothesis Testing: Type I and Type II

The quantifications of these errors in reality in statistical modeling of clinical, biomedical and population-based data are relevant for finding application in evidence-based scientific studies and application in care improvement and intervention mapping.

Type I or alpha error refers to an incorrect rejection of the null hypothesis, implying the rejection of the null hypothesis when indeed the null hypothesis is true.

When the null hypothesis is true and the investigator rejects the null hypothesis, a type I error is committed (false-positive).

Type II or beta error refers to erroneously failing to reject the null hypothesis when indeed it is false.

When the investigator fails to reject the null hypothesis when it is false, a type II error is committed (false-negative).

12.2.17 Hypothesis Testing and Type I Error Tabulation

	No Association	Association
No association	Correct (a)	Type II error (b)
Association	Type I error* (c)	Correct (d)

Notes and abbreviations. *p-value is the probability of a type I error. Because samples come from the population, the p-value plays a role in inferential statistics by allowing a conclusion to be drawn regarding the population or the universe of subjects. Since population parameters remain unknown but could be estimated from the sample, the p-value reflects the size of the study, implying how representative the sample is with respect to the universe or population of subjects upon which the sample was drawn.

12.2.18   Confidence Interval and Confidence Limit

The CI is determined by the quantification of precision or random error around the point estimate, with the width of the CI determined by random error arising from measurement error or imprecise measurement and sampling variability, and some cutoff value (95%). The CI simply implies that if a study were repeated 100 times and 100 point estimates and 100 CIs were estimated, 95 out of 100 CIs would contain the true point estimate (measure of association). It is used to determine statistical significance of an association. If the 95% fails to include 1.0 (null), then the association is considered to be statistically significant.

The CI reflects the degree of precision around the point estimate (OR/RR/RO/HR). If the range of RR, RO or OR (point estimate) values consistent with the observed data falls within the lower and upper CI, the data are consistent with the inference, implying the rejection of the null hypothesis. Therefore, when the null value (1.0), implying no association, is excluded from the 95% CI, one can conclude that the findings are statistically significant. Consequently, such data are not consistent with the null hypothesis of no association, implying that such an association cannot be explained solely by chance.

12.2.19   Application of CI in Assessing Evidence

While large studies may not necessarily convey clinical importance, small studies are often labeled "non-significant" because of the significance level being greater than 0.05. This is due to the low power of these studies, which precludes a detection of a statistically significant difference. The magnitude of effect (quantification of the association) and 95% CI, which may appear to be wide, indicating considerable uncertainty, are reliable interpretations of small and negative findings. The *p*-value interpretations of such studies are misleading, clearly wrong and foolhardy.

VIGNETTE 12.2: Passive Smoking and Bronchial Carcinoma: Point Estimate

Consider a study conducted to examine the role of passive smoking on lung carcinoma. If the OR is 1.56 and 95% CI = 1.4–1.9, can we claim that there is a statistically significant association between passive smoking and lung carcinoma?

Solution: Because the point estimate for the association lies within the upper and lower confidence limits, and 1.0 is not included, the observed result is statistically significant.

12.2.20 Bias (Systematic Error) and Sources of Bias

One has to determine if bias, which is systematic error, contributes to the observed results. What are the types of bias? In critical appraisal of clinical and biomedical research findings, creating a laundry list of biases is not a useful practice, but one should assess what systematic errors may possibly influence the result. Examples of bias are selection bias, prevalence or incidence bias (admission rate bias—Berkson's fallacy studying hospitalized patients as cases), nonresponse, volunteer bias, etc. Measurement validity may introduce recall bias, detection bias, information bias and compliance bias. Systematic error is likely to occur because of observer bias, subject bias or instrument bias. However, systematic errors are minimized by improving design and increasing accuracy.

12.2.21 Randomization and Blinding (Experimental and Clinical Trial)

We have to determine whether or not randomization was properly achieved. Also, was double blinding utilized?

12.2.22 Power (Rejecting a False Alternative Hypothesis) and Sample Size

Power measures the ability of the test to correctly reject the null hypothesis when the alternative hypothesis is true. This is presented mathematically as follows:

Statistical power = $1-\beta$.

Both alpha (type I) and beta (type II) errors are involved in sample size computation of a study. Lowering alpha decreases power because it makes it less likely to reject the null hypothesis, even where true differences exist. A small number is unlikely to show the difference between the two groups. Smaller sample sizes reduce power because the translation of sigma (σ) into standard error (SE) of the mean produces a larger SE for smaller samples. The sample size varies with the magnitude of the outcome effect expected. Thus, when the variance is large, the outcome effect, even if robust, will be obscured by the underlying variation. Conversely, when the variation is modest, even modest effect may be perceived clearly with a small sample size.

12.3 Quantitative Evidence Synthesis (QES) as Applied Meta-Analysis

This methodology, QES, developed by Holmes, L Jr. (2006) involves a systematic review as applied Meta-Analysis. The utilization of QES ensures a quantitative systematic review with a common effect size (CES) in providing a summary estimate as observed in the study on the epigenomic modulation involved in the glucocorticoid gene (NR3C1) receptor, thus allowing for the scientific statement of dense DNA methylation of NR3C1 in early life stress (ELS) and major depressive disorder (MDD) [10].

The search process involves the identification of relevant literature, selecting articles based on a set of predetermined inclusion criteria, and performing a study quality assessment. The qualitative synthesis of selected studies included data abstraction and summary. The QES included data extraction from eligible published literature, the pool assessment estimation, test for heterogeneity and the creation of forest plots.

The overarching objectives of QES are to (1) minimize random error and (2) marginalize measurement errors which have a huge effect on the point estimate by down-drifting away from the null. Because all studies have measurement errors, and some studies have more measurement errors than others, QES assesses the differences between studies that are due to measurement errors. Additionally, because studies in medicine and public health are often conducted with small samples, such samples have increased random errors. The QES, which is a method of summarizing the effect across studies, increases the study or sample size and, therefore, minimizes random error and enhances generalizability of findings. Furthermore, QES integrates results across studies to identify patterns and to some extent establish causation. In effect, the overall relevance of QES is to generate scientific data that is accumulative and reliable in improving health or other conditions upon which it is applied.

The methodology used in QES differs from that of traditional Meta-Analysis. While Meta-Analysis utilizes fixed- and random-effect methods, QES only employs the random-effect method and examines heterogeneity after and not before the pool estimates. The fixed-effect method is only applicable to QES when the combined studies or publications are from multicenter trial where the study protocol is identical. However, when studies are combined from different settings, observation and measurement errors induce significant variability in the observed estimates, limiting such combinations without adjusting for between-study variability. The random-effect method compensates for the between-stud variability, hence its unique application in QES.

Scientific endeavor makes sense of the accumulating literature in medicine and public health, given the confounding and contradicting results. QES reflects such attempts at study integration for public health and clinical decision-making. A unique feature of QES is temporality, in which findings in QES accumulate with time. For example, if QES was performed on the implication of epigenetics as a consequence of early childhood trauma and adult-onset MDD, this study must identify the time of conduct and continue to add findings and reanalyze the data for contrasting or negative findings with time. Subsequently, the emergence of new data on epigenetic modulation (physical, in utero, social, endocrine, neurobiologic, environment) informs the results of QES by shifting the direction of the previously observed data, implying a change in the results of QES and thus moving evidence in a different direction.

Science and scientific endeavors are not static but dynamic (continually shifting and modifying as new evidence emerges), implying the emergence of new data creating a shift in evidence. The scientific community cannot wait until evidence accumulates to such a point that no further addition is required with respect to evidence discovery in order to initiate an intervention. Consequently, QES can inform and generate the knowledge required in risk characterization (specific risk characterization), subclinical and clinical disease processes, disease prognosis, as well as control and disease prevention at the population level.

12.3.1   Search Engine and Strategies

The search engine implies an online database search involving MEDLINE via PubMed with search terms created based on medical subject headings (MeSH) and terms used, for example, in epigenetic literature reviews of ELS and MDD in order to maximize sensitivity:

(gene expression OR DNA methylation OR histone acetylation OR microRNA OR gene transcription OR siRNA OR mRNA OR histone methylation OR epigenotype AND early childhood trauma) OR (gene expression OR DNA methylation OR histone acetylation OR microRNA OR gene transcription OR siRNA OR mRNA OR histone methylation OR epigenotype AND schizophrenia) OR (gene expression OR DNA methylation OR histone acetylation OR microRNA OR gene transcription OR siRNA OR mRNA OR histone methylation OR epigenotype AND neuroendocrine development (cortisol, pituitary hypothalamus, HPA-axis, vasopressin, corticotropin hormone, CRF, ERA, glucocorticoid receptor gene, (NR3C1), brain derived neurotropic factor (BDNF), glucocorticoid receptor (GR)), GABA aminobutyric acid AND MDDs AND human). Additionally, hand searches through reference lists of relevant articles could be applied.

12.3.2 Eligibility Criteria

One author (ES) screened abstracts for inclusion in the full-text evaluation. Eligible articles had to meet the following criteria: (a) study published in certain language and with a certain duration; (b) study investigating, for example, epigenomic modulations and their associations with ELS and MDD; (c) study with a well-defined outcome, namely MDD and ELS; and (d) study that contains quantitative data, such as the parameter values (OR, risk ratio, relative risk). Studies with a loss to follow-up >25% or a sample size smaller than ten were excluded to lessen the likelihood of selection bias and sparse data bias, respectively (QES). Inclusion criteria are required in order to maximize incorporation of any potentially useful findings while limiting inclusion of irrelevant data.

12.3.3 Data Extraction Reliability: Kappa

Two authors (XX and XY) independently read the full texts (kappa = 9.3, indicative of excellent inter-rater agreement). Discrepancies in agreement were resolved through discussion between the study investigators. Studies included in the qualitative synthesis had to meet the inclusion criteria above, implying studies involving epigenomic modulation measured by DNA methylation and its association with ELS and MDD, for instance.

12.3.4 Study Variables

For example, study variables included in QES in the assessment of life stress (ELS) and MDDs as the response require a very careful assessment with respect to the scale of measurements of the specific variables. Epigenetic alterations as well as neuroendocrine markers of neurobehavioral dysfunctions remain independent variables, namely the glucocorticoid receptor gene (NR3C1) and the DNA methylation profile. Specifically, cellular function commences with the central dogma of molecular biology, namely: (a) replication as the origin of cellular function, (b) transcription, (C) RNA translation and (d) protein synthesis.

12.3.5 Data Collection and Processing

Data are collected from all eligible studies based on the outcome variables and specific research questions. For the qualitative synthesis, all available data concerning epigenetic markers and MDD as well as ELS must be obtained. For the QES, the abstracted data on DNA methylation percentage from ELS versus non-ELS are required for evidence of dense DNA methylation in ELS. Additionally, the same approach is applied in MDD with DNA methylation percentage as well as relative point estimates. Specifically, if data are not available on the measure of the outcome, QES cannot be performed, but if data are available, the precision measure of the parameter estimate using the 95% CI is estimated.

12.3.6 Study Quality Assessment

Two authors (XX and XY) are required to assess the eligible studies' quality based upon study design, sampling techniques, clarity of aims or purposes, and adequacy of statistical analysis. Studies are also assessed for any confounding factors that might have influenced the outcomes and any potential bias, including selection, information and misclassification bias. The QES study quality assessment technique required the application of the method of reporting for systematic reviews [PRISMA statement] [1–3, 10].

12.3.7 Statistical Analysis: Applied Meta-Analysis—QES

The QES analysis that involved the pooled estimate for the CES requires a performance prior to the heterogeneity test. For example, a template is required in the transformation of the proportion of epigenetic modulation and MDD cases into percentage, standard error and 95% CIs to enable the application of meta-analytic commands using STATA syntax or command, namely: *metan percent lower CI upper CI, label (namevar = study) random.*

12.3.8 QES Analytic Example: ELS and MDD

To test the hypothesis with respect to the implication of dense DNA methylation in ELS or MDD as well as MDD due to ELS, a random-effect analysis of Dersimonian-Laird is required. The Dersimonian-Laird method is applicable given significant studies' heterogeneity, while the fixed method could be employed in the absence of heterogeneity (homogenous studies). This procedure, namely the random-effect method, examines the between-study effect as well as the effect sizes of the combined studies, weighing each study for their contributions to the overall sample size involved in the pool estimate. In addition, the study precision was measured by the 95% CI. The effect size (ES) was estimated by testing the null hypothesis that the CES = 0, based on the standardized normal (z-statistic).

The heterogeneity test is performed to determine variability among studies overall and within each outcome category. The heterogeneity test is performed using $Q = (1/\text{variance\_i}) * (\text{effect\_i} - \text{effect\_pool})2$. The variance is estimated using: $\text{variance\_i} = (\text{upper limit} - \text{lower limit})/(2*z)2$. The test of heterogeneity reflects the variation in the ES that is attributable to the differences between study effect sizes.

12.3.9 QES Rationale and Purpose

The purposes of QES are: (I) to minimize random error and (II) to marginalize measurement errors, which have a huge effect on the point estimate by drifting away from the null. Small samples in epidemiological research studies have increased random errors. All studies have measurement errors and some studies have more measurement errors than others. Therefore, QES is useful in assessing the differences between studies that are due to measurement errors. QES is a method of summarizing the observed effect across studies. It increases the study or sample size, minimizing random error and enhancing the generalization of findings. Further, QES integrates results across studies to identify patterns and, to some extent, establish causation. As a result of the accumulating literature in medicine and public health, and given the confounding and contradicting claims, QES is an attempt to utilize study integration practices for public health and clinical decision-making.

A unique feature of QES is temporality, in which findings in QES accumulate with time. For example, if QES is performed on the impact of culturally competent care on pediatric care improvement, this finding must identify the time of conduct and continue to add studies and reanalyze the data for contrasting or negative findings with time. Subsequently, the emergence of new knowledge has had an impact on changing the results of QES and moving evidence toward a factual association.

Despite the fluidity of QES in enhancing knowledge as well as informing intervention, science and scientific endeavors cannot be static, but rather dynamic. The scientific community cannot wait until evidence accumulates to such a point that no further addition is required with respect to evidence discovery in order to start intervention. QES can inform and provide at any point in time the knowledge required in order to improve the care of our patients as well as control and prevent disease at the population level.

Quantitative Systematic Review: This is a method of combining the results from a number of studies of similar design to produce an overall estimate of effect, which incorporates the information provided by all the studies. The quantitative evidence synthesis (QES) is comparable to traditional meta-analysis since both methods aim at quantifying the summary effect of the individual studies. However, the two methods differ since QES applies biologic and clinical relevance to the interpretation of the pool estimates as well. It is a popular method of critically assessing the value of evidence used to support health interventions—evidence-based medicine, QES. It is useful in answering research questions whenever an investigation of a particular research subject presents with conflicting or contradictory results. For example, some research groups may report a statistically significant difference in the use of anti-androgens in prolonging the survival of men treated for loco-regional prostate cancer, while other groups report no statistically significant difference.

12.3.10   Meta-Analysis and Pool Analysis

Meta-Analysis is a method of summarizing, integrating and interpreting research studies that produces quantitative findings. It is a technique of encoding and analyzing the statistics that summarize research findings. If full datasets of studies of interest are available, a pool analysis is the preferred method. Because Meta-Analysis focuses on the aggregation and comparison of findings of different research studies, meaningful comparability is required. For example, studies assessing the association between selenium intake and prostate cancer can be compared with meta-analytic designs using prospective cohort or case-control studies but not mixed, given the differences in the point estimates generated by these two designs. Likewise, observational and experimental cannot be mixed in meta-analytic designs but can be compared separately.

Meta-Analysis represents each study's findings in the form of effect sizes or point estimates. An effect size encodes the quantitative information from each relevant study's findings. Studies that produce bivariate correlations cannot be combined with those that compared groups of subjects on the mean values of the dependent variables.

12.3.11   Meta-Analysis and QES—Methodology

A traditional meta-analytic process and QES as applied Meta-Analysis methods involve:

a   defining the research question
b   defining the criteria for studies to be included
c   identifying and retrieving the studies that meet the inclusion criteria
d   abstracting information
e   analyzing statistics (fixed-effect or random-effect analysis)
f   reporting results.

12.3.12   Statistical/Analytic Methods

Common analytic methods used in QES include fixed- and random-effect models.

12.3.13   Heterogeneity Test

The heterogeneity or homogeneity statistic tests whether the overall summary estimate is an adequate representation of the dataset, compares each of the individual study results with the summary estimate and examines the differences between the studies. The meta-analytic method is based on a weighted average of the differences of the results of each study and the summary estimate of the effect. If there is significant heterogeneity, the analysis may be repeated after excluding the studies that are particularly divergent. The heterogeneity statistics produce a $\chi 2$ value for each individual study, based on the comparison of that study's result to the summary result.

12.3.14   Fixed-Effect Model: Mantel-Haenszel and Peto

There are two commonly used fixed-effect methods: Mantel-Haenszel and Peto. The Mantel-Haenszel method attempts to derive the most useful summary estimate of effect from the data given in all the studies included in the analysis. This test is similar to the analysis of stratified data, where the stratification variable is the individual study. The Peto method utilizes a 2 × 2 table for the observed and expected, the chi-square value is obtained by Oi – Ei and the variance of the expected (Vi) is calculated.

12.3.15   Random-Effect Models: DerSimonian-Laird

The random-effect model assumes that the studies that have been included are a representative sample of a hypothetical larger population of studies. Where there is no heterogeneity between studies, the fixed-effect and random-effect models yield the same result. But where there is heterogeneity, the random-effect model may give a substantially different result. The most widely used random-effect models is the DerSimonian-Laird method. This method weighs the inverse of a combination of within-study variation and between-study variation; as this variance will be larger, the CI of summary measure of effect will be wider. With substantial between-study variance (heterogeneity), the DerSimonian-Laird method gives relatively more weight to the smaller studies (Figure 12.2).

12.3.16   Advantages and Disadvantages of Meta-Analysis and QES

While scientific evidence discovery is not completely and absolutely certain, advantages and disadvantages of QES are observed:

12.3.17   Advantages as Benefits

- QES utilizes structured research techniques to summarize and analyze a body of research studies.
- It represents key study findings (i.e., more differentiated from the conventional review process) that rely on qualitative summaries.
- It is capable of finding effects or associations that are obscured in qualitative reviews.

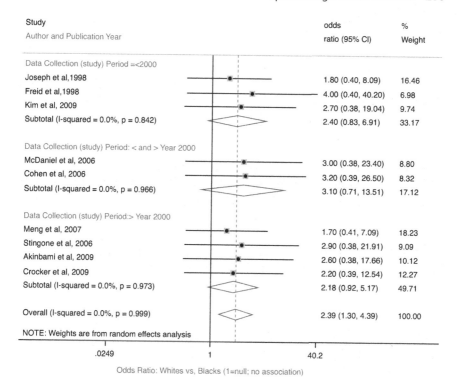

Odds Ratio: Whites vs, Blacks (1=null; no association)

FIGURE 12.2 Forest plot, illustrating the common effect size as diamond and the individual study effect size as square.

- It provides an organized and structured way of handling information from a large number of study findings under review.
- The homogeneity test, which indicates if a grouping of effect sizes is from different studies, shows more variation than would be expected from sampling error alone.
- QES is capable of performing meta-regression that is not feasible with other types of review.

12.3.18 Disadvantages as Limitations

- Time-consuming and requires specialized skills.
- Methodological issues—such as study mixing, different effect sizes or measure of effect.
- Publication bias.
- QES cannot overcome limitations of the individual studies that make up the sample size (k).

12.3.19 Bias

Bias was mentioned earlier. Please remember that bias is a type of error. It is a systematic error that occurs as a result of the investigator's design or conduct of the study that eventually causes inaccurate assessment of the association between the exposure and the outcome of interest.

12.3.19.1 Types of Bias

While the laundry list of errors is not what we advocate for a critical appraisal of scientific literature, the following are examples of bias that are commonly encountered in clinical research: recall bias (commonly encountered in a case-control study) refers to the inability to remember information regarding exposure, especially among the control, resulting in misclassification bias; misclassification bias (errors or mistakes in data acquisition that result in the wrong grouping of study subjects); information bias (record abstraction, interviewing, surrogate interviews, recall bias, surveillance, reporting); and selection bias.

12.3.19.2 Surveillance Bias

Because populations with disease are more closely monitored compared with those who do not have the disease, disease ascertainment may be better in the monitored population and may introduce surveillance bias (monitoring of one population [diseased] more than the other [disease-free]). This bias may lead to erroneous estimations of the effect of the disease in the monitored population, thus inflating the point estimate (RR, RO, OR, HR).

12.3.19.3 Controlling and Minimizing Bias

Biases can be controlled or minimized by accurate definition of items, methods of measurement, standardization of procedures, and quality control of data collection and processing.

12.3.20 Confounding

Confounding has been addressed in previous chapters. One of the issues in the validation of epidemiological research is assessing whether associations between exposure and disease derived from observational epidemiological studies are of a causal nature or not (because of systematic error, random error or confounding). Confounding refers to the influence or effect of an extraneous factor(s) on the relationship or associations between the exposure and the outcome of interest. Observational studies are potentially subject to the effect of extraneous factors, which may distort the findings of these studies. To be a confounding variable, the extraneous variable must be a risk factor for the disease being studied and associated with the exposure being studied but not a consequence of exposure.

Note that confounding occurs when the effects of the exposure are mixed together with the effects of another variable, leading to a bias, and if exposure X causes disease Y, Z is a confounder if Z is a known risk factor for disease Y and Z is associated with X, but Z is not a result of exposure X.

VIGNETTE 12.3

Consider a study to assess the association between coffee drinking (X) and pancreatic cancer risk (Y). The exposure variable is coffee drinking, and coffee drinking is known to be associated with cigarette smoking (Z). Likewise, cigarette smoking is a known risk factor for pancreatic cancer. If causal association is observed between coffee drinking and pancreatic cancer, this might be due to the confounding effect of smoking. Therefore, to be confounding, smoking must be a risk factor for pancreatic cancer and be associated with coffee drinking.

If a causal association, such as $X \rightarrow Y$, occurs, then this causal relationship may be due to Z (confounder).

Controlling for confounding is a method of producing an unconfounded effect (point) estimate:

---

1 During the design phase of the study: (a) restriction, (b) matching, (c) randomization.
2 During the analysis phase of the study: (a) restriction, (b) stratification (stratified analysis), (c) multivariable method (analysis) (Figure 12.3).

12.3.21 Study Validity: Characteristics

Outlined here are the characteristic and types of scientific research validity:

- Validity (internal validity) refers to the lack of bias and confounding in the design of an epidemiologic study.
- External validity refers to the generalization of the findings from a study to a larger population different from the population that was sampled.

  - External validity cannot be established without internal validity.

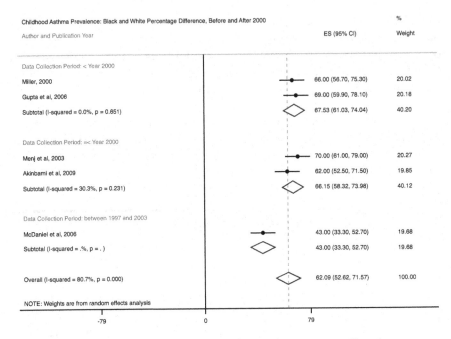

FIGURE 12.3   Forest plot. The diamond indicates the common effect size.

12.3.22   Elements and Characteristics of Confounders (Third Extraneous Variable)

A confounder is an agent or extraneous factor that accounts for differences in disease occurrence or frequency or the measure of effect between the exposed and the unexposed.

- It predicts disease frequency in the unexposed or referent population. For example, in the association between oral cancer and alcohol consumption, smoking is considered confounding if it is associated with both oral cancer and alcohol consumption.
    - A confounder is not qualified by this association only.
    - To qualify as a confounder, smoking must be associated with the occurrence of oral cancer in the unexposed or referent group, apart from its association with alcohol consumption.
    - Also, smoking must be associated with oral cancer among non-consumers of alcohol.
- If the effect of alcohol consumption is mediated through the effect of smoking, then it is not a confounder, regardless of whether there is an effect of exposure (alcohol consumption) on oral cancer (outcome or disease).

- Any variate that represents a step on the pathway between the exposure and disease does not represent a confounder but could be termed an intermediate variate.
  - Alcohol consumption → Smoking → Oral cancer.

- Surrogate confounders refer to factors associated with confounders. For example, in chronologic age and aging, chronologic age is a surrogate confounder.
- Characteristics of confounding variables:

  - An extraneous risk factor for disease.
  - Associated with the exposure in the source population or the population at risk from which the case is derived.
  - Not be affected by the exposure or disease, implying that it cannot be an intermediate in the causal pathway between the disease and exposure.

12.3.23   *Random Error and Precision*

12.3.23.1   *Random Error*

Basically, random error remains an unaccountable error that needs to be quantified. It refers to unsystematic errors that arise from an unforeseeable and unpredictable process, such as a mistake in assessing the exposure and disease and sampling variability (unrepresentative sample or chance).

12.3.23.2   *Precision*

This is the lack of random error. Precision, and hence a reduction in random error, may be induced by increasing the sample size, repeating measurements within a study and utilizing an efficient study design in order to maximize the amount of information obtained.

Precision (lack of random error) may be influenced by sampling, hypothesis testing and p-values, CI estimation, the probability distribution of random variables, and sample size and power estimation.

Systematic error may be present in a study despite the absence or reduction of random error (the study may be precise but findings are inaccurate). It is important to note that no matter the degree of random error marginalization, random error exists, implying some element of uncertainty in all studies, no matter the sampling technique utilized, study size or the magnitude of effect.

12.3.24   *Interaction*

As used in epidemiology, interaction is a biologic phenomenon indicating biologic interaction. Specifically, interaction occurs when the incidence rate of a disease or outcome in the presence of two or more risk factors differs from the incidence rate expected to result from their individual effects. This rate may be greater than what is expected (synergism) or less than what is expected (antagonism). Like the effect measure modifier, interaction is said to occur if there is a difference in the strata-specific risk point estimate (RR, OR) on the basis of the third variable.

Additive model: This occurs in association with effect if the effect of one exposure is added to the effect of the other (e.g., if those with neither exposure have an incidence of 2.0, while for those with a smoking history, the incidence is 8.0 and in those with a smoking history and heavy alcohol consumption, 16.0). The additive model assumes that the incidence will be X in those with both types of risk. What is X? X is 22. Because smoking adds 6.0 to those with no risk, it will be expected to add 6.0 to those with a history of alcohol drinking. The additive model is not accurate in describing the effect of exposure to two independent factors on disease causation.

Multiplicative model: This is the appropriate model for describing the effects of two independent factors or exposures in disease causation (e.g., if the absence of neither exposure has an incidence of 2.0 and those exposed to cigarette smoking have an incidence of 8.0, while those exposed to heavy alcohol consumption have an incidence of 16.0). The multiplicative model assumes that the incidence will be Y in those with both risks. What is Y? Y is 64. Because smoking multiplies the risk by four times in the absence of alcohol, we also expect it to multiply the risk in alcohol users by four (16×4). If so, the effect of exposure to both smoking and alcohol will be $16 \times 4 = 64$.

12.3.25 Effect Measure Modifier

Effect measure modification remains an appropriate epidemiologic concept in assessing heterogeneity of a third variable on the pathway of association. Suppose we wish to examine the data on the association between second primary thyroid cancer and radiation therapy for the first primary cancer in children, and to determine whether or not the effect of radiation on second primary thyroid cancer differs by the level of age or age group, with age as the third variable. Does age modify the OR of the association between radiation and second primary thyroid cancer? If it does, then the result of the association based on the overall estimate without stratum-specific result is invalid, flawed and misleading. Specifically, to examine the OR effect modification, one has to examine the OR by separate level of age or age groups, namely <0, 1–4, 5–9, 10–14 and 15–18 in the association between radiation and second primary thyroid cancer. Practically, if there is no association between radiation and second primary thyroid cancer in the pool analysis (age grouped lumped), the consideration of the stratified analysis by age group may lead to reliable and meaningful result and interpretation. The following steps should be taken in assessing the OR effect modification of age: (1) estimate the overall or crude OR, (2) use the C-M-H method to stratify the data by age, (3) observe the effect of age on the OR of the association between radiation and second primary thyroid cancer. If effect measure modification is observed, the pool estimate should not be reported but the stratum-specific OR in order to address this as a biologic phenomenon. Additionally, if there is only effect measure modification, the stratum-specific estimates differ from one another significantly and should be tested with the chi-square test of homogeneity [2, 3].

Consider another example of effect measure modifier. Is age a modifier in the association between ethnicity and hypertension? Differences are not observed between black and white men under the age of 35 with respect to hypertension incidence. After age 35, incidence tends to be two to three times higher in blacks relative to whites of the same age. Biologically, an effect measure modifier is the third variable that is not a confounder but enters into a causal pathway between the exposure and the disease of interest. For example, the relationship between lung cancer and cigarette smoking is modified by asbestos exposure because asbestos exposure has been known to increase the risk of dying by 92 times among smokers, whereas the risk of dying from lung cancer among those exposed to asbestos only is tenfold. Another example is the modifying effect of cigarette smoking and obesity on the association between oral contraceptives and myocardial infarction in women. Effect measure modifier and confounding have similarities. Both confounding and effect measure modifier involve a third variable and are assessed or evaluated by performing stratified analysis. Effect measure modifier also differs from confounding. In confounding, one is interested in knowing whether the crude measure of association (unadjusted point estimate) changes (distorted) and whether the stratum-specific and adjusted summary estimate differs from the crude or unadjusted estimate. In effect measure modification, one is interested in finding out if the association differs according to the third variable (the difference in stratum-specific estimates from one another).

VIGNETTE 12.4

Consider a case-control study of the effect of lycopene on prostate cancer stratified by BMI (normal versus overweight). The stratum-specific odds ratio for men with a BMI greater than or equal to 24.99 kg/m² = 2.2, and the stratum-specific odds ratio for men with normal BMI (<24.99 kg/m²) is 1.0. Does this illustration indicate the presence of effect modifier or confounding by BMI?

Solution: Because the stratum-specific odds ratio differs between men with normal and abnormal BMI, BMI is an effect measure modifier between lycopene and prostate cancer in men. In this example, the BMI needs to be described or explained in the causal pathway of prostate cancer and does not need to be adjusted for since it is not a confounder.

Question: Can the same variable (gender) be an effect measure modifier and confounder in the same setting (simultaneously)? Explore this possibility using the combined odds ratio and stratum specific odds ratio illustration.

12.3.26 Epidemiologic Causal Inference

Epidemiologic investigation is concerned with association as well as causal association. Simply, cause refers to whatever produces an effect (result, outcome, response variable). Cause may be understood as a factor if its operation increases the frequency of an event (outcome, result). Cause is also described as an event, condition or characteristic that preceded a health-related event and without which the event would not have occurred at all or would not have occurred until some later time. Causal inference in epidemiology involves two steps:

1 valid result—internal validity of the study (association that is not as a result of bias, confounding and random error) and
2 assessment of whether the exposure actually caused the effect (outcome, result).

Causal relationships may be

- necessary and sufficient (necessary if the outcome occurs only if the causal factor operated and sufficient if the operation of the causal factor always results in the outcome)
- necessary but not sufficient
- sufficient but not necessary
- neither sufficient nor necessary, implying that the operation of the causal factor increases the frequency of the causal factor, but the outcome does not always result and the outcome can occur without the operation of the causal factor.

The criteria commonly used to assess causal inference in epidemiologic studies follow those used by Bradford Hill [2, 3, 17].

12.3.27 Bradford Austin Hill's Criteria for Causal Inference (17)

12.3.27.1 Temporality

- The cause must precede the outcome (disease).
- Complete consensus among investigators and most relevant criterion.
- Easily established in prospective studies.

12.3.28 Strength of Association

- Measured by relative risk or odds ratio.
- Larger relative risk or odds ratio is more indicative of a stronger association.

12.3.29   Dose-Response (Biologic Gradient)

- Effect increases as the exposure level increases.

12.3.30   Consistency of Association

- Association is most likely to be causal if observed repeatedly by different persons, in different places, circumstances and times.

12.3.31   Plausibility

- Coherency with the current body of knowledge (existence of biologic or social model to explain the association).

12.3.32   Coherence

- Cause-and-effect interpretation of the data should not seriously conflict with generally known facts of the natural history and the biology of the disease.

12.3.33   Experiment

- If exposure causes a disease, the disease is expected to decline when the exposure is reduced or eliminated.

12.3.34   Analogy

- Similarities between the observed association and other associations.

12.3.35   Specificity

- A cause should lead to a single effect and vice versa.
- An association is specific when a certain exposure is associated with only one disease.

12.3.36   Component Cause Model (Causal Pies)

1 Sufficient cause: complete causal mechanisms that inevitably produce disease.
2 Component cause: each participating factor in a sufficient cause.
3 Necessary cause: a causal component that is a member of every sufficient cause.

The causal pie model [3, 6] indicates that a sufficient cause is not a single factor but rather a minimal set of factors that unavoidably produce disease, implying

implying that the termination of the action of a single causal component blocks the completion of a sufficient cause, thus preventing disease occurrence by that pathway.

VIGNETTE 12.5

Consider an epidemiologic investigation conducted to assess the association between exposure to sulfur and brain tumors in children. If the investigator wishes to compare the findings in this study with other evidence, which criteria, according to Bradford Hill, might be worth considering, and what sort of study design may provide a more valid and reliable comparison?

Solution: Evidence from one study may be compared with another in terms of Hill's criteria of consistency, plausibility, coherence and specificity. The most appropriate design would be prospective studies.

VIGNETTE 12.6

Consider an investigator who wishes to examine published studies on the evidence of estrogen replacement therapy in postmenopausal breast cancer. If s/he wishes to examine the features consistent with causation using the Bradford Hill criteria, which features should be taken into consideration?

Solution: Bradford Hill's features consistent with causation are (a) temporal sequence, (b) strength of association, (c) dose response, (d) consistency and (e) specificity.

VIGNETTE 12.7

Consider an investigation of epidemiologic causal inference that attempts to examine the study validity prior to assessing whether the exposure actually led to the disease. Which aspects of the study must the investigator consider in order to determine if the observed result was valid?

Solution: The first step in epidemiologic causal inference is to illustrate that the result was not due to (a) systematic error (bias), (b) confounding or (c) random error (Figure 12.4).

12.5 Summary

Epidemiologic and clinical research evidence requires the disentangling of bias, random errors, and confounding prior to sustaining the internal and

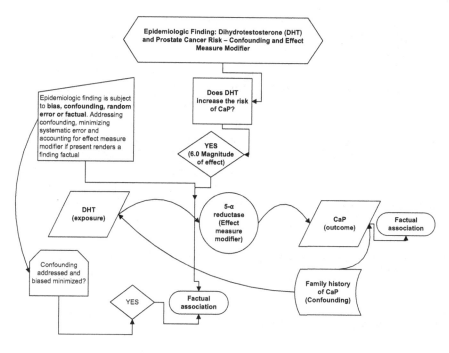

FIGURE 12.4   Confounding as explanatory model in the association between exposure and outcome.

external validity of the study. A single study, no matter how scientifically valid, rarely establishes causal inference. The claim of causality or causal inference involves a combination of criteria, one of which is the combination of studies for the summary effect, termed Meta-Analysis, quantitative systematic review or QES.

QES is contingent on the validity of the individual studies that form the basis of the summary point estimate. The more homogeneous the studies are, the more likely it is that the summary point estimates will reflect the effect of the intervention studied. There are two commonly used methods of summary effect in Meta-Analysis: the fixed-effect and random-effect models. The fixed-effect model is used when the test of heterogeneity indicates homogeneity of the studies combined, while the random-effect model is appropriate if heterogeneity of studies is assumed.

The search for causal inference in epidemiologic studies relies primarily on the assessment of the internal and external validity of studies. The external validity process involves the assessment of the statistical stability or significance level in order to determine whether or not the result is representative of the population from which the sample arose. The test of significance (statistical stability) simply asserts that a random sample represents the population, and hence the result from the sample can then be generalized to the target population. Traditionally, this level of significance is set at 5% error tolerance should one reject the null hypothesis if indeed the null hypothesis is true. Once the obtained probability value is less than 0.05, the null hypothesis is rejected since the obtained result is unlikely to be explained by chance only. With this claim (statistical significance establishment), researchers are required to examine the significant association in the data in the light of bias and confounding, since significance does not rule out the possibility of bias and confounding. Therefore, a result can be statistically significant but clinically and biologically irrelevant, as the finding may be driven by measurement or observation bias and confounding.

The internal validity of the studies involves the assessment of studies for temporality (cause-and-effect relationship, magnitude of association, dose-response relationship, consistency and specificity). The external validity should be assessed but not unless the internal validity is achieved, implying the de-emphasis of the p-value.

12.5.1 Critical Appraisal of Scientific Literature

A. **Research Question**: Assess the clarity and relevance of the question.

B. **Design Process:** Examine the appropriateness of the design to the proposed study question.

C. **Outcome Measure/Variable**: Is the outcome or response variable well determined and is the measure clinically relevant?

D. **Predictor/Independent Variable**: Assess how the exposures were determined and the appropriateness of the exposures in influencing the response.

E. **Analysis**: Is the analytic method appropriate with respect to the scales of measurement of the outcome and predictor variables as well as the design of the study? What are the assumptions behind the test? Sample size and power estimation? Errors?

F. **Systematic Error (Bias)**: *Assessment and minimization*: were biases recognized and addressed?

G. **Results and Interpretation**: Are the findings clinically relevant (effect size)? If negative findings were reported, did the authors document the power of the study?

H. **Discuss and Limitations:** Findings supported by previous publication as well as biologic, biomedical sciences, public health, clinical medicine and population-based explanation of current findings.

I. **Study Implications**: Will the findings impact medicine, public health and clinical practice?

12.6   Questions for Review

1 Suppose you are appointed as the director of a clinical taskforce to establish the guidelines for the assessment and treatment of avascular necrosis associated with sickle cell disease, and you intend to base this guideline on the Meta-Analysis or systematic quantitative review.

   a What will your inclusion and exclusion criteria be?
   b What method of Meta-Analysis will you employ if the studies indicate heterogeneity, and why?
   c What are the limitations of this approach in establishing clinical guidelines?

2 A study was conducted to examine the role of paternal exposure to cigarette smoking and asthma in children. The result was found to be consistent with a causal relationship.

   a If genetic predisposition was also a likely explanation, can we affirm a conclusion regarding a causal relationship?
   b In terms of internal validity and causation, comment on the

   i consistency of this study with other evidence
   ii specificity
   iii biologic plausibility
   iv coherency of the effect with the distribution of the exposure and the outcome.

3 Discuss the role of QES in epidemiologic causal inference.
4 Differentiate between effect measure modifiers, biologic interactions, statistical interactions and confounding. Discuss how to assess for effect measure modifiers and confounding. Can a variable be both an effect measure modifier and a confounding? If that is the case, how will you handle the inference and report the findings?
5 Comment on the assessment of random error, bias and confounding in the establishment of study validity.

   a How relevant is the assessment of bias and confounding if the result of a study is statistically insignificant?
   b What is the significance of probability value in the interpretation of study finding if the sample studied was not a random sample?

6 If a QES is anticipated to be conducted on differential DNA methylation at Acute Lymphoblastic Leukemia (ALL) diagnosis, how could the following strategies be addressed?

   a Search terms, search engine and strategies
   b Study eligibility and quality assessment

    c PRISMA structure

    d Analysis including meta-regression

    e Interpretation and discussion

    f Strengths, limitations and recommendation

References

1 Holmes L Jr et al. DNA methylation of candidate genes (ACE II, IFN-γ, AGTR 1, CKG, ADD1, SCNN1B and TLR2) in essential hypertension: a systematic review and quantitative evidence synthesis. *Int. J. Environ. Res. Public Health.* 2019;16(23):4829. doi: 10.3390/ijerph16234829.

2 Elwood M. *Critical Appraisal of Epidemiological Studies in Clinical Trials,* 2nd ed. (New York: Oxford University Press, 2003).

3 Holmes L Jr. *Applied Epidemiologic Principles and Concepts.* (Boca Raton, FL: Taylor & Francis Publisher, 2018).

4 Aschengrau A, Seage III GR. *Essentials of Epidemiology.* (Sudbury, MA: Jones & Bartlett, 2003).

5 Lipsey MW, Wilson D. *Practical Meta-Analysis.* (Thousand Oaks, CA: Sage Publications, 2001).

6 Rothman KJ. *Epidemiology: An Introduction.* (New York: Oxford University Press, 2002).

7 Szklo M, Nieto J. *Epidemiology: Beyond the Basics.* (Sudbury, MA: Jones & Bartlett, 2003).

8 Lehmann EL. *Testing Statistical Hypothesis,* 2nd ed. (New York: Wiley, 1989).

9 Murray GD. Statistical guidelines for British journal of surgery. *Br. J. Surg.* 1991;78:782–784.

10 Holmes L Jr et al. Aberrant epigenomic modulation of glucocorticoid receptor gene (NR3C1) in early life stress and major depressive disorder correlation: Systematic review and quantitative evidence synthesis. *Int. J. Environ. Res. Public Health.* 2019;16(21):4280.

11 Gore SM et al. The lancet's statistical review process: Areas for improvement by authors. *Lancet.* 1992;340:100–102.

12 DerSimonian R, Laird N. Meta-analysis in clinical trials. *Control Clin. Trials.* 1986;7:177–188.

13 Jones DR. Meta-analysis: weighing the evidence. *Stat. Med.* 1995;14:137–139.

14 Lau J et al. Quantitative synthesis in systematic reviews. *Ann. Intern. Med.* 1997;127:820–826.

15 Olkin I. Meta-analysis: Reconciling the results of independent studies. *Stat. Med.* 1995;14:457–472.

16 Gordis L. *Epidemiology,* 3rd ed. (Philadelphia, PA: Elsevier Saunders, 2004).

17 Hill AB. The environment and disease: Association or causation? *Proc. R. Soc. Med.* 1965;58:295–300.

18 Kadhim M, Thacker M, Kadhim A, Holmes L Jr. Treatment of unicameral bone cyst: Systematic review and meta analysis. *Child Orthop.* 2014;8(2):171–91. doi: 10.1007/s11832-014-0566-3.

Laboratory Techniques and
Epigenomic Mechanistic
Process in Epidemiologic
Principles, Concept
and Application

13

EPIGENOMIC LABORATORY PROCEDURES

Mechanistic Process and Techniques

13.1 Introduction

Epigenetic and epigenomic laboratory procedures involved the application of several laboratory techniques depending on the nature and process of aberrant epigenomic modulation. The approach involves the following: (a) DNA immunoprecipitation-sequencing (DIP-seq), (b) chromatin immunoprecipitation-sequencing (ChIP-seq), (c) an assay for transposase-accessible chromatin using sequencing (ATAC-seq), (d) single-cell ATAC-seq (scATAC-seq) and single-cell multiome. These processes basically involve the main epigenomic modulation mechanistic processes, mainly DNA methylation, histone acetylation, phosphorylation, non-coding RNA, etc.

13.1.1 DNA Immunoprecipitation-Sequencing (DIP-seq)

DIP-seq is an antibody-based technology used to profile the genome-wide distribution of DNA-associated epigenetic marks such as 5-methylcytosine (5mC), 5-hydroxymethylcytosine (5hmC), 5-formylcytosine (5fC) and 5-carboxylcytosine (5caC). The Epigenomics Development Laboratory and Recharge Center offers DIP-seq services using genomic DNA (2.5–10 µg) isolated from cell lines, fluorescence-activated cell sorting (FACS)-purified cells, buffy coat samples, tissues and formalin-fixed, paraffin-embedded (FFPE)-archived tissues.

13.1.2 Chromatin Immunoprecipitation-Sequencing (ChIP-seq)

ChIP-seq is a valuable and widely used epigenetic approach for studying genome-wide protein-DNA interactions in cells and tissues. The Epigenomics

DOI: 10.4324/9781003094487-16

Development Laboratory and Recharge Center offers standard or Tn5 transposase-based ChIP-seq services, depending on sample size (50,000 to 10 million cells). Suitable samples include cell lines, FACS-purified cells, whole blood, buffy coat samples, peripheral blood mononuclear cells (PBMC), frozen tissues, FFPE tissues and spike-in normalization.

13.1.3 Assay for Transposase-Accessible Chromatin Using Sequencing (ATAC-Seq)

The ATAC-seq provides information about open and accessible regions of chromatin that are indicative of active regulatory regions. Sample types suitable for this assay are around 50,000 cells or equivalent and include cell lines, buffy coat samples, sorted cells and frozen tissues.

13.1.4 Single-Cell ATAC-Seq (scATAC-Seq) and Single-Cell Multiome

The scATAC-seq provides information about genome-wide chromatin accessibility of thousands of individual cells in parallel, allowing identification of subpopulations of cells within a heterogeneous population that would otherwise be lost in standard bulk ATAC-seq. Sample types suitable for this assay include cell lines and sorted cells, requiring approximately 50,000–100,000 cells. The single-cell multiome combines scATAC-seq and scRNA-seq assays to accomplish simultaneous profiling of gene expression and chromatin accessibility from the same cell.

13.2 Epigenetics/Epigenomics—Mechanistic Process (Modulation) and Techniques

Epigenomic epidemiology in disease determinants involves the understanding of aberrant epigenomic modulations at specific population levels and the application of such findings in induction therapy prior to the standard of care. There are studies, especially in malignant neoplasms such as acute lymphoblastic leukemia (ALL), that have observed aberrant epigenomic modulation in impaired gene expression, protein synthesis and abnormal cellular proliferation. Specifically, the epigenomic modulation process involved DNA methylation, histone modification, different chromatin structure states, affiliated protein compositions and gene expression changes associated with transcriptional activity. DNA methylation is a major epigenomic mechanistic process in the evaluation of specific epigenetic conditions as normal or aberrant, catalyzed by three different DNA methyltransferases (DNMTs): DNMT1, DNMT3a and DNMT3b, which involve the methyl group, CH_3. The methylation process involves the binding of the methyl groups to the 5' position of cytosine (5C), resulting in 5-methylcytosine (5mC) [1–4].

In a mammalian genome, DNA methylation primarily occurs at cytosine residues, followed by guanine residues, which are symbolized as CpG dinucleotides, with "p" as phosphate. The DNMT1 is essential for genomic imprinting, heterochromatin formation and gene silencing. During X chromosome inactivation, DNA methylation plays a crucial role in long-term silencing, thereby affecting cell memory [5–7]. The DNMT3a and DNMT3b are essential in embryonic development and play a crucial role in de novo methylation in the genome [8, 9]. However, studies have connected DNA methylation and transcription factor binding variants with tumors, changes in the amount of lipid access in the blood—leading to cardiovascular disorders—as well as T2D. The observed implication of DNA methylation in malignant neoplasms, cardiovascular diseases (CVDs) and T2D was observed in several assays performed with ChIP and microarray analysis [2, 7]. This approach remains relevant in the understanding of the aberrant epigenomic mechanistic process involving DNA methylation and gene silencing and its implications for disease development, prognosis and mortality.

In addition to DNA methylation, covalent histone modifications remain an additional epigenomic mechanistic process which consists of histone proteins with a nucleosome (core), N-terminus domain and C-terminus domain. The histone modification involves the N-terminus tails that undergo post-translational modifications such as acetylation, methylation, ubiquitylation and phosphorylation on specific residues. The observed or identified modification signals transcription, repair and replication. In effect, histone variations or modifications involve chromatin functionality, resulting in either activation or repression depending on different residues that undergo modifications [9–14]. For example, lysine 4 trimethylation on histone H3 (H3K4me3) influences transcriptionally active gene promoters [7, 8], while trimethylation of H3K9 (H3K9me3) and H3K27 (H3K27me3) occurs on transcriptionally suppressed gene promoters [15, 16]. There is a wide range of histone modifications identified, constituting a complex gene regulatory network critical for cell physiological activity. The histone modifications are dynamically regulated by enzymes that add and remove covalent changes to the histone proteins. Regarding histone enzymes, histone acetyltransferases (HATs) and histone methyltransferases (HMTs) are associated with the addition of acetyl or methyl groups, respectively, while histone deacetylases (HDACs) and histone demethylases (HDMs) are related to the removal of either acetyl or methyl groups. Specifically, the changes in histone patterns can result in transcriptional activation or silencing. For example, H3K4me2, H3K4me3, H3R17me, H3K36me3 and H4R3me are involved in transcriptional activation, while transcriptional silencing involves H3K9me3, H3K27me3, H4K20me1 and H4K20me3 (8) implicated in malignant cells. The variations in methylation patterns of H3K9 and H3K27 are related to anomalous gene silencing in different types of cancer [17–19]. In addition, several studies have observed various HMTs involved in abnormal silencing of tumor suppressor genes (TSGs) such as p53, EZH2 and p27. For example, the overexpression of EZH2 (an H3K27 HMT) is observed in breast and prostatic adenocarcinoma, while elevated levels of G9a (an H3K9 HMT) area found in hepatic carcinoma [20–22].

Cancer progression is also associated with site-specific demethylases along with overall methylation patterns. For example, LSD1 (lysine demethylase) can potentially remove histone activating and suppressing markers such as H3K4 and H3K9 methylation, thereby serving as a co-repressor or co-activator. Complex interactions exist between DNA methylation and histone modifications. Other than conducting their mutually exclusive purposes, histone modifications and DNA methylation interact at numerous levels to modulate gene expression changes and chromatin organization. Available data have implicated epigenetic interaction and aberrant modulation in disease causation. Additionally, the association of both gene hypermethylation and hypomethylation as well as histone modifications has been implicated in CaP development [1, 2].

Specifically, several HMTs and HDMs also impact DNA methylation levels by modulating the stability of DNMT proteins directly or indirectly, thus engaging HDACs and methyl-binding proteins to silence genes with chromatin condensation. Studies have implicated a close association of various HMTs such as G9a/GLP (mediating H3K9 methylation), SUV39H1 (mediating H3K9 methylation) and PRMT5 (mediating H4R3 methylation) by specifically recruiting DNMTs to stably silence genomes and further direct DNA methylation at specific genomic targets (such as pericentric heterochromatin).

DNA methylation discriminates promoters from enhancers through a H3K4me1-H3K4me3 seesaw mechanism, and suggests its possible function in the inheritance of chromatin marks after cell division, an aberrant effect correlated with cancer and aging. Some studies have observed DNA methylation as influential in H3K9 methylation by regulating effector proteins such as Methyl-CpG-binding protein 2 (MeCP2), eventually creating a restrictive chromatin state. Some studies have observed a bidirectional relationship between DNA methylation and transcription, wherein an NGS approach on the oocyte transcriptome and methylome analyses displayed a consistent pattern for CGIs that are methylated in the oocyte, which need to be transcribed and reduced by the active promoter-associated histone H3 lysine 5 methylation (H3K4me3).

Additionally, elongation of the RNA Pol II transcript has also made significant contributions to the intragenic aggregation of Histone H3 lysine 36 methylation (H3K36me3), which enhances DNMT3A activity (50). Therefore, complex histone modifications such as lysine methylation contribute to the alterable and dynamic regulation of gene expression in comparison to DNA methylation. In effect, DNA methylation and histone modification paradigms can strengthen epigenetic regulation by modulating gene expression activity which can further assist in determining and maintaining cellular identity and functionality [1, 21–26]. These studies play a crucial role in bringing to the forefront various fundamental biological insights and have resulted in the generation of a tremendous amount of experimental data.

From an epigenomic epidemiology perspective, it remains pivotal to design central database (DB) repositories to better interpret and analyze the data using various computational approaches, including machine learning (ML) approaches and other robust methods such as data mining, text mining and many others, in the understanding of this mechanistic process.

13.3 Computational Techniques for DNA Methylation Analysis and Histone Modifications Analysis

13.3.1 Computational Techniques for DNA Methylation Analysis

Numerous studies have reported various ML methods such as predictive modeling methods for determining DNA methylation patterns. Currently, ML has eased epigenetic studies such as DNA methylation due to its massive database and low power input. In general, biological and molecular data are obtained as raw datasets. To make biological interpretations, the raw datasets need to be annotated with class labels. Various ML techniques such as active learning (ACL), deep learning (DL) and imbalanced class learning (ICL) have been employed in various cancer-related studies for genomic mapping to methylation patterns. All of these methods have exhibited various applications in biological datasets [27, 28].

13.3.2 Bisulfite Conversion-Based Methods

The protocol of bisulfite sequencing (BS-Seq) begins with the treatment of denatured DNA with bisulfite, during which the nonmodified cytosine is converted to uracil; although methylated cytosines remain stable without undergoing any changes, leading to the identification of 5-methyl Cytocine (5mC) resolution. As a result, the genomic regions treated with bisulfite are amplified by site-specific polymerase chain reaction (PCR), cloned and subjected to Sanger sequencing [29–33]. Additionally, sequencing reads are evaluated periodically and visualized as a matrix with each clone's CpG material depicted as a row. After the treatment with bisulfite, the sequencing library is subjected to PCR amplifications which extend the sequencing of the adapter, thereby allowing clonal amplification and sequence. Recent advancements in next-generation sequencing (NGS) systems have enhanced the performance and reliability of this method, thereby reducing the costs associated with experimental procedures [34]. Whole-genome bisulfite sequencing (WGBS) is by far the most informative technology that targets the whole genome, which in turn makes it the most expensive technology for base resolution. The process begins with the creation of genomic DNA libraries that are further subjected to bisulfite conversion, following sequencing and aligning to the reference genome. Even though BS-seq is by far the most direct assay, exhibiting the highest methylation detection resolution, this approach is specifically restricted to various studies which aim to answer specific questions related to comprehensive DNA methylation profiling. In the reduced representation of bisulfite sequencing (RRBS) method, the genome is digested by Msp1 (a methylation-insensitive restriction enzyme), and specific DNA fragments approximately ranging from 100 to 300 bps are selected to generate a fragment library using NGS platforms. These shortlisted DNA fragments are considered as the input for the library construction using adapters (methylated) and are further subjected to bisulfite conversion.

Although RRBS covers only 12% of CpGs, the CpGs are enormously enriched in CpG islands. The method has been applied in an experiment to detect methylome profiling in plants, which is termed plant-reduced representation bisulfite sequencing (plant-RRBS), using optimized double restriction endonuclease digestion, fragment end repair and adapter ligation, followed by bisulfite conversion, PCR amplification and NGS. While the results have produced tens of millions of reduced representation bisulfide sequencing (RRBS) methylated regions using multiple samples, this application is limited due to the high cost of performing the assays with large patient samples.

13.3.3   Histone Modifications Profiling and Next-Generation Sequencing

The underlying beliefs for mapping these genome-wide posttranslation modifications involve an NGS methodology such as ChIP [35–37].

Chromatin Immunoprecipitation (ChIP): The process begins by either integrating histones biologically with DNA via the intervention of a cross-linking reagent (such as formaldehyde) or releasing the histones in their native form by nuclease addition which results in the digestion of genomic DNA (gDNA) at unprotected linker sequences. The protein/DNA mixture is subjected to immunoprecipitation after gDNA fragmentation using antibodies raised against posttranslational modification. Subsequently, during the process of immunoprecipitation, DNA fragments associated with histone peptides are subjected to purification and library construction followed by direct sequencing. Single-cell ChIP-sequencing in different stem cells and progenitor cells has led to the identification of population subgroups that are differentiated based on variations in pluripotent chromatin signatures and primer distinction. Studies have suggested that direct sequencing of ChIP fractions has remarkable benefits over alternative techniques such as ChIP-chip, where fragments obtained from ChIP are potentially determined by hybridization to the microarray. However, the study also reported that in ChIP-seq, fragments of the DNA are sequenced explicitly rather than being hybridized on an array. Unlike hybridization, ChIP-Seq does not have background noise which arises during the hybridization process due to the higher frequency of inconsistently matched sequences [36].

Genome-Wide ChIP-Seq: This process has been applied to histone-modification profiles, including mapping of H3K4 acetylation and H3K4 tri-methylation, H3K9 acetylation and H3K27 methylation, which have been used, for example, in defining breast cancer subtypes and recognizing special players in tumorigenesis. Previous data have reported the use of NGS in breast cancer studies. This was conducted using cell-based models transcribing three oncogenes, resulting in reductions in histones H3K9me2 and H3K9me3, as well as elevations in the demethylases for H3K9me1 and H3K9me2 (with KDM3A being relevant events in breast cancer). Recent advancements in technologies have offered innovative and more efficient NGS platforms such as the Illumina Genome Analyzer, and SOLiD offers significant advantages by offering parallel processing of shorter reads and facilitating direct library construction from the immuno-precipitated products, unlike early methods of ChIP such as capillary sequencing [23–26].

The process of library construction for Illumina Genome Analyzer and SOLiD is very similar to typical approaches to whole genome shotgun sequencing. This process begins with the repair of the disheveled ends (within low nanogram range) of the enriched fragmented DNA and further linking the resulting fragments on either the A-tailed end in Illumina Genome Analyzer or the blunt end in SOLiD DNA fragments. The adapter-ligated product is later amplified with PCR primers and conjugated to the adapter sequences. Additionally, in SoLiD, the inclusion of two independent adapter sequences during ligation enables the inclusion of 50% of adapted fragments in PCR amplification [33].

Unlike SoLiD, Illumina genome Analyzer library preparation utilizes adapters which are partially analogous, generating a "fork" in the adapter which is ultimately resolved during PCR. Either of these platforms facilitates enhanced spatial resolution which is crucial for epigenome characterization, which comprises posttranslational modifications of chromatin and nucleosome positioning. Further investigation demonstrated the role of histone modifications during cell differentiation by profiling seven lysine trimethylation marks in mouse ES cells, encompassing both pluripotent and lineage-committed cells. Furthermore, ChIP-seq has been implemented in conjugation with Roche 454 pyrosequencing for generating histone variant H2A.Z maps in yeast as well as common fruit fly. These studies have significantly observed the advantages of NGS methodologies in histone modification profiling [25, 26].

The NGS technology has fundamentally pioneered DNA methylation and histone modification research, leading to the determination of new approaches which can potentially extend understanding and characterization of epigenetic machinery at a global level. In addition, the efficacious assessment of datasets generated by various research facilities employing common DNA profiling and histone modification techniques involves the application of experimental and computational method specifications to facilitate significant relationships between these experiments.

13.3.4 Epigenomic Modulation Research Efficiency

Investigators have made extensive use of computational methods ranging from different databases designed specifically for the demonstration of epigenetic machineries such as DNA methylation and histone modifications. Furthermore, in-depth use of NGS technologies has significantly contributed toward DNA methylation profiling and histone modification profiling at a relatively affordable price as utilized in the ALL epigenomic mechanistic process. This is a very significant aspect of medical diagnostics and therapeutics, particularly with respect to oncology studies. Additionally, such massively parallel high-throughput sequencing technologies offer promising results to decipher the existence and trends of epigenomic modulations as well as their effects on the different processes of physiology, pathology and therapeutics. However, some challenges do exist for the NGS in that it can be technologically demanding.

In this direction (NGS), there is a need to create statistically validated quality methods for the assessment of data quality and thereafter an effort toward enrichment-dependent epigenomic profiles which are mainly used in genomic studies, hence epigenomic studies initiatives and reliable directions. In the future, as the epigenomic datasets increase, bioinformatics-based methodologies will remain to be utilized in ensuring accurate and reliable evidence discovery in this perspective of aberrant epigenomic modulations and induction therapy initiated prior to the standard of care.

13.4 Questions for Review

1 Describe epigenomic mechanistic processes and illustrate the mechanisms involved in aberrant epigenomic modulations.
2 What are the laboratory techniques utilized in epigenomic modulation identification and characterization?
3 Should you wish to illustrate aberrant epigenomic modulations of pediatric ALL genes, what laboratory technique could be utilized in this context?
4 Discuss the chromatin immunoprecipitation (ChIP) laboratory process.
5 What is the next-generation sequencing (NGS) approach in DNA methylation of ALL genes? Please provide the advantages and disadvantages of this laboratory procedure.
6 Describe the bisulfite conversion-based methods in DNA methylation and provide the advantages and disadvantages of this laboratory technique.

References

1 Holmes L Jr et al. DNA Methylation of candidate genes (ACE II, IFN-γ, AGTR 1, CKG, ADD1, SCNN1B and TLR2) in essential hypertension: A systematic review and quantitative evidence synthesis. *Int. J. Environ. Res. Public Health.* 2019;16(23):4829. doi: 10.3390/ijerph16234829.

2 Holmes L Jr et al. Aberrant epigenomic modulation of glucocorticoid receptor gene (NR3C1) in early life stress and major depressive disorder correlation: Systematic review and quantitative evidence synthesis. *Int. J. Environ. Res. Public Health.* 2019;16(21):4280.

3 Kumar S, Singh AK, Mohapatra T. Epigenetics: History, present status and future perspective. *Indian J. Genet. Plant Breed.* 2017;77:445–632.

4 Chakravarthi BV, Nepal S, Varambally S. Genomic and epigenomic alterations in cancer. *Am. J. Pathol.* 2016;186(7):1724–1735.

5 Zhu P, Li G. Structural insights of nucleosome and the 30-nm chromatin fiber. *Curr. Opin. Struct. Biol.* 2016;36:106–1015.

6 Lai WK, Pugh BF. Understanding nucleosome dynamics and their links to gene expression and DNA replication. *Nat. Rev. Mol. Cell Biol.* 2017;18(9):548–562.

7 Baylin SB, Jones PA. Epigenetic determinants of cancer. *Cold Spring Harb. Perspect. Biol.* 2016;8(9):a019505.

8 Banik A, Kandilya D, Ramya S, Stünkel W, Chong YS, Dheen ST. Maternal factors that induce epigenetic changes contribute to neurological disorders in offspring. *Genes.* 2017;8(6):150.

9 Kundaje A, Meuleman W, Ernst J, Bilenky M, Yen A, Heravi-Moussavi A et al. Integrative analysis of 111 reference human epigenomes. *Nature.* 2015;518(7539):317–330.

10 Mensaert K, Denil S, Trooskens G, Van Criekinge W, Thas O, De Meyer T. Next-generation technologies and data analytical approaches for epigenomics. *Environ. Mol. Mutagen.* 2014;55(3):155–170.

11 Irigoyen A, Jimenez-Luna C, Benavides M, Caba O, Gallego J, Ortuño FM, et al. Integrative multiplatform meta-analysis of gene expression profiles in pancreatic ductal adenocarcinoma patients for identifying novel diagnostic biomarkers. *PLoS One.* 2018;13(4):e0194844.

12 Peng A, Mao X, Zhong J, Fan S, Hu Y. Single-cell multi-omics and its prospective application in cancer biology. *Proteomics.* 2020;20:e1900271.

13 Hoang NM, Rui L. DNA methyltransferases in hematological malignancies. *J. Genet. Genomics.* 2020;47(7):361–372.

14 Lewsey MG, Hardcastle TJ, Melnyk CW, Molnar A, Valli A, Urich MA, et al. Mobile small RNAs regulate genome-wide DNA methylation. *Proc. Natl. Acad. Sci. U.S.A.* 2016;113(6):E801–E810.

15 Bird AP. CpG-rich islands and the function of DNA methylation. *Nature.* 1986;321(6067):209–213.

16 Corujo D, Buschbeck M. Post-translational modifications of H2A histone variants and their role in cancer. *Cancers.* 2018;10(3):59.

17 Kouzarides T. Chromatin modifications and their function. *Cell.* 2007;128(4):693–705.

18 Ricketts MD, Han J, Szurgot MR, Marmorstein R. Molecular basis for chromatin assembly and modification by multiprotein complexes. *Protein Sci.* 2019;28(2):329–343.

19 Bernstein BE, Meissner A, Lander ES. The mammalian epigenome. *Cell.* 2007;128(4):669–681.

20 Woo H, Ha SD, Lee SB, Buratowski S, Kim T. Modulation of gene expression dynamics by cotranscriptional histone methylations. *Exp. Mol. Med.* 2017;49(4):e326.

21 Lubecka K, Kurzava L, Flower K, Buvala H, Zhang H, Teegarden D et al. Stilbenoids remodel the DNA methylation patterns in breast cancer cells and inhibit oncogenic NOTCH signaling through epigenetic regulation of MAML2 transcriptional activity. *Carcinogenesis.* 2016;37(7):656–668.

22 Hu Z, Zhou J, Jiang J, Yuan J, Zhang Y, Wei X, et al. Genomic characterization of genes encoding histone acetylation modulator proteins identifies therapeutic targets for cancer treatment. *Nat. Commun.* 2019;10(1):1–17.

23 Cedar H, Bergman Y. Linking DNA methylation and histone modification: Patterns and paradigms. *Nat. Rev. Genet.* 2009;10(5):295–304.

24 Wen K-x, Miliç J, El-Khodor B, Dhana K, Nano J, Pulido T, et al. The role of DNA methylation and histone modifications in neurodegenerative diseases: A systematic review. PLoS One. 2016;11(12):e0167201.

25 Nowacka-Zawisza M, Wiśnik E. DNA methylation and histone modifications as epigenetic regulation in prostate cancer. *Oncol. Rep.* 2017;38(5):2587–2596.

26 Eisenberg CA, Eisenberg LM. G9a and G9a-like histone methyltransferases and their effect on cell phenotype, embryonic development, and human disease. In: *The DNA, RNA, and Histone Methylomes.* (New York: Springer, 2019, pp. 399–433).

27 Hyun K, Jeon J, Park K, Kim J. Writing, erasing and reading histone lysine methylations. *Exp. Mol. Med.* 2017;49(4):e324.

28 Stewart KR, Veselovska L, Kelsey G. Establishment and functions of DNA methylation in the germline. *Epigenomics.* 2016;8(10):1399–1413.

29 Dai H, Wang Z. Histone modification patterns and their responses to environment. *Curr. Environ. Health Rep.* 2014;1(1):11–21.

30 Bernstein BE, Stamatoyannopoulos JA, Costello JF, Ren B, Milosavljevic A, Meissner A et al. The NIH roadmap epigenomics mapping consortium. *Nat. Biotechnol.* 2010;28(10):1045–1048.

31 Adams D, Altucci L, Antonarakis SE, Ballesteros J, Beck S, Bird A, et al. BLUEPRINT to decode the epigenetic signature written in blood. *Nat. Biotechnol.* 2012;30(3):224–226.

32 Zhou X, Maricque B, Xie M, Li D, Sundaram V, Martin EA, et al. The human epigenome browser at Washington University. *Nat. Methods.* 2011;8(12):989–990.

33 Li D, Hsu S, Purushotham D, Sears RL, Wang T. WashU epigenome browser update 2019. *Nucleic Acids Res.* 2019;47(W1):W158–W65.

34 Consortium EP. The ENCODE (ENCyclopedia of DNA elements) project. *Science.* 2004;306(5696):636–640.

35 Lauss M, Visne I, Weinhaeusel A, Vierlinger K, Noehammer C, Kriegner A. MethCancerDB–aberrant DNA methylation in human cancer. *Br. J. Cancer.* 2008;98(4):816–817.

36 Dodd IB, Micheelsen MA, Sneppen K, Thon G. Theoretical analysis of epigenetic cell memory by nucleosome modification. *Cell.* 2007;129(4):813–822.

37 Atlas E. Epigenome wide atlas. 2018.

14

EPIGENOMIC STUDIES PERSPECTIVE

Malignant Neoplasm, Prostatic Adenocarcinoma— Prostate Cancer CaP

14.1   Introduction

Prostate cancer (CaP) remains the second leading cause of cancer mortality among US males, with blacks/African Americans having the highest mortality compared with their white counterparts, while CaP mortality is lowest among Asian Americans. Since CaP therapeutics do not provide a reliable explanation for the disproportionate burden of mortality among blacks/African Americans (AA) males, aberrant epigenomic modulations remain a feasible pathway in this mortality racial/ethnic differential. With CaP incidence, prognosis and survival, subpopulation differentials reflect aberrant epigenomic modulations driven by education level, low socioeconmic status (SES), late screening, uninsured and underinsured, air pollutants, toxic waste, clinician/implicit bias, etc. These adverse environments signal epigenomic modulations that are aberrant, resulting in transcriptome marginalization, implying inverse gene expression, impaired protein synthesis and cellular dysfunctionality as abnormal cellular proliferation.

14.1.1   Specific Malignancies and Epigenomic Modulations as Aberrant

DNA methylation remains a relevant and significant regulator of gene transcription and expression, with the implication of this epigenomic mechanistic process in carcinogenesis being a current direction in malignant neoplasms as well as other pathologies. DNA hypermethylation represses transcription of CpG-rich promoter regions of tumor suppressor genes such as p53 and p27, resulting in gene silencing. DNA methylation is a covalent chemical modification, resulting in the binding of a methyl ($-CH_3$) group at the carbon-5 position

DOI: 10.4324/9781003094487-17

of the cytosine ring. This DNA methylation is catalyzed by DNA methyltransferase (DNMT) in the context of the sequence 5'-CG-3', termed the CpG dinucleotide. CpGs are nonrandomly distributed, and an estimated 1% of human DNA comprises short, CpG-dense sequences termed CpG islands [1]. Within the unmethylated state, chromatin at the CpG island regions can be molded into active conformations, thus facilitating the loading of RNA polymerases onto gene promoters. However, an estimated 60–90% of CpG dinucleotides are methylated in the adult genome, implying the spontaneous deamination of 5-methylcytosine to thymine and thereby chromatin structure transformation or alteration, adversely influencing the transcriptome. Additionally, an estimated 50% of all genes in humans have CpG islands or shores, implicated in both housekeeping genes and genes with tissue-specific patterns of expression. Specifically, the promoter region's CpG islands are usually unmethylated in all normal tissues, regardless of the transcriptional activity of the gene [2, 3].

14.1.2 DNA Methyltransferase and DNA Methylation

With respect to DNA enzymes, there are three active DNMTs which have been identified, namely DNMT1, DNMT3A and DNMT3B. DNMT1 has a principal role in the maintenance of the cell methylation profile and, to a lesser extent, de novo methylation of tumor suppressor genes. This de novo activity of DNMT1 has been observed to be stimulated by aberrant DNA structures. Specifically, DNMT3A and DNMT3B have both maintenance and de novo methylation activities and are observed to be responsible for the wave of methylation that occurs during embryogenesis. Notwithstanding the observed methylation process or pathway, it has been demonstrated that DNMTs physically bind to several histone modifiers, including histone deacetylases (HDACs) and EZH2. The formation of multicomponent epigenomic regulatory complexes observed in DNA methylation and histone modification machineries functions in a highly cooperative manner in regulating chromatin structure as well as gene expression [3, 4].

14.2 Malignant Neoplasm—Prostatitc (CaP): Hypermethylation in Prostate Cancer (CaP)

Prostatic adenocarcinoma cells commonly have promoter DNA hypermethylation as a means of gene repression in the incidence and prognosis of the neoplastic phenotype. This modulation silences substantial classic tumor-suppressor gene functions, including hormone signaling, DNA repair, cell adhesion, cell-cycle control and apoptosis [4, 5]. Tumor suppressor genes frequently altered in other human cancers such as PTEN, RB1 and TP53 are not observed as hypermethylated in CaP, although allelic loss and point mutations are observed in advanced CaP stages [1].

14.2.1 DNA Repair Genes and Aberrant Epigenomic Modulation

The pathologic pathway of CaP has been observed in CpG island hypermethylation involving the glutathione S-transferase (GSTP1) gene. The GSTP1 gene is implicated in the metabolism, detoxification and elimination of potentially genotoxic foreign compounds, reflecting the protection of cells from DNA damage and cancer development through abnormal cellular proliferation. The CpG island promoter region spanning the GSTP1 gene becomes methylated in the majority of prostatic adenocarcinomas. The observed GSTP1 gene is expressed and unmethylated in all normal tissues [6]. However, in CaP as indicated earlier, it remains hypermethylated. There are no mutations or deletions observed in this GSTP1 gene with respect to CaP; however, this gene is inactivated and both alleles are commonly methylated, indicative of a normal genome but aberrant epigenomic modulation of GSTP1. Further, promoter methylation of GSTP1 is absent in normal epithelium and 6.4% in proliferative inflammatory atrophy, 70% in high-grade prostatic intraepithelial neoplasia as well as 90% in CaP [7]. The GSTP1 methylation appears to discriminate between benign and premalignant/malignant prostate and persists through all stages of CaP, and can be detected in circulating tumor cells (CTCs) [8]. The GSTP1 gene encodes the π-class glutathione S-transferase (GST), an enzyme involved in detoxifying electrophilic and oxidant carcinogens [9]. Specifically, the implied loss of π-class GST function sensitizes prostatic epithelial cells to cell and genome damage caused by dietary carcinogens and inflammatory oxidants, indicative of the contributory effect of diet and lifestyle on CaP development [10].

With respect to the DNA repair protein methylguanine DNA methyltransferase (MGMT), this protein deletes the alkyl adducts from the O6 position of guanine. However, this MGMT expression is decreased in some tumor tissues and in cell lines, enhancing carcinogenesis as tumor development. Specifically, the loss of expression of the MGMT is rarely due to deletion, mutation or rearrangement of the MGMT gene; however, the methylation of discrete regions of the CpG islands of MGMT, associated with the silencing of the gene in cell lines, is implicated in aberrant epigenomic modulation. Specifically, MGMT DNA hypermethylation is observed in CaP incidence and progression.

14.2.1.1 Tumor Suppression Genes and Aberrant Epigenomic Modulation

The adenomatous polyposis coli (APC) is a relevant tumor suppressor gene that participates in different molecular pathways and causes epigenomic aberration in malignant neoplasm. This hypermethylation of APC has been observed as a biomarker for CaP prognosis, with the DNA methylation in APC associated with higher CaP mortality relative to unmethylated CaP patients.

The APC, as observed in colorectal cancer cells, prevents the transcription of gene products that promote cell proliferation and survival rather than normal cell differentiation and apoptosis. The DNA hypermethylation of APC reflects the transcriptome, implying cell vulnerability, hence malignant neoplasm.

The retinoic acid receptor beta (RARβ) and PDLM4 have been implicated as tumor suppressor genes in human CaP cell and xenograft models. These RARβ and PDLM4 promoters are highly hypermethylated during CaP progression. Mainly, retinoid acid (RA) exerts its biological effect through two families of nuclear receptors: RA receptors (RAR α, β, γ) and retinoid X receptors (RXR α, β, γ), which are ligand-dependent transcription factors of the steroid/thyroid hormone nuclear receptor superfamily. The RARβ2 gene is located in chromosomal region 3p24 and has been observed to harbor a CpG-rich region in its promoter with CaP hypermethylation [11]. Specifically, RARβ2 hypermethylation has been estimated at 97.5% among CaP patients, 94.7% in high-grade prostatic intraepithelial neoplasia (HGPIN) and 23.3% in benign prostatic hyperplasia (BPH), with methylation levels significantly higher in CaP relative to HGPIN and BPH. In addition, the inactivation of the tumor suppressor gene RASSF1A has been associated with hypermethylation of its CpG-island promoter region [11]. Selective promoter methylation of the RASSF1A promoter, but not of RASSF1C, is implicated in 53% of CaP as well as in higher Gleason score and serum PSA [11, 12]. Simply, the RASSF1A protein has been observed to adversely impact cell proliferation by RAS-linked pathways, inhibiting the accumulation of cyclin D1 and implying cell cycle arrest [13].

14.2.1.2 Cell Adhesion Genes and Cell Cycle and Proapoptotic Genes

E-cadherin (CDH1) is a relevant suppressor of invasion. Decreased CDH1 expression has been observed in extensive metastases and CaP survival disadvantages, with a 5′ CpG island of CDH1 densely methylated in CaP cells. Increased hypermethylation of the CDH1 promoter has been observed in association with fibroblastic cell morphology characteristic of epithelial-to-mesenchymal transition in non-prostate malignancies. CD44 encodes another integral membrane protein involved in matrix adhesion and signal transduction. In CaP, CD44 hypermethylation is observed in 78% of patients compared to only 10% of patients without malignancy [13].

The protein encoded by the CCND2 gene also encodes the protein involved in the cell cycle. Specifically, cyclin D is a regulatory subunit of CDK4 or CDK6, implying the cell cycle transition from G1 to S phase. The DNA hypermethylation of CCND2 is significantly higher in CaP (32%) compared to normal prostate tissues (6%), p <0.05. Additionally, there are substantial similarities between the DNA hypermethylation of CCND2 and the hypermethylation of RARβ, GSTP1, CDH13, RASSF1A and APC genes [14]. Specifically, the DNA hypermethylation of CCND2 observed in invasive CaP correlates with clinicopathologic features of CaP and other tumor aggressiveness [12].

14.2 CaP: Aberrant Epigenomic Modulation Mechanistic Process

14.2.1 DNA Hypomethylation in CaP

Hypomethylation is a second methylation defect that is observed in a wide variety of malignancies, including CaP and breast tumors [15]. Since hypermethylation alterations seem to precede hypomethylation changes, which are generally detected in malignancies at a higher stage and histologic grade and occur heterogeneously during CaP progression and metastasis [16]. Hypomethylation is observed due to the diminished methylation of abundant repetitive sequences that are densely methylated in normal cells, such as LINE-1 retrotransposons [12, 15]. Specifically, hypomethylation has been hypothesized to contribute to oncogenesis through multiple mechanisms, including but not limited to the activation of oncogenes such as c-MYC, d H-RAS, latent retrotransposons and chromosome instability [17]. Current studies have illustrated an association between family of regulator gene and prto-oncogene that code for transription factor (MYC) overexpression in CaP tissues and CaP progression. The MYC is involved in androgen-dependent growth and is implicated in androgen-independent growth in CaP cells [18–20].

14.2.2 Histone Modification and Modulations

Histone modification is an additional mechanistic process in epigenomic modulation. The main regulators or enzymes in histone modification are HDACs, histone acetyltransferases (HAT) and histone methyltransferases. Collectively, HDACs and HATs determine the acetylation status of histones. Histones, although considered "DNA-packaging" proteins, remain dynamic regulators of gene activity that undergo many posttranslational chemical modifications, such as acetylation, methylation or phosphorylation. The N-terminal tails of histone proteins, which protrude out of the nucleosome, are rich in positively charged amino acids that are subject to various reversible posttranslational modifications. The status of acetylation and methylation of specific lysine residues contained within the tails of nucleosomal core histones is observed to play a crucial role in regulating chromatin structure and gene expression. Histone modifications, as well as DNA methylation, play a significant role in nuclear architecture organization, which is involved in regulating transcription and other nuclear processes. Specifically, the alterations of histone modification patterns have the potential to affect the structure and integrity of the genome and to disrupt normal patterns of gene expression, which remains as causal inference in malignant neoplasm.

Mainly, the histone acetylation mediated by HATs correlates with transcriptional activation, and the histone deacetylation mediated by HDACs is linked to gene silencing. Specifically, through the removal of acetyl groups from histones, HDACs create a nonpermissive chromatin conformation that prevents the transcription of genes that encode proteins involved in tumorigenesis. Further, histone methylation on arginine and lysine has been observed to be affiliated with either gene activation or suppression, depending on the amino acid position and the number of methylated residues [19].

14.2.2.1 Histone Modification in CaP

With respect to CaP cell lines, methylation of lysine 9 in histone 3 (H3K9) is linked to repression of AR genes [20], while histone H3K4 methylation is linked with AR gene activation in CRPC cell lines and tissues [21]. H3K4 is significantly methylated at the AR enhancer of the protooncogene UBE2C gene in CRPC, which leads to AR binding and UBE2C gene expression [21]. HDAC6 regulates AR hypersensitivity and nuclear localization, mainly via modulating TRAP1 acetylation [22]. Available evidence indicates histone modification as a relevant contributor to prostate tumorigenesis. In effect, changes in global levels of individual histone modifications are predictive of the clinical outcome of CaP independently of other features such as tumor stage, preoperative prostate-specific antigen levels and capsule invasion. Specifically, global methylations of H3K4 and histone H3 lysine 18 acetylation (H3K18Ac) have been observed as predictors of recurrence in low-grade CaP patients. Additionally, DAB2IP is a novel GTPase-activating protein for modulating the Ras-mediated signal pathway and tumor necrosis factor (TNF)-associated apoptosis as implicated by CaP. The loss of DAB2IP expression is frequently detected in metastatic CaP. The epigenetic/epigenomic silencing of DAB2IP is a significant mechanistic pathway in which EZH2 activates Ras and NF-κB, implying metastasis [23–25].

14.2.3 Laboratory Techniques: Diagnostic, Prognostic Markers

The direction for laboratory techniques requires: (a) methylation as a diagnostic and prognostic marker for CaP and (b) histone modification as a diagnostic and prognostic marker for CaP.

14.2.4 Epigenomic Therapy as Therapy Induction Prior to Standard Therapy

The direction in epigenomic therapy involves the identification of epigenomic markers such as aberrant epigenomic modulations involved in tumor suppressor genes, cell adhesion genes, etc., and the application of induction therapy such as DNA demethylase and HDAC prior to the recommended tumor standard of care like chemotherapeutic agents. The example of induction therapy in CaP prior to the application of the standard of care involves hypomethylating agents in CaP as induction therapy. With respect to these novel agents as epigenomic induction therapy in cancer therapeutics, implying the efficacy of DNA methylation inhibitors in malignant neoplasms, these directions remain to improve cancer therapeutics at the population level as well as individual patient care.

14.3   Summary

DNA methylation remains a relevant and significant regulator of gene transcription and expression, with the implication of this epigenomic mechanistic process in carcinogenesis being a current direction in malignant neoplasms as well as other pathologies. However, DNA hypermethylation represses transcription of CpG-rich promoter regions of tumor suppressor genes such as p53 and p27, resulting in gene silencing. The DNA methylation is a covalent chemical modification, resulting in the binding of a methyl ($-CH_3$) group at the carbon-5 position of the cytosine ring. This DNA methylation is catalyzed by DNMT in the context of the sequence 5'-CG-3', termed the CpG dinucleotide.

With respect to CaP, prostatic adenocarcinoma cells commonly have promoter DNA hypermethylation as a means of gene repression in the incidence and prognosis of the neoplastic phenotype. This modulation silences substantial classic tumor-suppressor gene functions, including hormone signaling, DNA repair, cell adhesion, cell-cycle control and apoptosis. The tumor suppressor genes frequently altered in other human cancers such as PTEN, RB1 and TP53 are not observed as hypermethylated in CaP, although allelic loss and point mutations are observed in advanced CaP stages.

The pathologic pathway of CaP had been observed in CpG island hypermethylation involving the glutathione S-transferase (GSTP1) gene. The GSTP1 gene is implicated in the metabolism, detoxification and elimination of potentially genotoxic foreign compounds, reflecting the protection of cells from DNA damage and cancer development as abnormal cellular proliferation.

The understanding of aberrant epigenomic modulations in prostatic tissues and the application of the risk determinants in these aberrations facilitate the application of induction therapy prior to the standard of care in CaP therapeutics.

14.4   Questions for Review

1 Discuss the risk factors as environmental determinants in prostate cancer (CaP).
2 Describe the genes involved in CaP.
3 What are the tumor suppressor genes in CaP?

4 During the conduct of an epigenomic study on subpopulation differentials in CaP genes with respect to the environment, which epigenomic modulation process could be applied?

5 With respect to ALL malignancy, identify epigenomic modulation or mechanistic process in specific gene implication in ALL incidence.

References

1 Holmes L Jr et al. DNA Methylation of candidate genes (ACE II, IFN-γ, AGTR 1, CKG, ADD1, SCNN1B and TLR2) in essential hypertension: A systematic review and quantitative evidence synthesis. *Int. J. Environ. Res. Public Health.* 2019;16(23):4829. doi: 10.3390/ijerph16234829.

2 Holmes L Jr et al. Aberrant epigenomic modulation of glucocorticoid receptor gene (NR3C1) in early life stress and major depressive disorder correlation: Systematic review and quantitative evidence synthesis. *Int. J. Environ. Res Public Health.* 2019;16(21):4280.

3 National Center for Biotechnology Information KRT13-Keratin 13 (Human), NCBI Gene=3860. Available online: https://pubchem.ncbi.nlm.nih.gov/gene/KRT13/human [Accessed 2 May 2023].

4 López-Jaramillo P, Camacho PA, Forero-Naranjo L. The role of environment and epigenetics in hypertension. *Expert Rev. Cardiovasc. Ther.* 2009;11:1455–1457. doi: 10.1586/14779072.2013.846217.

5 Boslaugh SE. *The SAGE Encyclopedia of Pharmacology and Society.* (Saunders Oaks, CA: SAGE Publications, 2016). Centers for Disease Control and Prevention.

6 Fernández-Sanlés A, Sayols-Baixeras S, Curcio S, Subirana I, Marrugat J, Elosua R. DNA methylation and age-independent cardiovascular risk, an epigenome-wide approach. *Arter. Thromb. Vasc. Biol.* 2018;38:645–652. doi: 10.1161/ATVBAHA.117.310340.

7 Schiano C, Vietri MT, Grimaldi V, Picascia A, De Pascale MR, Napoli C. Epigenetic-related therapeutic challenges in cardiovascular disease. *Trends Pharmacol. Sci.* 2015;36:226–235. doi: 10.1016/j.tips.2015.02.005.

8 Song JZ, Stirzaker C, Harrison J, Melki JR, Clark SJ. Hypermethylation trigger of the glutathione-S-transferase gene (GSTP1) in prostate cancer cells. *Oncogene.* 2002;21(7):1048–1061.

9 Nakayama M, Bennett CJ, Hicks JL et al. Hypermethylation of the human glutathione S-transferase-π gene (GSTP1) CpG island is present in a subset of proliferative inflammatory atrophy lesions but not in normal or hyperplastic epithelium of the prostate: a detailed study using laser-capture microdissection. *Am. J. Pathol.* 2003;163(3):923–933.

10 Lee WH, Morton RA, Epstein JI et al. Cytidine methylation of regulatory sequences near the π-class glutathione S-transferase gene accompanies human prostatic carcinogenesis. *Proc. Natl. Acad. Sci. U. S. Am.* 1994;91(24):11733–11737.

11 Singal R, Van Wert J, Bashambu M. Cytosine methylation represses glutathione S-transferase P1 (GSTP1) gene expression in human prostate cancer cells. *Cancer Res.* 2001;61(12):4820–4826.

12 Rouprêt M, Hupertan V, Catto JWF et al. Promoter hypermethylation in circulating blood cells identifies prostate cancer progression. *Int. J. Cancer.* 2008;122(4):952–956.

13 Ellinger J, Bastian PJ, Jurgan T et al. CpG island hypermethylation at multiple gene sites in diagnosis and prognosis of prostate cancer. *Urology.* 2008;71(1):161–167.

14 Nakayama M, Gonzalgo ML, Yegnasubramanian S, Lin X, De Marzo AM, Nelson WG. GSTP1 CpG island hypermethylation as a molecular biomarker for prostate cancer. *J. Cell. Biochem.* 2004;91(3):540–552.

15 Padar A, Sathyanarayana UG, Suzuki M et al. Inactivation of cyclin D2 gene in prostate cancers by aberrant promoter methylation. *Clin. Cancer Res.* 2003;9(13):4730–4734.

16 Henrique R, Costa VL, Cerveira N et al. Hypermethylation of Cyclin D2 is associated with loss of mRNA expression and tumor development in prostate cancer. *J. Mol. Med.* 2006;84(11):911–918.

17 Bedford MT, Van Helden PD. Hypomethylation of DNA in pathological conditions of the human prostate. *Cancer Res.* 1987;47(20):5274–5276.

18 Nelson WG, Yegnasubramanian S, Agoston AT et al. Abnormal DNA methylation, epigenetics, and prostate cancer. *Front Biosci.* 2007;12:4254–4266.

19 Yegnasubramanian S, Haffner MC, Zhang Y et al. DNA hypomethylation arises later in prostate cancer progression than CpG island hypermethylation and contributes to metastatic tumor heterogeneity. *Cancer Res.* 2008;68(21):8954–8967.

20 Mathews LA, Crea F, Farrar WL. Epigenetic gene regulation in stem cells and correlation to cancer. *Differentiation.* 2009;78(1):1–17.

21 Wang Q, Li W, Zhang Y et al. Androgen receptor regulates a distinct transcription program in androgen-independent prostate cancer. *Cell.* 2009;138(2):245–256.

22 van Ree JH, Jeganathan KB, Malureanu L, Van Deursen JM. Overexpression of the E2 ubiquitin-conjugating enzyme UbcH10 causes chromosome missegregation and tumor formation. *J. Cell Biol.* 2010;188(1):83–100.

23 Ai J, Wang Y, Dar JA et al. HDAC6 regulates androgen receptor hypersensitivity and nuclear localization via modulating Hsp90 acetylation in castration-resistant prostate cancer. *Mol. Endocrinol.* 2009;23(12):1963–1972.

24 Chen H, Toyooka S, Gazdar AF, Hsieh JT. Epigenetic regulation of a novel tumor suppressor gene (hDAB2IP) in prostate cancer cell lines. *J. Biol. Chem.* 2003;278(5):3121–3130.

25 Min J, Zaslavsky A, Fedele G et al. An oncogene-tumor suppressor cascade drives metastatic prostate cancer by coordinately activating Ras and nuclear factor -kappaB. *Nat. Med.* 2010;16(3):286–294.

15

PEDIATRIC ACUTE LYMPHOBLASTIC LEUKEMIA (ALL)

Aberrant Epigenomic Modulation Surrogate

This study investigates the conjoint effect of urbanity and tumor immunophenotype on survival disadvantage of males and blacks/African Americans with pediatric acute lymphoblastic leukemia (ALL): SEER (1973–2015).

15.1 Introduction

Translational epidemiologic data indicate an increasing pediatric cancer incidence in the United States, with an annual rate of 0.6% since 1975 [1, 2]. However, there has been survival improvement due to advances in cytogenetics and enhancing therapeutics. An estimated 0.24% probability of cancer development before the age of 15 years, implying 1 in 408 children being diagnosed with cancer before 20 years of age, has been observed [2, 3]. Leukemias are the most commonly diagnosed pediatric cancer, accounting for an estimated one third (34%) of childhood malignant neoplasms, with an estimated prevalence of four cases per 100,000 children aged 0–19 years [4]. Whereas ALL is the most commonly diagnosed malignant neoplasm in this age group, survival is remarkable, with a five-year relative survival rate estimated at 85–88% [4].

ALL comprises B-cell, T-cell and other as immunophenotype. T-cell ALL reflects an estimated 10–25% of incident pediatric ALL, while B-ALL accounts for 75–85% of ALL cases [5]. This hematologic malignancy, namely T-ALL, is due to cytogenetic and molecular dysfunctions as well as an adverse environment resulting in the dysregulation of the oncogenic, tumor suppressor and growth/developmental pathways involved in the regulation of normal thymocyte differentiation and maturation. The dysregulation of this pathway results

DOI: 10.4324/9781003094487-18

in an alternation in normal cell growth and hence abnormal cell proliferation, hence T-ALL [6]. The lymphoblasts which reflect early thymic progenitors differentiate by the process of somatic rearrangement of T-cell receptor (TCR) genes. An estimated 50% of patients with T-ALL have been associated with chromosome rearrangements that involve T-cell receptor genes, mainly T-cell receptors α and δ (14q11), T-cell receptor β (7q34) or T-cell receptor γ (7p14.1.) [7, 8]. Specifically, the completely differentiated T-lymphocyte is both functional and self-tolerant, a necessary and robust requirement resulting in an approximately 95% attrition rate of mature T-lymphocytes. In addition, an estimated 5% migrate from the thymus and circulate in the blood and through lymphatic and non-lymphatic organs [8, 9]. Simply, T-ALL is a malignancy of the lymphoblast involved in the T-lymphocytes lineage.

Relative to B-ALL, T-ALL is biologically more aggressive and is characterized by genomic instability and excessive epigenomic aberrations, adversely impacting normal T-cell development, differentiation and maturation. Specifically, transcription factor inhibition, dysregulation of cell-cycle regulators CDKN2A (p16)/2B(p15), and upregulation or hyperactivity of Notch (Drosophila) homolog 1, translocation-associated (NOTCH1) signaling have been implicated in T-ALL. An estimated 50–60% of T-ALL cases have been observed with activating mutations of NOTCH1 [5, 6]. However, much remains to be understood in this malignancy, given the implication of JAX/STAT signaling dysregulation.

The cytogenetics of ALL and leukomogenesis involve cell cycle dysregulation due to excess kinase activation and tumor suppressor gene inactivation, which are required in programed cell death. Simply, ALL develops from dysfunctional lymphoid stem cells and results from abnormal proliferations of lymphoid B-cell precursors (BCPs) and/or T cells with arrested maturation, implying leukemic transformation. T-ALL is clinically characterized by abnormal white blood cells in the blood and bone marrow, uncontrolled accumulation of T-cell progenitors and disruption of immune responses [10]. The T-ALL cytogenetics is indicative of the several mutations involving the proliferative genes (TAL 1, TLX1, TLX3, NKX2-1, LYL1, IL-7R, JAK1, JAK3, STAT5 and FBXW7) and tumor suppressor genes (PTEN, KRAS, RB1, HOXA5, HOXA6) due to chromosomal defects such as the 9p deletion that results in CDKN2A (p16) and CDKN2B (p15) inactivation [6, 8, 9]. Specifically, the aberration of the cyelin-dependent inhibitor 2A/2B (CDKN2A/2B), which occurs as a result of chromosome 9 deletion (9p21.3), is indicated in about 30% of pediatric T-ALL and has been observed in an estimated 88% of pediatric T-ALL leukomogenesis [9]. This gene is a negative regulator of the cell cycle during G1 progression by downregulating CDK4 kinase as well as stabilizing TP53, which is the protein required for the tumor suppressor gene p53 degradation [7, 8, 10, 11]. Whereas T-ALL cytogenetics has provided some reliable data on the management of ALL, the several aberrant epigenomic modulations in T-ALL explain the increased relapses and decreased survival in this immunophenotype relative to B-ALL.

Whereas B-ALL has been observed with reliable prognostic predictive values, an estimated 20% of incident B-ALL or BCP-ALL remains cytogenetically undetermined and is termed B-other [5, 8]. The B-other subtype of B-ALL indicates poorer survival due to limited understanding of the minimal residual disease (MRD) at diagnosis, restricting clinical decision-making with respect to therapeutics [10]. The understanding of the cytogenetics in B-other provides a pathway for adequate information accumulation on MRD and reliable clinical decision-making, thus narrowing the survival gap between B-ALL and B-other as a component of ALL-unspecified in this study.

Despite the improvement in pediatric ALL survival, racial and sex disparities exist and continue to persist [12]. While incidence of ALL is higher among whites relative to blacks/African Americans (AA), black/AA children continue to experience survival disadvantage relative to whites and Asians/Pacific Islanders [13–16]. Epidemiologic and clinical data on pediatric ALL incidence indicate increasing trends and percent change variabilities by subpopulations, namely race, ethnicity, age, geographic locale, income and sex. The sex variance in incidence and survival implicates males with increased incidence and poorer survival relative to females. While the cumulative incidence (CmI) of pediatric ALL is higher among whites, the annual percent change (APC), implying a positive trend, is higher among blacks, especially black males [12]. The understanding of pediatric ALL specific risk, cytogenetics and aberrant epigenomic modulations will enhance specific-risk characterization, induction therapy development and treatment effect homogeneity, thus addressing dose escalation and chemotoxicity observed in T-ALL relapses and equitable subpopulation therapeutics.

Whereas the survival disadvantage of males and blacks relative to females and whites has been observed, there are no reliable explanations for the indicated variances with respect to immunophenotype and environment interaction or mediating effect. Additionally, few studies have examined the role of area of residence in survival, which may play a role in the prognosis as well as survivability, given the contributions of physical and social environment interaction with molecular events, including genomic and epigenomic instabilities. In effect, immunophenotype and environment interaction as a surrogate for epigenomic modulation provide reliable information for future epigenomic investigations of aberrant gene and environment interaction as a function of gene expression in leukomogenesis.

The current study utilized a novel research strategy, namely signal amplification and specific-risk characterization, in survival variability predictions. We aimed to assess cumulative incidence and temporal trends in pediatric ALL, as well as rate and risk stratification by ALL immunophenotype and environment interaction as a conjoint effect, and to determine the immunophenotype and urbanity interaction survival risk difference as a potential explanation of the male and black ALL survival disadvantage.

15.2   Materials and Methods

15.2.1   Data Use and Institutional Review Board (IRB) Approval

This study involved secondary data analysis from the United States National Health Institute (NIH), National Cancer Institute (NCI) and Surveillance Epidemiology and End Results (SEER) dataset (1973–2015). The SEER data are a preexisting and public access database for researchers in population-based cancer projects. The utilization of these data required preapproval from the NCI. In addition, prior to the conduct of this study, an Institutional Review Board (IRB) approval was obtained from the Nemours Healthcare System for Children.

15.2.2   Study Design

The contributory effect of ALL immunophenotype as an explanatory or predictive model in sex on pediatric ALL survival was examined as the main model stipulation in this study. Additionally, we examined temporal trends, namely percent change (PC) and annual percent change (APC), as well as age-adjusted incidence rate and rate ratio by age at tumor diagnosis and sex. A retrospective cohort design was used to assess these aims, despite the potential for exposure or outcome misclassification bias in the proposed design. However, this design is appropriate, given the availability of both the exposure and outcome variable data prior to the study's conduct. In ensuring the internal validity of this study, a signal amplification and specific risk characterization model was employed, which allowed for a critical appraisal of confoundings and effect measure modifiers prior to model building risk and predisposing factors quantification and generalizability.

15.2.3   Data Source

The data from the National Cancer Institute's (NCI) Surveillance, Epidemiology and End Results (SEER) Program were used in this study. The SEER program is a cancer registry operated and managed by the NCI within NIH. The registry began in 1973 with nine SEER areas termed registries. In 1992, the registry expanded to include four additional registries, and in 2005, the registry was further expanded and included five additional registries, rendering the current registry in SEER at 18. In the evolution of the database, the commonly identified registries include 9, 11, 13, 17 and 18. The information collected and stored in the SEER registries includes cancer diagnosis, patient demographics, primary tumor site, tumor morphology and stage at diagnosis, prognostic factors, treatment modalities, follow-up period, vital status as well as some social determinants of health (group-level education, income, area of residence). This registry remains the most comprehensive source of population-based data which includes cancer stage at the time of diagnosis as well as patient survival. The selection of the registries for the SEER program is based on the ability of cancer centers to provide high-quality clinical, laboratory, population-based and other variables to SEER.

15.2.4 Patient Sample and Study Population

The study participants involved cancer cases 0–19 years of age with ALL diagnosed between 1973 and 2015. As a tumor registry, the sample for assessment was consecutive, meaning the evaluation of all pediatric patients with ALL in the registry. This approach renders the process into a probability sample, implying random variables in the assessment of time as a function of survival with respect to ALL immunophenotype. In effect, a random variable implies an evaluation based on an unbiased sample with an equal and known probability of being included in the study, as well as the enhanced ability to generalize the findings beyond the study sample to the targeted population, pediatric ALL.

15.2.5 Sample Size and Power Estimations

This study was based on preexisting data with a sample size of n = 18,720, thus requiring statistical power estimation, which is the ability of the study to detect a minimum difference between independent or paired samples, should such an example truly exist. The power estimation was based on the sample size (n = 18,720), type 1 error tolerance of 5% (0.05) and effect size of 20% (0.20), implying a hazard ratio difference of 20% comparing the immunophenotype as well as urbanity with respect to survival. Using the Cox proportional hazard model in determining the point estimates, namely the hazard ratio (HR), we estimated the power which is the ability to detect the minimum difference (20%) in survival between T- and B-ALL immunophenotypes, and rural compared to metropolitan and urban cases, should such a difference really exist, $1-\beta = 98.2\%$.

15.2.6 Study Variables

The response variable was time as a function of survival, given that the response variable, namely ALL mortality, is not very well understood in time-to-event data modeling. With this characterization, ALL survival or mortality remains a primary outcome variable despite the implication of time as a respondent attribute. Other predictor variables were areas of residence, such as rural, urban and metropolitan, as exposure functions of survival. This variable was transformed into a dichotomous scale, namely rural/urban and metropolitan. The sociodemographic variables assessed included poverty level and education as group-level variables. The race variable, namely black, white, Native American/Alaskan native, Asian/Pacific Islanders and others, as along with sex (male or female), constituted other main independent variables as well as predictors of survival. Additionally, urbanity, sex and race were treated as effect measure modifiers, also broadly termed interaction. The mortality variable captured as vital status in SEER, being the primary outcome affiliated with the survival months, was measured on a binary scale, implying dead (1) or alive (0). The ALL immunophenotype was treated as a categorical variable, while sex was handled as a dichotomous and nominal variable. The race variable was measured on a nominal scale, while the age at tumor diagnosis was measured on a categorical scale, implying 0, 1–4, 5–9, 10–14 and 15–19 age groups. The main independent, explanatory or predictor variable was a construct based on discrete variables combination. Stata fits such a construct: egen urbanity = rowmax (residence area immunophenotype).

15.2.7 *Statistical Analysis*

A pre-analysis screening was performed to identify outliers and missing variables as well as "unknown" and "unavailable" fields in the dataset. To summarize the categorical, nominal, binary or dichotomized variables, we used frequency and percentages. The survival months as a continuous variable were summarized using the median survival. The selection of the median survival was based on the understanding that the mean survival months are not feasible since all events did not occur at the end of the study, which could have rendered the mean survival an inappropriate measure of the summary statistic related to survival time. To examine the relationship between the qualitative or discrete variables in relation to ALL immunophenotype and urbanity, a chi-square statistic was used and Fisher's exact to compensate for the small expected cell count. Further, the chi-square was applicable while assessing the relationship between race and sex with other study variables such as education and income or poverty level as categorical variables. The mortality experience with overall cases, ALL immunophenotypes, urbanity and immunophenotype and urbanity conjoint effects was examined using a binomial regression model for risk prediction.

To examine the survival function for the ALL immunophenotype and urbanity interaction, the Kaplan-Meier survival curve was used. This model examined the overall survival proportion as well as subgroup survival proportions, while the Nelson Aalen cumulative hazard was used to assess the risk of dying among patients with ALL, given immuno-phenotype and urbanity interaction. Similarly, the predictive margins plots were used to illustrate the mortality by urbanity. To test the equality of survival by sex and ALL immunophenotype, the log-rank test was employed.

The examination of survival by immunophenotype and urbanity interaction, the main study hypothesis, was performed using the Cox proportional hazard model, while the Schonfeld global test was used to assess the Cox proportional hazard model assumption, implying that the hazard rate (HR) remains constant over time. To control for confounding in the risk of dying following immunophenotype and urbanity interaction, a multivariable Cox proportional hazard model was built, which allowed for the balancing of the confounding effect of the assessed variables as potential confounders while observing the risk of dying as a result of T-ALL or B-ALL immunophenotype and urbanity interaction. To enter the multivariable model, all potentially confounding variables were assessed for the magnitude of confounding using Cox-Mantel stratification analysis, and any variable with a difference of 10% or higher (>10%) between the crude and adjusted risk ratio was retained in the model.

The type 1 error tolerance for the univariable Cox model was set at 5% (95% CI), while 1% (99% CI) was set for the multivariable model. All tests were two tailed, and the entire analyses were performed using Stata/MP, 15.1 (STATA-Corp, College Station, Texas).

15.3 Results: Study Findings as Epigenomic Surrogate (Urbanicity and Immunophenotype Survival)

15.3.1 ALL Cumulative Incidence (CmI)

The study characteristics stratified by race and acute lymphoblastic leukemia (ALL) immunophenotype are described in Table 15.1. The subpopulations by race reflect white, black/African American (AA), Asian/Pacific Islander and American Indians/Alaska native (AI/AN), as well as others. These subpopulations are illustrated with the immunophenotype, namely T-ALL, B-ALL and other, non-specified (ONS). Although not on the table, B-ALL was less commonly diagnosed in blacks (55.8%) compared to whites (62.0%). In contrast, T-ALL was more diagnosed in blacks (15.8%) relative to whites (7.9%). In addition, the T-ALL diagnosis was intermediate among Asians/Pacific Islander/American Indians (9.8%). Further, ALL otherwise non-specified (ONS) was intermediate among blacks (28.4%), and lowest among Asian/Pacific Islander/American Indian (21.3%), but slightly highest among whites (30.1%). Relative to white females, white males were diagnosed more with T-ALL (26.3% v. 73.7%). Similarly, among blacks, males had a higher cumulative incidence (CmI) of T-ALL relative to females (66.7% versus 33.3%). The age group at ALL diagnosis with the highest CmI of T-ALL among whites was

TABLE 15.1 Study characteristics by race and Acute Lymphoblastic Leukemia (ALL) immunophenotype, SEER (1973–2015)

	White			Black			AI/API/AN			Other		
	B-cell	T-cell	ALL-NOS	B-cell	T-cell	ALL-NOS	B-cell	T-cell	ALL-NOS	B-cell	T-cell	ALL-NOS
	N(%)	N(%)	N(%)	N(%)	N(%)	N(%)	N(%)	N(%)	N(%)	N(%)	N(%)	N(%)
Sex												
Female	4,412(45.1)	329(26.3)	2,073(43.6)	330(43.1)	72(33.3)	198(50.1)	473(45.3)	39(26.3)	137(42.4)	52(43.7)	3(37.5)	19(47.5)
Male	5,362(54.9)	920(73.7)	2,680(56.4)	435(56.9)	144(66.7)	192(49.2)	572(54.7)	109(73.6)	186(57.6)	67(56.3)	5(62.5)	21(52.5)
Age												
<1	262(2.7)	13(1.0)	173(3.6)	34(4.4)	4(1.9)	20(5.1)	41(3.9)	5(3.4)	7(2.2)	4(3.4)	0(0.0)	3(7.5)
1–4 years	4,542(46.5)	249(19.9)	2,222(46.7)	316(41.3)	30(13.9)	157(40.3)	515(49.3)	22(14.9)	163(50.5)	67(56.3)	5(62.5)	15(37.5)
5–9 years	2,362(24.2)	415(33.2)	1,140(24.0)	194(25.4)	62(28.7)	90(23.1)	248(23.7)	43(29.0)	84(26.0)	29(24.4)	2(25.0)	13(32.5)
10–14 years	1,367(14.0)	328(26.3)	710(14.9)	144(18.8)	75(34.7)	70(17.9)	139(13.3)	41(27.7)	42(13.0)	13(10.9)	0(0.00)	5(12.5)
15–19 years	1,241(12.7)	244(19.5)	508(10.7)	77(10.1)	45(20.8)	53(13.6)	102(9.8)	37(25.0)	27(8.4)	6(5.0)	1(12.5)	4(10.0)
Mortality												
Alive	8,415(86.1)	982(78.6)	3,251(68.4)	627(82.0)	152(70.4)	233(59.7)	883(84.5)	113(76.3)	233(72.1)	115(96.6)	8(1000)	33(82.5)
Dead	1,359(13.9)	267(21.4)	1,502(31.6)	138(18.0)	64(29.6)	157(40.3)	162(15.5)	35(23.6)	90(27.9)	4(3.40)	0(0.00)	7(17.5)
Malignancy												
No	41(0.4)	7(0.6)	14(0.3)	6(0.8)	0(0.00)	0(0.00)	9(0.9)	1(0.7)	2(0.6)	0(0.00)	0(0.00)	0(0.00)
Yes	9,733(99.6)	1,242(99.4)	4,739(99.7)	759(99.2)	216(100.0)	390(100.0)	1,036(99.1)	147(99.3)	321(99.4)	119(100.0)	8(100.0)	40(100.0)
Insurance												
Medicaid	2,740(28.1)	233(18.7)	142(3.0)	283(37.2)	62(28.7)	9(2.4)	195(18.7)	25(17.0)	11(3.4)	42(35.3)	4(50.0)	1(2.6)
Uninsured	196(2.0)	14(1.10)	13(0.3)	33(4.30)	7(3.20)	0(0.00)	15(1.400)	0(0.00)	0(0.00)	20(16.8)	1(12.5)	0(0.00)
Private	2,424(24.9)	286(23.0)	129(2.7)	139(18.3)	36(16.7)	9(2.4)	355(34.0)	51(34.7)	9(2.8)	31(26.0)	2(25.0)	2(5.1)
Urbanicity												
Rural	76(.78)	17(1.4)	53(1.1)	5(0.7)	2(0.9)	0(0.0)	1(0.1)	0(0.0)	0(0.00)	0(0.00)	0(0.00)	0(0.00)
Metro	8,951(91.8)	1,120(90.1)	4,143(88.2)	715(94.0)	197(91.2)	373(97.6)	979(93.8)	142(96.6)	373(97.6)	116(97.5)	7(87.5)	38(97.4)
Urban	718(7.4)	106(8.5)	499(10.6)	41(5.4)	17(7.9)	9(2.4)	64(6.1)	5(3.4)	9(2.4)	3(2.5)	1(12.5)	1(2.6)

Abbreviations and Notes: AI/AN/API= American Indian/Alaska native/Asia and Pacific Islanders, ALL-NOS=acute lymphoblastic leukemia –not otherwise specified, implying other ALL. First malignancy refers to first primary malignancy as distinctive from second primary malignancy. Malignancy is indicative of first malignant neoplasm.

5–9 years (33.2%), followed by 10–14 years (23.6%). However, among blacks, the age group with the highest CmI of T-ALL was 10–14 years (34.7%), followed by 5–9 years (28.7%). Invariably within these two racial groups, T-ALL was most diagnosed between 5 and 14 years of age.

15.3.2 Pediatric ALL Urbanity and Immunophenotype Interaction and Sex

There was sex variance in urbanity and immunophenotype interaction. Regarding rural area and immunophenotype interaction, the CmI of T-ALL was higher among males relative to females (0.14% v. 0.05%). With respect to metropolitan and immunophenotype interaction, CmI of B-ALL was higher among females relative to males (60% v. 55.3%), while T-ALL was higher among males compared to females (10.0% versus 5.0%). Concerning urban area and immunophenotype interaction, the CmI of T-ALL was higher among males (0.9%) relative to females (0.4%), $\chi^2(8) = 186.4$, p <0.001. The B-ALL exhibits an improved survival, indicative of survival advantage relative to T-ALL (Figure 15.5). In addition, the Kaplan-Meier (KM) survival curve distinctively demonstrates the survival advantage of B-cell ALL relative to T-cell ALL and ALL-unspecified (Figure 15.5).

15.3.3 ALL Urbanity and Immunophenotype Interaction and Race

There was an association between race and the conjoint effect of tumor immunophenotype and urbanity or interaction. With respect to B-cell and rural/urban areas, the CmI of B-ALL was higher in whites relative to blacks (0.48 versus 0.36), while T-ALL was lower among whites relative to blacks (0.11 versus 0.15). Regarding the metropolitan and immunophenotype interaction, the racial distribution varied, with lower B-ALL cumulative incidence observed in blacks relative to whites (52.4 vs. 57.0), while T-ALL CmI was higher in blacks relative to whites (14.4% vs. 7.1%) and ALL-other (28.0% vs. 26.6%) as well. With respect to urban area and immunophenotype interaction, the CmI for B-ALL was higher among whites relative to blacks (4.6% versus 3.0%), while T-ALL was higher among blacks relative to whites (1.2% versus 0.7%), $\chi^2(16) = 210.9$, p <0.001.

15.3.4 Pediatric ALL Mortality, Race and Age

With respect to race, mortality from pediatric ALL was higher among blacks (26.2%) compared to whites (19.8%), $\chi^2(3) = 52.6$, p <0.001. The CmI was highest among infants (48.2%), intermediate among age groups, 10–14 years (27.5%) and 15–19 years (38.0%), but lowest among age groups, 1–4 years (12.4%) and 5–9 years (16.6%), $\chi^2(4) = 1,200$, p <0.001.

15.3.5   ALL Mortality by Immunophenotype, Race, Health Insurance Coverage, Urbanity

A substantial mortality variance was observed in ALL immunophenotype. Regardless of race or sex, mortality outcome was higher in T-ALL relative to B-ALL. The predictive margins of mortality by immunophenotype of pediatric ALL illustrated an excess mortality of children diagnosed with ALL-non-specified (ALL-NOS). Likewise, relative to B-ALL, there was an excess predicted mortality among children with T-ALL (Figures 15.1 and 15.2). The prediction of ALL mortality by urbanity from the margins plot indicates excess mortality among urban cases with the higher point estimate, in contrast to the Kaplan-Meier survival curve, which illustrates survival advantage with the upper curve (Figure 15.3).

With respect to insurance, black children were covered more by Medicaid relative to whites (26.0% versus 19.9%), while white children had more private insurance relative to blacks (18.1% versus 13.5%). Among whites, children diagnosed with B-ALL received more Medicaid (28.1%) compared to T-ALL (18.7%). Similarly, blacks diagnosed with B-ALL were associated with more Medicaid (37.2%). Relative to blacks diagnosed with B-ALL, private insurance coverage was higher among their white counterparts (18.3% v. 23.0%). Although not in the table, private insurance was associated with 7.2% ALL mortality, while Medicaid or public insurance was associated with 10.8% mortality, implying an estimated 3% increased risk of dying, given public insurance coverage among cases with ALL, $\chi^2(3) = 886.2$, p <0.001.

15.3.6   Urbanity and Tumor Immunophenotype in ALL Mortality

With respect to urbanity and ALL mortality, metropolitan areas were associated with a 1% decreased risk of dying (RR, 0.99, 95% CI, 0.72–1.36), while there was a clinically meaningful 19% increased risk of dying for patients in urban areas relative to rural (RR, 1.19, 95% CI, 0.86–1.65). The cumulative incidence (CmI) of pediatric ALL mortality was lowest among children diagnosed with B-cell immunophenotype (14.2%), intermediate among T-cell immunophenotype (22.6%) and highest among ALL-other, implying ALL, non-specific (31.9%), $\chi^2(2) = 735.7$, p <0.001.

In a predictive model without time as a function of survival, implying the CmI of dying relative to B-ALL immunophenotype, there was a significant 59% increased risk of dying among children with T-ALL (risk ratio (RR) = 1.59, 95% CI, 1.44–1.76). The error bars illustrate margin plots of the predicted risk of dying following pediatric ALL diagnosis. Without an overlap in the confidence limits, comparing the ALL immunophenotype, there is a significant risk of dying, given T-ALL diagnosis relative to B-ALL. Cases with ALL, otherwise, non-specified (ALL-other) were more than twice as likely to die compared to B-ALL cases (RR = 2.24, 95% CI, 2.12–2.38). There was a racial variation in CmI mortality, with blacks relative to whites observed with a significant 32% excess risk (RR = 1.32, 95% CI, 1.20–1.45).

15.3.7 Urbanity and Tumor Immunophenotype Interaction or Conjoint Effect

This section compares ALL period prevalence by metropolitan and urban areas. There were percentage variance by race and immunophenotype. With respect to B-ALL and metropolitan area, there were less blacks relative to whites (52.4% versus 57%), while in contrast there were more blacks with ALL-other residing in the metropolitan area (14.4% versus 7.1%). Relative to whites, more blacks were diagnosed with T-ALL (28% versus 28%), $\chi^2(10)$ = 203.5, p <0.001. While females were more diagnosed with B-cell in the metropolitan area relative to males (60% versus 55%), males were more diagnosed with ALL-other (10% versus 5%), $\chi^2(5)$ = 186.1, p <0.001.

15.3.8 Mortality and Survival Difference by Urbanity and Immunophenotype

This section demonstrates the crude and unadjusted predictors of pediatric ALL mortality. There were significant associations between urbanity, immunophenotype, race and sex, and ALL mortality (Table 15.2). Relative to metropolitan areas, cases residing in urban areas were significantly 19% more likely to die (RR, 1.19, 95% CI, 1.08–1.30). In addition, compared to B-ALL, T-ALL and ALL-Other were 59% (RR, 1.59, 95% CI, 1.44–1.76) more likely to die, while ALL-other were three times as likely to die (RR = 2.24, 95% CI, 2.12–2.38).

The predictors of survival, namely tumor immunophenotype, urbanity, race, sex and urban-immunophenotype interaction, are demonstrated in this section. Survival disadvantage was associated with T-ALL, ALL-other, urban areas, blacks, males and urban areas-immunophenotype interaction. Compared to B-ALL, T-ALL and ALL-other were 54% (HR = 1.54, 95% CI, 1.37–1.74) and 81% more likely to die (HR = 1.81, 95% CI, 1.69–1.95), and compared to whites, blacks were 42% more likely to die (HR = 1.42, 95% CI, 1.27–1.58). Also, relative to females, males were 30% more likely to die (HR = 1.30, 95% CI, 1.21–1.39). The interaction or conjoint effect of immunophenotype and urbanity indicated a dose-response risk of dying for metropolitan-B-ALL to rural/urban area-ALL other. Compared to B-ALL cases in metropolitan areas, cases in T-ALL-metropolitan, ALL-other-metropolitan, B-ALL-rural/urban area, T-ALL-rural/urban area and ALL-other-rural/urban area were 5%, 54% (HR = 1.54, 95% CI, 1.36–1.75), 62%, 79% (HR = 1.79, 95% CI, 1.66–1.92) and two times as likely to die (HR = 2.06, 95% CI, 1.78–2.39) respectively.

TABLE 15.2 Univariable Model of Pediatric ALL Survival by Immunophenotype, SEER (1973–2015).

Variable	B-ALL			T-ALL			ALL-Unspecified		
	HR	95%CI	p	HR	95%CI	p	HR	95%CI	p
Race									
White	1.0	referent	referent	1.0	referent	referent	1.00	referent	referent
Black	1.36	1.13–1.62	0.001	1.57	1.08–2.08	0.0002	1.39	1.17–1.65	0.0001
AI/AN/API	1.12	0.95–1.33	0.182	1.14	0.78–1.66	0.501	0.87	0.70–1.08	0.22
Other	0.33	0.13–.89	0.028	–	–	–	0.51	0.23–1.13	0.097
Sex									
Female	1.00	referent	referent	1.00	referent	referent	1.00	referent	referent
Male	1.28	1.16–1.42	0.0001	1.03	0.81–1.32	0.804	1.33	1.21–1.47	0.0001
Age									
<1	1.00	referent	referent	1.00	referent	referent	1.00	referent	referent
1–4 years	0.11	0.09–0.14	0.0001	0.39	0.20–0.76	0.006	0.25	0.20–0.30	0.0001
5–9 years	0.18	0.15–0.22	0.0001	0.27	0.14–0.52	0.0001	0.34	0.28–0.42	0.0001
10–14 years	0.28	0.31–0.46	0.0001	0.39	0.20–0.75	0.005	0.58	0.45–0.70	0.0001

(Continued)

TABLE 15.2 (Continued)

	B-ALL			T-ALL			ALL-Unspecified		
15–19 years	0.65	0.54–0.79	0.0001	0.48	0.25–0.92	0.028	0.86	0.69–1.08	0.196
Insurance									
Medicaid	1.00	referent	referent	1.00	referent	referent	1.00	referent	referent
Uninsured	2.76	0.81–1.73	0.38	1.18	0.81–1.73	0.38	2.29	0.69–7.62	0.175
Private	3.79	0.54–0.79	0.001	0.66	0.54–0.79	0.0001	0.74	0.39–1.39	0.347
First Malignancy									
No	1.00	referent	referent	1.00	referent	referent	1.00	referent	referent
Yes	0.37	0.22–0.60	0.0001	0.71	0.18–2.86	0.632	0.35	0.19–0.64	0.001
Urbanicity									
Rural	1.00	referent	referent	1.00	referent	referent	1.00	referent	referent
Metro	1.10	0.57–2.12	0.774	4.5	0.63–32.0	0.133	0.88	0.55–1.40	0.583
Urban	1.17	0.59–2.31	0.649	5.4	0.73–39.6	0.097	1.00	0.62–1.60	0.977

Notes and abbreviations: The significance level, type I error tolerance was set at 5% (95% Confidence interval (CI)). HR=Hazard ratio as the measure of effect or point estimate in survival modeling. AI/AN/API, American Indian/Alaska native/Asia and Pacific Islanders. *p* = probability value for random error quantification as type I error tolerance.

15.3.9   Multi-Variable and Multilevel Modeling

This section demonstrates the multivariable modeling of the conjoint exposure of urbanity and immunophenotype (Table 15.3). After controlling for sex, race, tumor grade, age, education and tumor primaries, survival disadvantage was associated with T-ALL, ALL-other, urban areas, blacks, males and urban areas-immunophenotype interaction. Compared to metropolitan area (MeT)-B-ALL, MeT-T-ALL and MeT-ALL-other were 4% (adjusted HR (aHR) = 1.04, 99% CI, 0.87–1.26)) and 15% (aHR = 1.15, 99% CI, 1.01–1.31) more likely to die respectively. In addition, relative to MeT-B-ALL, there was a 23% increased risk of dying in rural/urban-B-ALL (aHR = 1.23, 99% CI, 0.86–1.76) and an 82% increased mortality risk in rural/urban-T-ALL (aHR = 1.82, 99% CI, 1.85–2.49), while the risk of dying was twice as likely in rural/urban-ALL-other (aHR = 2.14, 99% CI, 1.85–2.49). The survival disadvantage of

TABLE 15.3 Multi-variable modeling of the exposure function of tumor immunophenotype in racial differences in pediatric ALL survival, SEER (1973–2015).

Models and Variables	Race			
	Black		Others	
	aHR	99% CI	aHR	99% CI
T-ALL				
Model I				
Race	1.54	1.10–2.30	1.03	0.63–1.71
Model II				
Model I + age, education, insurance	1.60	1.11–2.33	1.13	0.68–1.87
Model III				
Model II + income	1.61	1.10–2.36	1.12	0.68–1.86
Model IV				
Model III + urbanicity	1.61	1.10–2.39	1.13	0.68–2.39
B-ALL				
Model I				
Race	1.32	1.05–1.67	1.11	0.89–1.38
Model II				
Model I +age, education	1.30	1.03–1.66	1.17	0.94–1.46
Model III				
Model II + income	1.30	1.03–1.66	1.17	0.94–1.47
Model IV				
Model III + urbanicity	1.30	1.03–1.66	1.17	0.94–1.47

Abbreviations and notes: CI, confidence interval; aHR, adjusted hazard ratio. Type I error tolerance was set at 1% (99% CI) for models II–IV, while the type I error tolerance for model I was set at 5% (95% CI). p = probability value for random error quantification as type I error tolerance.

blacks and males persisted despite controlling for tumor prognostic factors and sociodemographic and social determinants of health. Relative to whites, there was a significant 35% increased risk of dying (aHR = 1.35, 99% CI, 1.16–1.47). Similarly, compared to females, males were 24% more likely to die (aHR = 1.24, 99% CI, 1.14–1.36).

15.4 Discussion

Albeit the dramatic improvement in pediatric ALL survival in the United States and elsewhere, some subpopulations continue to experience survival disadvantages, namely blacks and male patients. The observed subpopulation variances remain to be explained for pediatric ALL optimal care transformation. This study was proposed to examine the conjoint effect of tumor immunophenotype and urbanity on pediatric acute lymphoblastic leukemia (ALL) survival and to assess whether or not the persistently observed survival disadvantage of male and black children with ALL is explained in part by this interaction. To assess these variabilities and rationale, we utilized a retrospective cohort design of prospectively collected data on tumor diagnosis, prognostic factors, sociodemographics and social determinants of health. Using percent change, annual percent change and the Cox proportional hazard model, we examined the cumulative incidence, incidence trends and survival. Additionally, we determined the prognostic factors in survival variability by urbanity and ALL immunophenotype interaction. There are a few relevant findings from these population-based data on a representative sample of US children with ALL. First, incidence trends continued to increase in pediatric ALL from 1973 through 2015, and were higher among blacks relative to whites despite a higher cumulative incidence among whites. Second, the ALL incidence was higher among males relative to females, as were the increased T-ALL and ALL-NOS cases among male children compared to females. Third, survival was poorer among blacks and males relative to whites and females. Fourth, T-ALL illustrated poorer survival relative to B-ALL, regardless of sex or race. Further, the survival disadvantage of blacks and male children is explained in part by immunophenotype and urbanity interaction, indicative of survival disadvantage of children with ALL in rural/urban areas.

This retrospective cohort assessment of more than four decades of pediatric ALL data clearly demonstrated increased cumulative incidence (CmI) among males and whites relative to female and blacks, despite higher annual percent change among blacks. The observed excess incidence of pediatric ALL among whites and males has been shown previously [12–15]. The increase in the cumulative incidence of pediatric ALL among whites is not fully understood, but may be due to improvements in diagnostics or changes in tumor nosology as well as differential DNA methylation of candidate genes in pediatric ALL. Overall, while survival in pediatric ALL has dramatically improved, incidence continues to rise [12, 17] regardless of subpopulations characteristic with ALL. Additionally, the observed increase in cumulative incidence of pediatric ALL among whites may be explained by black children being underdiagnosed due to limited access to cancer treatment and preventive services, as well as differences in exposure to potential carcinogens [18, 19] and aberrant epigenomic modulations. Understanding the epigenomic modulations and the mechanistic processes in the gene and environment interaction in leukemic genes may facilitate specific risk characterization and induction therapy with demethylase building blocks prior to primary therapies in the treatment of pediatric ALL, thus narrowing subpopulation risk differences in ALL mortality [20, 21].

Available data on relapsed and remission T-ALL DNA methylation (mDNA) and mRNA sequencing correlation and the stratification of such aberrant epigenomic modulation of the candidate genes involved in leukemic transformation (STAT5, MLL11, RB1, PTEN, IL-7R, KRAS, TLX1, TLX3, NKX2-1, LYL1, IL-7R, JAK1, JAK3, etc.) by sex and race will provide a further and more comprehensive explanation of the observed sex and racial disparities in ALL survival.[23–25] Basically, as observed earlier, epigenomic modulation reflects the gene and environment interaction involving the CpG island at the enhancer-promoter gene region, but does not involve DNA sequence (mutational alteration in the underling DNA) [26–28]. Normal hematopoietic cell development, differentiation and maturation require tightly controlled regulation of DNA methylation, histone modification and non-coding RNA expression: mDNA $\rightarrow$ epigenomic modulation $\rightarrow$ (1) gene expression, (2) genomic stability maintenance and (3) cellular differentiation [28]. The detection of aberrant modulation requires systematic analysis of DNA methylation and histone protein modifications such as acetylation and the correlated gene expression via mRNA sequencing [22, 28]. Such initiatives will lead to specific risk characterization, induction therapy through demethylases, transcription factors or protein accessibility, gene expression or upregulation, implying enhanced treatment response. Subsequently, given the restricted explanatory model of T-ALL in male-female and black-white differences in pediatric ALL survival, an urgent epigenomic investigation of ALL, B-other, ALL-NOS and T-ALL relapse cases is required, which will involve candidate signaling pathway genes such as NOTCH1 and cell cycle regulator genes (CDKN2A (p16) and CDKN2B (p15)), bisulfite pyrosequencing and mRNA sequencing for mDNA and inverse gene expression correlation via next-generation sequencing (NGS). Therefore, to provide further explanation in the observed survival disadvantage of male and black children with ALL, the DNA methylation analysis implying the detection of epigenetic marks will require subpopulation samples, namely sex, race and urbanity [22, 23].

Cancer epigenetics/epigenomic research is in an exciting phase of translational epigenomics, where novel epigenome therapeutics such as induction therapy are being developed for application in clinical settings [22, 25, 28]. A range of different epigenetic "marks" or "signatures" can activate or repress gene expression. While aberrant epigenomic alterations are associated with most clinical conditions, epigenetic dysregulation has a substantial and significant causal role in ALL etiologies, prognoses, relapses and survival. Specifically, epigenetically disrupted stem or progenitor cells have an early role in neoplastic transformations, while lesions or aberrations of epigenetic regulatory mechanisms controlling gene expression in cancer remain a contributing factor in ALL prognosis and mortality. The reversibility of epigenetic marks provides the possibility that the activity of key cancer genes and pathways can be regulated as a therapeutic approach. The growing availability of a range of chemical agents which can affect epigenome functioning will lead to a range of epigenetic-therapeutic approaches for cancer and intense interest in the development of second-generation epigenetic drugs such as demethylase agents as induction therapy. Such initiatives will imply greater specificity and efficacy in clinical settings, thus enhancing precision medicine initiatives and optimizing care across all subpopulations of children with ALL, especially blacks and males. In effect, subpopulation differences in these lesions or aberrations remain a possibility, rendering pediatric ALL sex and racial disparities in survival a history.

Aberrant or differential DNA methylation (mDNA) has been observed in malignant neoplasms as implicated in tumor suppressor gene [29], cardiovascular diseases [30] and preterm birth [31]. The increase in the observed aberrant epigenomic modulations among blacks/African Americans (AA) implies a relatively excess psychosocial stress [32, 33] and adverse environmental factors such as air pollutants [34] experienced by this subpopulation in the United States. Available epidemiologic and population-based data have implicated psychosocial stress and air pollutants in breast cancer, hypertension and preterm births, with these conditions more likely to be diagnosed among blacks/AA [35–39]. Specifically, dense mDNA of exon F1 in the CpG regions of the glucocorticoid receptor gene (NR3C1) has been observed in early life stress, early adversity and major depressive episodes [28, 40].

Despite the strength of this study and its novelty in identifying ALL immunophenotype with respect to survival variability between males and female children, blacks and whites, as well as immunophenotype and urbanity interaction, there are some limitations. First, the current study was based on preexisting data, which, despite its source (NCI, SEER), may be predisposed to selection, information and misclassification biases. However, the inherent misclassification bias may be non-differential, thus minimizing the potential for biased estimates of the effect of ALL immunophenotype on male-female risk differences as well as immunophenotype and urbanity interactions in ALL survival.

Second, these findings may be limited due to the inability to assess treatment data, such as radiation, chemotherapy and bone marrow transplant. The SEER dataset requires this treatment information as a prognostic factor in assessing survivability in malignancies. The NCI's inability to provide these essential and necessary data renders population-based cancer studies in the United States less reliable in treatment assessment and subsequent therapeutic mapping for cancer care improvement. Third, these findings may be limited, or restricted by unmeasured and residual confoundings. However, it is highly unlikely that the findings of survival disadvantage with T-ALL, ALL-other immunophenotype, blacks, urban areas and males are driven solely by unmeasured as well as residual confoundings, since no matter how sophisticated a statistical software used in controlling for confounding, residual confounding persists [41].

15.5   Conclusion as Inference

In summary, pediatric ALL incidence trends continue to increase, with higher cumulative incidence among males and whites as well as a survival disadvantage for male and black children in a representative sample of US pediatric ALL. The T-ALL immunophenotype predicts the survival disadvantage of male and black children with ALL. Further, the conjoint effect of urbanity and immunophenotype demonstrated the survival disadvantage of children in rural/urban areas relative to metropolitan areas, indicative of environmental interactions. Aberrant DNA methylation of the CpG islands of the candidate genes in ALL results in gene silencing, adversely impacting cell signaling, transcription, cell cycle, apoptosis and cell adhesion. These findings are suggestive of the need to assess epigenomic programming and mechanistic processes associated with T-ALL, B-other and ALL-NOS gene and environment interactions and the correlated gene expression in order to specifically characterize risk and initiate induction therapy, as well as minimize T-ALL relapse and subsequent male-female and black-white disparities gap narrowing in pediatric ALL survival.

15.6   Questions for Review

1 Describe ALL with respect to the risk and predisposing factors in incidence or development.
2 What is epigenomic surrogate study?
3 Discuss the data acquisition and application in this study.
4 Examine the statistical analysis utilized in this study and identify, if applicable, the disadvantages and limitations in this modeling.
5 Discuss the study's limitations and provide a recommendation for research improvement.

References

1 Siegel RL, Miller KD, Jemal A. Cancer statistics, 2018. *CA Cancer J. Clin.* 2018; 68(1):7–30. [PubMed Abstract]

2 Noone AM, Howlader N, Krapcho M et al. (eds). SEER Cancer Statistics Review, 1975–2015, National Cancer Institute. Bethesda, MD, https://seer.cancer.gov/ csr/1975_2015/, based on November 2017 SEER data submission, posted to the SEER web site, April 2018.

3 Jemal A, Ward EM, Johnson CJ et al. Annual report to the nation on the status of cancer, 1975–2014, featuring survival. *J. Natl. Cancer Inst.* 2017;109(9):djx030. [PubMed Abstract]

4 American Cancer Society (ACS). Childhood Leukemia Survival Rates. Available at: https://www.cancer.org/cancer/leukemia-in-children/detection-diagnosis-staging/survival-rates.html [Accessed 7 Feb. 2018].

5 Williger T, Abdul-Hay M. Acute lymphoblastic leukemia: a comprehensive review and 2017 update. *Blood Cancer J.* 2017;7(6):e577. Published online 2017 Jun 30. doi: 10.1038/bcj.2017.53.

6 Graux C, Cools J, Michaux L, Vandenberghe P, Hagemeijer A. Cytogenetics and molecular genetics of T-cell acute lymphoblastic leukemia: From thymocyte to lymphoblast. *Leukemia.* 2006;20;1496–1510.

7 Girardi T, Vicente C, Cools J, De Keersmaecker K. The genetics and molecular biology of T-ALL. *Blood.* 2017;129(9):1113–1123.

8 Iacobucci I, Mulligan CG. Genetic basis of acute lymphoblastic leukemia. *J. Clin. Oncol.* 2017;35(9):975–983.

9 Karrman K, Johansson B. Pediatric T-cell acute lymphoblastic leukemia. *Genes Chromosomes Cancer.* 2017;56(2):89–116.

10 Mohsen M, Uludag H, Brandwein JM. Advances in biology of acute lymphoblastic leukemia (ALL) and therapeutic implications. *Am. J. Blood Res.* 2018;8(4): 29–56. Published online 2018 Dec 10.

11 Muñoz-Fontela C, Mandinova A, Aaronson SA, Lee SW. Emerging roles of p53 and other tumour-suppressor genes in immune regulation. *Nat. Rev. Immunol.* 2016;16(12):741–750.

12 Holmes L Jr, Hossain J, Desvignes-Kendrick M et al. Sex variability in pediatric leukemia survival: Large cohort evidence. *ISRN Oncol.* 2012;2012:439070. doi: 10.5402/2012/439070. Epub 2012 Apr 3.

13 Hunger SP, Mulligan CG. Acute lymphoblastic leukemia in children. *N. Engl. J. Med.* 2015;373(16):1541–1552.

14 Bhatia S. Disparities in cancer outcomes: lessons learned from children with cancer. *Pediatr. Blood Cancer.* 2011;56:994–1002.

15 Barrington-Trimis JL, Cockburn M, Metayer C, Gauderman WJ, Wiemels J, McKean-Cowdin R. Trends in childhood leukemia incidence over two decades from 1992 to 2013. *Int. J. Cancer.* 2016;140(5):1000–1008.

16 Dama E, Pastore G, Mosso ML, Maule MM, Zuccolo L, Magnani C et al. Time trends and prognostic factors for survival from childhood cancer: A report from the childhood cancer registry of piedmont (Italy). *Eur. J. Pediatr.* 2006;165:240–249.

17 National Cancer Institute. Cancer in Children and Adolescents. [online] NCI. Available at: https://www.cancer.gov/types/childhood-cancers/child-adolescent-cancers-fact-sheet [Accessed 15 Sept. 2018].

18 Fitzgerald JC, Li Y, Fisher BT, et al. Hospital variation in intensive care resource utilization and mortality in newly diagnosed pediatric leukemia. *Pediatr. Crit. Care Med.* 2018;19:e312–e320.

19 Jung J, Park K, Kim S, Kim J. Synergistic therapeutic effect of diethylstilbestrol and CX-4945 in human acute T-lymphocytic leukemia cells. *Biomed. Pharmacother.* 2018;98: 357–363.

20 Ward, E., DeSantis, C., Robbins, A., Kohler, B. and Jemal, A. (2014). Childhood and adolescent cancer statistics, 2014. [online] Wiley Online Library. Available at: https://onlinelibrary.wiley.com/doi/abs/10.3322/caac.21219 [Accessed 29 Jun. 2018].

21 Snodgrass R, Nguyen L, Guo M, Vaska M, Naugler C, Rashid-Kolvear F. Incidence of acute lymphocytic leukemia in Calgary, Alberta, Canada: a retrospective cohort study. *BMC Res. Notes.* 2018;11:104.

22 Holmes L, Chavan P, Blake T, Dabney K. Unequal cumulative incidence and mortality outcome in childhood brain and central nervous system malignancy in the USA. *J. Racial Ethn. Health Disparities.* 2018;5(5):1131–1141.

23 Kehm, RD, Spector LG, Poynter, JN, Vock DM, Altekruse SF, Osypuk TL. Does socioeconomic status account for racial and ethnic disparities in childhood cancer survival? *Cancer.* 2018;124(20):4090–4097. doi: 10.1002/cncr.31560.

24 Holmes L, Jr., Opara F, Desvignes-Kendrick M, Hossain J. Age variance in the survival of united states pediatric leukemia patients (1973–2006). *ISRN Public Health.* 2012; Article ID 721329.

25 Feller A, Schmidlin K, Bordoni A, Bouchardy C, Bulliard J, Camey B et al. Socioeconomic and demographic disparities in breast cancer stage at presentation and survival: A Swiss population-based study. *Int. J.Cancer.* 2017;141:1529–1539.

26 Goggins WB, Lo FF. Racial and ethnic disparities in survival of US children with acute lymphoblastic leukemia: evidence from the SEER database 1988–2008. *Cancer Causes Control.* 2012;23(5):737–743.

27 MacLennan I. Autoimmunity: Deletion of autoreactive B cells. *Curr. Biol.* 1995;5(2):103–106.

28 Holmes L Jr, Shutman E, Chinaka C, Deepika K, Pelaez L, Dabney KW. Aberrant epigenomic modulation of glucocorticoid receptor gene (NR3C1) in early life stress and major depressive disorder correlation: Systematic review and quantitative evidence synthesis. *Int. J. Environ. Res. Public Health.* 2019;16(21). pii: E4280. doi: 10.3390/ijerph16214280.

29 Wang S, Dorsey TH, Terunuma A, et al. Relationship between tumor DNA methylation status and patient characteristics in African Americans and European American women with breast cancer. *PLoS One.* 2012;7(5):e37928.

30 Zhong J, Colicino E, Lin X, et al. Cardiac autonomic dysfunction: particular air pollution effects are modulated by epigenetic immunoregulation of Toll-like receptor 2 and dietary flavonoid intake. *J. Am Heart Assoc.* 2015;4(1):e001423.

31 Shroeder JW, Conneely KN, Cubells JC, et al.Neonatal DNA methylation patterns associated with gestational age. *Epigenetics.* 2011;6(12):1498–1504.

32 Turner RJ, Avison WR. Status variations in stress exposure: implications for the interpretation of research on race, socioeconomic status, and gender. *J. Health Soc. Behav.* 2003;44(4):488–505.

33 Hatch SL, Dohrenwend BP. Distribution of traumatic and other stressful life events by race/ethnicity, gender, SES and age: a review of the research. *Am. J. Community Psychol.* 2007;40(3–4):313–332.

34 Pratt GC, Vadali ML, Kvale DL, Ellickson KM. Traffic, air pollution, minority and socio-economic status: addressing inequities in exposure and risk. *Int. J. Environ. Res. Public Health.* 2015;12:5355–5372.

35 Wang C, Chen R, Cai J, et al. Personal exposure to fine particulate matter and blood pressure: A role of angiotensin converting enzyme and its DNA methylation. *Environ Int.* 2016;94:661–666.

36 Parikh PV, Wei Y. PAHs and PM 2.5 emissions and female breast cancer incidence in metro Atlanta and rural Georgia. *Int. J. Environ. Health Res.* 2016;3123:1–9.

37 Ritz B, Yu F, Chapa G, Fruin S. Effect of Air pollution on preterm birth among children born in Southern California between. *Epidemiology.* 2000;11(5):502–511.

38 Steptoe A, Kivimäki M, Lowe G, Rumley A, Hamer M. Blood pressure and fibrinogen responses to mental stress as predictors of incident hypertension over an 8-year period. *Ann. Behav. Med.* 2016;50(6):898–906.

39 Williams DR, Mohammed SA, Shields AE. Understanding and effectively addressing breast cancer in African American women: Unpacking the social context. *Cancer.* 2016;122(14):2138–2149.

40 Palma-Gudiel H, Córdova-Palomera A, Eixarch E, Deuschle M, Fañanás L. Maternal psychosocial stress during pregnancy alters the epigenetic signature of the glucocorticoid receptor gene promoter in their offspring: A meta-analysis. *Epigenetics.* 2015;10(10):893–902.

41 Holmes L, Chan W, Ziang Z, Du XL. Effectiveness of androgen deprivation therapy in prolonging survival of older men treated with locoregional prostate cancer. *Prostate Cancer Prostatic Dis.* 2007;10:388–395.

16

CARDIOVASCULAR DISEASE (CVD)

DNA Methylation of Candidate Genes (ACE II, IFN-γ, AGTR1, CKG, ADD1, SCNN1B and TLR2) in Essential Hypertension

16.1 Introduction

Hypertension, which reflects elevated systolic and diastolic blood pressure, has been physiologically linked to elevated cardiac output, implying stroke volume, heart rate and increased peripheral resistance, which is an obstacle to blood flow. Epidemiologic and animal studies have illustrated the role of a sedentary lifestyle, a high-fat diet and sodium intake in predisposition to vascular constriction and volume loading. Additionally, available translational epidemiologic data have implicated race in the complex and multifactorial etiologic pathway of essential hypertension, with blacks/African Americans (AA) being disproportionally affected [1]. For example, a diet rich in the methyl group (CH3) such as processed red meat or stress as an environmental stimulus results in elevated blood pressure via epigenomic mechanistic processes such as DNA methylation, histone acetylation, DNA hydroxymethylation and DNA phosphorylation. Stress or social adversity induction in animal and human models has been shown to result in changes in the catecholamine pathway, implying the enzymatic regulation of blood pressure involving factors such as tyrosine hydroxylase and dopamine decarboxylase, which are associated with no epinephrine and epinephrine elaboration vasoconstriction. Specifically, the DNA methylation of the promoter region of candidate genes involved in hemostasis and hemodynamics due to social stress, physical inactivity or diet results in the inhibition of the gene transcription factor, impaired gene expression and abnormal protein synthesis, leading to disease development. For example, vasoconstriction occurs as a result of the conversion of angiotensin I to angiotensin II, a potent vasoconstrictor, due to the elaboration of the angiotensin I converting enzyme (ACE I) [2]. Specifically, the upregulation

DOI: 10.4324/9781003094487-19

of the ACE II gene, due to the aberrant DNA methylation process, results in vasoconstriction, increased peripheral resistance and hypertension (HTN).

Social signal transduction due to isolation, a social stressor or discrimination reflects the fight or flight notion of the sympathetic nervous system (SNS) by the elaboration of norepinephrine and the beta adrenergic receptor activation, explicit in essential or primary HTN [3]. Adverse social environments such as racial discrimination, unstable social status and psychosocial stressors serve as triggers of neural and endocrine activities, influencing the cellular response system and therefore resulting in the activation of the intracellular signal transduction pathways and the subsequent repression or activation of transcription factors that are involved in the transcription of the gene-bearing response element (GBRE).

The DNA methylation mechanism of several candidate genes involved in this quantitative evidence synthesis (QES) requires studies that have observed epigenomic signatures associated with the transcription factor inhibition at the 5 prime cytosine residue of the cytosine-phosphate-guanine (CpG) gene promoter region, resulting in the development of 5-methyl-cytosine (5mC) [4], implying DNA silencing without alternation in the DNA sequence. This process requires the excessive elaboration and availability of the DNA methyltransferase that accelerates the process of methylation by recruiting the methyl group (CH3) from the S-adenosyl methionine (SAM) to the CpG island and shores on DNA. Additionally, the transcription factor inhibition influences the gene that codes for the RNA polymerase involved in mRNA translation and subsequent gene expression and protein synthesis [5]. In general, DNA methylation involving 5mC correlates with gene repression or downregulation at the enhancer or promoter region.

The pathophysiology of hypertension reflects the cardiac output, implying stroke volume and heart rate (myocardium contractility) as well as peripheral resistance, which infers that the obstacle to the flow of blood, the specific candidate genes in these pathways and their influence on the hypertension mechanistic process were examined and incorporated into the QES. In examining the peripheral resistance and its contribution to hypertension, the ACE II gene was assessed for hypermethylation. The function of this gene is to facilitate the conversion of angiotensin I to angiotensin II, which is a vasoconstrictor, inducing hypertension. Specifically, the DNA methylation of this gene, which implies impaired or inhibited transcription factors at the promoter region of the gene, resulted in gene repression and angiotensin-converting enzyme upregulation.

The TLR2 (CD282, TIL4) identified as a toll-like receptor 2 gene encodes for the toll-like receptor (TLR) which is involved in pathogen recognition and innate and non-adaptive immune response activation. The TLRs activation by the pathogen-associated molecular patterns (PAMPs) results in the upregulation of signaling pathways that modulate a host's inflammatory response [5]. Simply, the TLR2 plays a role in the inflammatory response, facilitating the immune system's ability to recognize and respond to a pathogenic microbe or antigen. The epigenomic mechanistic process in TLR2 methylation involves the binding of the 5-cytosine at the promoter or enhancer region of the gene with the methyl group (CH3) due to the facilitating effect of the DNA methyltransferase and the subsequent inhibition of the transcription factor required for the gene product through gene expression and subsequent impaired protein synthesis (inappropriate mRNA translation). The observed DNA methylation affects an individual's response to stress, associated with an inflammatory response. Specifically, the methylation of TLR2 may result in the up- or downregulation of the gene product, implying an abnormal inflammatory response and the subsequent accumulation of pharmacologic mediators of inflammation, resulting in arteriosclerosis, arterial stenosis, plaque formation and occlusion of blood flow (peripheral resistance). The cardiac compensation to peripheral resistance reflects increased cardiac contractility and the subsequent elevation of the cardiac output, leading to hypertension.

Interferon gamma (IFN-γ) is a cell signal associated with increased elaboration, giving viral infections an innate antiviral response. The insult to tissue or microbe colonization that results in antigenicity may provoke IFN-γ release and subsequent pharmacologic mediators of inflammation. The hypomethylation of this gene is indicative of the inhibition of this responses and the subsequent accumulation of the mediators of inflammation that could be caused by a stressful environment resulting in hypertension.

The AGTR1 gene (angiotensin II receptor, type 1) encodes for the angiotensin II receptor (AT1 receptor). The AT1 receptor is a protein involved in the renin-angiotensin system that regulates blood pressure (BP), fluid and salt balance [6]. Specifically, this receptor acts as a vasopressor and regulates aldosterone secretion. This receptor binds with angiotensin II, stimulating chemical signals that result in vascular constriction and HTN. In addition, this binding results in aldosterone production, hence the increased renal absorption of salt and water with increased extracellular fluid, resulting in BP elevation. The hypomethylation of the angiotensin II receptor has been assessed to predict hypertension. This protein molecule plays a role in binding with angiotensin II and subsequent cellular functions, namely vasoconstriction. The hypomethylation of AGTR1 implies the lower availability of the methyl group at the CpG island with increasing 5-cytosine, resulting in transcription factor activation and subsequent gene expression due to the decreased availability of DNA methyltransferase. The consequence of this gene expression leads to the upregulation of the receptor and the availability of the angiotensin-converting enzyme II binding, resulting in vasoconstriction.

The ACE gene—angiotensin-I-converting enzyme—encodes for angiotensin-converting enzyme, which regulates BP and NaCl as well as H_2O balance [7]. This enzyme cleaves Angiotensin I to Angiotensin II, a potent vasoconstrictor, elevating the BP. The ACE cleaves bradykinnin, a vasodilator, thus inactivating this molecule or protein and elevating the BP and hence the essential HTN. The protein encoded by this gene belongs to the angiotensin-converting enzyme family of dipeptidyl carboxydipeptidases and has considerable homology to the human angiotensin-1-converting enzyme. This secreted protein catalyzes the cleavage of angiotensin I into angiotensin II. The organ- and cell-specific expression of this gene suggests that it may play a role in the regulation of cardiovascular and renal function, as well as reproductive processes.

Other candidate genes involved in HTN include: (a) SCNN1A (sodium channel epithelial 1 alpha subunit) gene, which encodes for the epithelial sodium channel (ENaC) complex. The ENaC transports sodium into cells, and a decreased ENaC may result in excess volume or fluid in some organs. The mutation (deletion, restriction shortening) in this gene had been observed in psuedohypoaldesterionism type 1 (PHA1), characterized by hyponatremia (low Na level), hyperkalemia (high K level) and severe dehydration. SCNN1B is the same as the alpha unit with impairment in this beta unit associated with sodium channel disruption and fluid balance as well as impaired Na reabsorption-hyponatremia. (b) The TIMP3 gene (22q12.3) encodes matrix metalloproteinases inhibitor proteins which are peptidases involved in degeneration of the extracellular matrix. TIMP3 expression results from mitogenic stimulation while its mutation has been observed in autosomal dominant disorders, namely Sorsby's fundus dystrophy. (c) GKG, the glucokinase gene, encodes a number of hexokinase family proteins. This gene encodes hexokinase phosporylate glucose to produce glucose-6-phosphate. CKG functions by providing G6P for the synthesis of glycogen. CKG mutation resulting in an alteration in enzyme activity is associated with diabetes and hyperinsulinemic hypoglycemia. (d) The Adducin1 (ADD1) gene encodes cytoskeletal proteins. These proteins are encoded by three genes, namely alpha, beta and gamma, and they bind with high affinity to Ca (2+)/Calmodulin [8]. (e) The Keratin 13 (KRT 13) gene (17q21.2) encodes the production of keratin protein-fibrous proteins that form the structural framework of epithelial cells. The KRT13 gene partners with the Keratin 14 (KRT4) gene (17q21.2) to form intermediate filaments, which function by protecting the mucosa from being damaged by friction or everyday physical stress [9]. The CAPG gene (2p11.2) encodes a member of the gelosin/villin family of actin regulatory protein. The encoded protein reversibly blocks the barbed ends of F-actin filaments in a Ca^{2+}-dependent manner and hence contributes to the control of actin-based motility in non-muscle cells [10].

Clinical and population-based data during the last three decades have implicated several biomarkers in HTN causal pathways. Recently, epigenomic studies have explored the heritable changes to gene activity regulation unrelated to the DNA sequence, with these changes being rapid but reversible modifications and often in response to environmental changes [11].

Seven of the top ten leading causes of death in the United States are attributable to chronic disease, which are influenced by epigenomic modulations. Cardiovascular diseases (CVDs) in the United States remain the leading cause of mortality, accounting for 23% of all deaths, and have been linked in several studies to modifications such as hyper- and hypomethylation of phosphodiester-linked CpG sites or acetylation of histone proteins [12–14]. Hypertension, diabetes, hypercholesterolemia and obesity continue to increase in the United States by the age of 20 and older, despite a reduction in smoking [12], which explains other predispositions to CVDs, including but not limited to adverse environment and gene interactions. The observed CVD morbidity and mortality risk is highest among blacks/African Americans, males, in an advanced age, and individuals with low socio-economic status [12]. The cardiovascular risk, which was age-independent, observed differential mDNA profiles, with eight cytosine-phosphate-guanine (CpG) indicating differential mDNA patterns. These CpGs correlated with smoking and some were associated BMI (body mass index). In addition, the risk scores based on these mDNA patterns were related to CVD outcomes and serve as predictive indices [13]. The majority of US annual healthcare expenditure (86% of $2.7 trillion) is on the treatment of chronic diseases [15]. The management of chronic disease has been a major focus of organizations including the CDC (Centers for Disease Control and Prevention) and legislatures such as the Affordable Care Act (ACA) in 2010. With the projected increasing number of Americans living with chronic conditions, a further understanding of chronic disease's etiological pathways is fundamental to providing timely and effective care [16], requiring an evidence-based approach in addressing the causes of HTN, namely social gradient and gene interaction.

Within multifactorial models of disease, gene-gene interactions and gene-environment interactions via epigenomic modifications exist with varying degrees of effect and heritability [17]. The likelihood of engaging in health-promoting behaviors may themselves be epigenetically influenced [18]. Epigenomic modifications of the DNA can entail various chemical additions that alter the three-dimensional structural organization of the DNA, RNA and proteins. The three most commonly examined modifications impacting chronic disease revolve around health-promoting behaviors [19]. The epigenomic mechanistic processes that may influence cardiovascular pathologies that can influence HTN include methylation of CpG sites [20, 21], varied functional groups to histone proteins [22] and binding of non-coding micro-RNA (miRNA) to target mRNAs [23, 24].

Epigenomics remains a comparatively new field of study within genetics, computational biology, computer programing, environmental science and public health. Studies on epigenomic pathways in disease causation could result in protective factor identification leading to healthy behaviors and improved outcomes in chronic disease, the leading cause of death in the United States.

Current methods for epigenomic investigations are often limited to clinical trials or epigenome-wide association studies (EWAS), which identify individual modification sites such as individual CpG methylation islands and miRNA sequences. These methods often yield inconsistent findings when analyzing epigenomic modulations or epigenomic signatures in chronic disease outcomes, particularly for specific sites and their individual roles in regulatory pathways. The current study aimed to assess the DNA methylation of candidate genes and miRNA binding in HTN for evidence-based data informing intervention mapping, with the perspective of narrowing the subpopulation or racial/ethnic disparities in HTN incidence and mortality.

16.2 Experimental Section

16.2.1 Design

This study involved a systematic review and applied meta-analysis termed quantitative evidence synthesis (QES). This design was used to provide evidence on the implication of epigenomic alterations driven possibly by social stress, isolation, diet or physical inactivity in HTN development. The search included relevant literature identification with article selection based on study quality assessment performance. The qualitative synthesis of selected studies included data abstraction and synopsis. The QES included data extraction from eligible published literature, the pooled assessment estimation, the test for heterogeneity and the creation of forest plots.

16.2.2 Design Description and Rationale

The overarching objectives of QES were to (1) minimize random error and (2) marginalize measurement errors, which have a substantial effect on the point estimate by down-drifting away from the null or toward the null. Since all studies have measurement errors and some studies have more measurement errors than others, QES assesses the differences between studies that are due to measurement errors. Additionally, because studies in medicine and public health are often conducted with small samples, such samples have increased random errors and hence restricted generalizability. The QES, which is a method of summarizing the effect across studies, increases the study or sample size and therefore minimizes random error and enhances the generalizability of findings. Furthermore, QES integrates results across studies to identify patterns and to some extent establish causation. In effect, the overall relevance of

QES is to generate scientific data that are cumulative and reliable in improving health or other conditions upon which it is applied.

The methodology used in QES differs from that of traditional meta-analysis. While meta-analysis utilizes fixed- and random-effect methods, QES only employs the random-effect method and examines heterogeneity after and not before the pool estimates. The fixed-effect method is only applicable to QES when the combined studies or publications are from a multicenter trial where the study protocol is identical. However, when studies are combined from different settings, observation and measurement errors induce significant variability in the observed estimates, limiting such a combination without adjusting for between-study variability. The random effect method compensates for the between-study variability, hence its unique application in QES.

Scientific endeavor makes sense of the accumulating literature in medicine and public health, given the confounding and contradicting results. QES reflects such attempts at study integration for public health and clinical decision-making. A unique feature of QES is temporality, in which findings in QES accumulate with time. For example, if QES was performed on the implication of epigenetic modification, such as DNA methylation and histone acetylation, with respect to hypertension development, this study must identify the time of conduct, continue to add findings and reanalyze the data for contrasting or negative findings with time. Subsequently, the emergence of new data on epigenomic modification, gene expression and posttranslation histone acetylation or methylation has an impact on changing the results of QES and moving evidence in a different direction.

Science and scientific endeavors are not static but dynamic, implying evidence transformation following the emergence of new data. The scientific community cannot wait until evidence accumulates to such a point that no further addition is required with respect to evidence discovery in order to initiate an intervention regarding epigenomic intervention mapping for specific risk characterization in predisposing factors associated with HTN. Consequently, QES can inform and provide at any point in time the knowledge required in order to understand the disease process, characterize risk, improve prognosis, as well as control and prevent disease at patient and population levels.

16.2.3 Search Engines and Strategies

An online database search of Google Scholar and MEDLINE via PubMed in June 2018 was conducted. Search terms were created based on medical subject headings (MeSH) and terms used in epigenomic literature reviews of HTN in order to maximize sensitivity: (gene expression OR DNA methylation OR histone acetylation OR microRNA OR gene transcription OR mRNA OR histone methylation OR epigenotype) AND hypertension (angiotensin-converting enzyme, C-reactive proteins, fibrinogen, plasminogen activator inhibitor I, aldosterone renin, B-type, natriuretic peptide, homocysteine, N-terminal proatrial natriuretic peptide, catecholamines pathways, enzymes involved in catecholamines pathways, dopamine decarboxylase, tyrosine hydroxylase) OR (gene expression OR DNA methylation OR histone acetylation OR microRNA OR gene transcription OR mRNA OR histone methylation OR epigenotype) AND hypertension (angiotensin-converting enzyme, C-reactive proteins, fibrinogen, plasminogen activator inhibitor I, aldosterone renin, B-type, natriuretic peptide, homocysteine, N-terminal proatrial natriuretic peptide, catecholamines pathways, enzymes involved in catecholamines pathways, dopamine decarboxylase, tyrosine hydroxylase) AND epigenetic modification (gene expression OR DNA methylation OR histone acetylation OR microRNA OR gene transcription OR mRNA OR histone methylation OR epigenotype) AND (hypertension OR angiotensin-converting enzyme OR C-reactive proteins OR fibrinogen OR plasminogen activator inhibitor I OR aldosterone renin OR B-type OR natriuretic peptide OR homocysteine OR N-terminal proatrial natriuretic peptide OR catecholamines pathways OR enzymes involved in catecholamines pathways OR dopamine decarboxylase OR tyrosine hydroxylase) OR (gene expression OR DNA methylation OR histone acetylation OR microRNA OR gene transcription OR mRNA OR histone methylation OR epigenotype) AND (hypertension OR angiotensin-converting enzyme OR C-reactive proteins OR fibrinogen OR plasminogen activator inhibitor I OR aldosterone renin OR B-type OR natriuretic peptide OR homocysteine OR N-terminal proatrial natriuretic peptide OR catecholamines pathways OR enzymes involved in catecholamines pathways OR dopamine decarboxylase OR tyrosine hydroxylase) AND epigenetic modification.

Additionally, we performed hand searches through reference lists of relevant articles. Such articles were identified in advance based upon their investigation of epigenomic modifications on hypertension.

16.2.4 Eligibility Criteria

Eligible articles had to meet the following criteria: study published in English from January 1, 2000 to June 1, 2018, study investigates hypertension and epigenomic changes, study has a well-defined outcome, namely hypertension, and study contains quantitative data, such as the parameter values (odd ratio, risk ratio, relative risk). Studies with a loss to follow-up >25% or a sample size smaller than ten were excluded to lessen the likelihood of selection bias and sparse data bias, respectively. Inclusion criteria were developed in order to maximize an inclusion of any potentially useful findings while limiting the inclusion of irrelevant data. When a study was identified that alluded to the existence of quantitative data but did not disclose any of it in the article itself, we contacted the authors via e-mail in an effort to obtain additional data. One researcher screened abstracts for inclusion in the full-text evaluation.

Two researchers independently read the full texts and extracted the data into a QES data sheet, with kappa = 0.98, 98%, implying strong or high inter-rater reliability. Discrepancies in agreement were resolved through a discussion between the study investigators. The final list of studies included in the qualitative and quantitative syntheses was the product of this discussion following the initial independent review. Studies included in the qualitative synthesis had to meet the above inclusion criteria. Studies included in the QES had to meet the inclusion criteria, implying studies with epigenomic modification measured by either DNA methylation or histone acetylation and hypertension.

16.2.5 Study Variables

The study variables included essential hypertension as the response variable while epigenomic alterations as well as biomarkers of hypertension as independent variables. Other study variables included age and sex.

16.2.6 Data Collection

Data was collected from all eligible studies based upon the outcome variables and the specific research questions. For the qualitative synthesis, all available data concerning hypertension and epigenomic markers were obtained through the data collection strategy. For the QES, we abstracted data on the proportion of those with and without hypertension given epigenomic modification. Where data were not available on the measure of the outcome, we estimated that based on the absence or presence of epigenomic changes and the outcome being hypertension.

16.2.7 Study Quality Assessment

Two researchers assessed the eligible studies' quality based upon the study design, sampling techniques, hypotheses, clarity of aims or purposes, and adequacy of statistical analysis. Studies were also assessed for any confounding factors that might have influenced the outcomes and any potential bias, including selection, information and misclassification biases. The study quality assessment technique was in line with the preferred method of reporting for systematic reviews (PRISMA statement).

16.2.8 Statistical Analysis

A descriptive or exploratory analysis was performed to examine qualitative scale measurement data for frequencies and percentages. The inferential statistics, namely QES analysis that involved the pooled estimate or the common effect sizes, was performed prior to the heterogeneity test. In addition, we created a template to transform the proportion of epigenomic modification and hypertensive cases into percentage, standard error and 95% confidence intervals to enable the application of the meta-analytic command using STATA, namely metan percent lowerci upperci, label (namevar = study) random.

To test the hypotheses with respect to the implication of epigenomic modification in hypertension, we used the random-effect analytic method of DerSimonian-Laird [25]. The DerSimonian-Laird method was applicable given significant studies on heterogeneity. This procedure, namely the random-effect method, examined the between-study effect as well as the effect sizes of the combined studies or the common effect size in relation to the individual effect sizes, weighing each study for their contribution to the overall sample size involved in the pooled estimate. In addition, the precision of the common effect size was measured by the 95% confidence interval. The effect size heterogeneity was estimated by testing the null hypothesis that the common effect size = 0 based on the standardized normal (z-statistic). Additionally, a meta-regression was performed to assess the subgroup effects of the candidate genes on either hypo- or hyper-DNA methylation in essential or idiopathic HTN. This process allowed for the examination of potential confoundings in applied meta-analytic designs, facilitating the subgroup heterogeneities in result interpretations involving the overall, individual and subgroup effect sizes.

The heterogeneity test was performed to determine variability among studies based on the individual study effect sizes in relation to the common effect size (diamond). Using $Q = (1/variance\_i) \times (effect\_i - effect\_pool)2$, we determined the heterogeneity in this QES. The variance was estimated using $Variance\_i = ((upper\ limit - lower\ limit)/2 \times z))2$. The test of heterogeneity reflected the variation in the effect size (ES) that is attributable to the differences between studies' effect sizes. The significance level was set at 5% (0.05 type I error tolerance) and all tests were two-tailed. The entire analyses were performed using STATA 15.0 (StataCorp, College Station, TX, USA).

16.2.9   *Results as Findings from the Data*

These data represent epigenomic aberrations in essential hypertension from the perspective of predisposition, given the gene-environment interaction that characterizes epigenomic modulation or epigenomic lesions of the candidate genes involved in hemodynamics and homoestatsis. The epigenomic moduation reflects ongoing changes within the gene promoter region that does not affect the DNA sequence, but alters the transcription and the subsequent gene expression such as repression. The impairment in this modulation, termed an epigenomic aberration or lesion, induces an alteration in plasticity, resulting in a decreased response to cellular damage and inflammation. Specifically, such alteration affects hemodynamics and hemostasis, resulting in sodium and fluid imbalance and the subsequent HTN.

We examined studies on DNA methylation that involved the methylation of the gene enhancer or promoter region, mainly the CpG islands, which affects transcriptional activities as well as the transcription factor's inability for mRNA to translate and consequently express the gene, impacting protein synthesis (Table 16.1). Such limitations or inabilities eventually result in abnormal protein synthesis as initially observed, implying a disease process, am impaired prognosis and subsequent mortality. Since hypertension involves several biomarkers resulting in vasoconstriction as reflected in increased peripheral resistance, increased stroke volume and increased heart rate, the genes associated with these biomarkers were the main focus of this aberrant epigenomic modulation in HTN.

16.2.10   DNA Hypomethylation of HTN Candidate Genes

With DNA methylation being the most commonly used epigenomic mechanistic process and current epigenomic detection technology, namely bisulfite pyrosequencing, we examined published literature for either hypo- or hypermethylation in order to observe patterns and identify epigenomic causal pathways or associations in HTN. Figure 16.1 presents the overall or common effect size of DNA hypomethylation of the candidate genes, namely ACE2, IFN-γ, TLR2, SCNN1A/1B, GCK, ADD1 and AGTR1, involved in HTN, as well as the meta-regression of these individual or specific genes. The mechanism of epigenomic modulation in these studies solely involved the DNA methylation of the cytosine-phosphate-guanine (CpG) 1, 4, 6 and 8, with respect to the TLR2 gene as well as the promoter region of ACE2, mainly CpG2 and CpG 5. Seven studies observed DNA hypomethylation as an exposure function of hypertension. The sample size for these studies was 1,105, while the mechanism of epigenomic modulation was DNA methylation at the CpG islands by bisulfite pyrosequencing. The pooled estimate (the common effect size) for the hypomethylation indicated a common effect size (CES) = 2.3%, 95%, CI = 2.51–7.07. The variabilities between the common effect sizes and the individual effect sizes were estimated, $I^2 = \chi^2(7) = 107$, 54.5, p <0.001, indicative of substantial variances. The observed CES was significantly different from zero (0), z = 3.87, p <0.001, negating the null hypothesis of a zero common effect size.

16.2.11   Dense DNA Methylation of HTN Candidate Genes

This section, as the forest plot, demonstrates five studies that observed hypermethylation, implying the dense DNA methylation of hemostasis and hemodynamics genes, namely ACE2, SCNN1B, IFN-γ and CKG, as an exposure function in HTN causation and prognosis. The hypermethylation ranged from 0.65% to 16.0% with respect to the individual effect sizes in the forest plot.

TABLE 16.1 DNA methylation (mDNA) process and selective candidate genes in essential Hypertension (e-HTN)

Author, (Year), Study	Specimen/ Source/ Sample	Methylation Process	Patient/Subject Characteristics	Methylation Profile/ Status
Mao, T. et al. (2017) TLR2 Hypo-mDNA in e-HTN	Blood sample–antecubital vein	Bisulfite pyrosequencing of TLR2 CpGs.	96 controls and 96 incident essential HTN cases	Hypo-methylation and increased transcription
Mao, S. et al. (2016) SCNN1A Dense mDNA in e-HTN	Peripheral blood sample	Sodium bisulfite pyrosequencing technology of 6 CpG dinucleotides of SCNN1A.	60 incident and 60 prevalent cases and 60 comparable controls	Hyper-methylation, 16% incident case and 15% prevalent case relative to controls
Zhang, L. et al. (2013) ADDI Hypo-mDNA in e-HTN	Overnight fasting-peripheral blood sample	Bisulfite pyrosequencing of α-adducin (ADD1) gene of 5 CpGs promoter	33 essential HTN (14 males and 19 females) and 28 controls (14 males/ females)	Hypo-methylation with sex differential and stable findings in males
Zhong, Q. et al. (2016) SCNN1B Hypo-mDNA in e-HTN	Peripheral blood sample	Bisulfite pyrosequencing of SCNN1B gene at 6 CpG sites	98 controls, 94 incident and 94 prevalent HTN cases	DNA hypomethylation, inverse correlation with HTN
Fan, R. et al. (2017) ACE2 Dense mDNA in e-HTN	12 h overnight fasting blood sample-antecubital vein from	Bisulfite pyrosequencing of ACE2 at 5 CpG inucleotides (1–5)	96 patients with essential HTN and 96 comparable controls	Dense DNA methylation–effect of sex on methylation profile
Bao, X.J. et al. (2018) IFN-γ gene in e-HTN	peripheral blood DNA	Bisulfite pyrosequencing of IFN-γ gene of 6 CpG sites	96 cases of HTN and 96 comparable controls	Hypo-methylation

Notes and abbreviations: e-HTN, essential hypertension; CpG, cytosine-phosphate-guanine; INF-γ, interferon gamma; mDNA, DNA methylation; TLR2, Toll like receptor 2; SCNN1A, sodium channel epithelial 1 alpha subunit; CpG3, cytosine-phosphate-guanine, specific site 3.

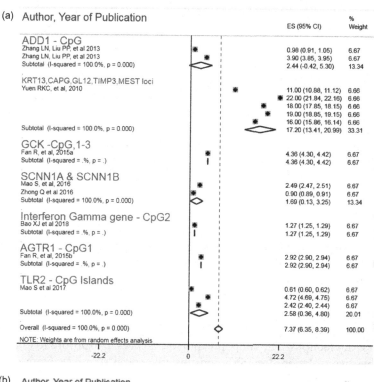

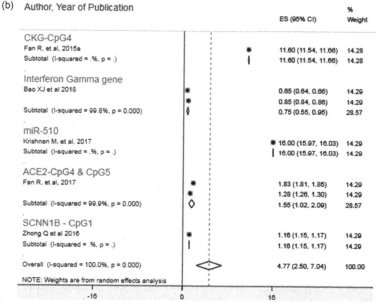

FIGURE 16.1 Forest plot on the common effect size (CES) in the association between DNA methylation (mDNA) of specific genes in essential hypertension (HTN).

The sample size for the hypermethylation was 1,105, implying a reasonable study size for a statistically stable finding of the effect of DNA methylation on the HTN causal pathway. The combined or pooled summary estimates for hypermethylation, although imprecise in terms of precision parameters, indicated a substantial common effect size (CES) = 6.0%, 95% CI = 0.002–11.26. The variabilities between the common effect sizes and the individual effect sizes were estimated, heterogeneity $(I^2) = \chi^2 (10) = 2610.3$, p <0.001. The observed common effect size was significantly different from zero, z = 11.96, p <0.001, negating the null hypothesis of a zero common effect size.

16.2.12 Discussion

Hypertension as a chronic disease involving the cardiovascular system, mainly cardiac output and peripheral resistance, is associated with several biomarkers, genes and gene products. However, subpopulation genetic heterogeneity does not explain the racial/ethnic differences in essential HTN incidence, prognosis and mortality. A possible explanation of racial/ethnic, sex and age differences in this manifestation is provided in greater part by the hemostasis and hemodynamics genes and endogenous as well as exogenous environments, which include social adversity, social isolation, diet, physical activities and persistent stress interactions. The subpopulation differences in exposure to objective and subjective isolation, low SES and unstable social status facilitate our understanding of the alteration in neural activities that results in vasoconstriction and subsequent increased peripheral resistance. With recent advances in epigenomic modulations in disease causation, prognosis and survival, there is an urgent need for evidence-based data on further understanding of the biologic mediation of psychosocial etiologies of HTN via the gene as well as interaction between physical, chemical and social environments.

The purpose of the current study was to examine published literature on DNA methylation as the most commonly utilized epigenomic mechanistic process in HTN causal pathways, implying that DNA methylation of the candidate genes involved in HTN was a biomarker of causation and prognosis. An applied meta-analytic design termed quantitative evidence synthesis (QES) was utilized with the intent to provide scientific evidence on the influence of mDNA on gene expression and the subsequent under-expression or upregulation of genes involved in cardiac output and peripheral resistance. There are a few relevant findings from this QES. First, biomarkers of homeostasis and hemodynamics were identified, along with their gene correlates. Second, DNA methylation of the candidate genes in cardiac output (stroke volume and heart rate) and peripheral resistance was observed in HTN causal pathways. Third, DNA hypermethylation of ACE, ACE2, SCNN1B, IFN-γ and CKG was observed in essential HTN. Fourth, DNA hypomethylation of ACE2, IFN-γ, TLR2, SCNN1A/1B, GCK, ADD1 and AGTR1 correlated with HTN.

There are several postulated risk factors in HTN, implying a multifactorial etiology as well as environmental differences in HTN predisposition. The postulated risk factors in HTN include race, sex, diet, medication, drugs, alcohol, high sodium ingestion, smoking, a sedentary lifestyle, overweight/obesity, stress, social isolation and physical inactivity, as well as a family history of HTN. The subpopulation variances in lifestyle and living conditions interacting with the genes, as observed in epigenomic modulation, provided an additional understanding of HTN risk and predisposition. While some of these risks have been established in HTN, risk synergism is more pronounced in subpopulations or individuals with aberrant epigenomic modulation of the candidate genes involved in hemodynamics.

We demonstrated that ACE gene upregulation increased the risk of HTN, given its role in vasoconstriction and sodium/water imbalance. This affirmation supports previous literature on sodium loading, fluid retention and decreased volume depletion in HTN [26]. The DNA methylation of ACE has a biologic underpinning in converting angiotensin I to angiotensin II, a potent vasoconstrictor, resulting in increased peripheral resistance and arterial stenosis, leading to elevated blood pressure or hypertension (HTN). The DNA hypomethylation was observed in IFN-γ gene, implying innate antiviral response inhibition, which increased the inflammatory process and mediators, thus enhancing arterial plague, arteriosclerosis, arterial stenosis and HTN. This explanation is supported by studies that implicate chronic inflammation in HTN [27]. In contrast, a study observed hypermethylation of the interferon gamma gene. Similarly, the DNA hypomethylation of the SCNN1B gene may result in sodium channel disruption and fluid imbalance. Depending on the dysregulation, sodium channel disruption may induce hypo- or hypertension. Additionally, the DNA hypo-methylation of the AGTR1 gene may predispose to hypertension by increasing the receptor for the potent vasoconstrictor, angiotensin II.

The observed DNA hypomethylation of TLR2 CpG1 and GCK CpG4 in HTN [28] is indicative of the inherent inability of this gene to elaborate the inflammatory cytokine in response to tissue damage, with such cellular insufficiencies resulting in vascular damage and microvascular compromization signaling disrupting homeostasis and hemodynamics. The observed aberrant epigenomic modulation of the TLR2 island is supported by studies that implicated depression in the pathogenesis of HTN. The hypomethylation of TLR2 cytosine-phosphate-guanine (CpG) results in accumulated inflammation, arterial stenosis, and subsequent elevated or increased peripheral resistance. The observed TLR2 CpGs hypomethylation directly correlated with IL-6 gene hypomethylation. The hypomethylation of IL-6, CpG2 and CpG3 induced inflammation and endothelial dysfunction, elevating blood pressure. This epigenomic modulation of IL-6 gene affirms the implication of smoking, alcohol and gender in HTN predisposition, where hypomethylation of IL-6, CpG2 and CpG3 was observed in males, smoking and alcohol [29].

The hypo-methylation of ADD1, implying aberrant epigenomic modulation, results in upregulation and increased expression of α-adducin, leading to increased activities of the Na+-K+pump, inducing sodium reabsorption, volume expansion and subsequent HTN. The observed inverse correlation between SCNN1B DNA methylation and essential HTN, implying hypomethylation, may be due to the upregulation of the protein expression of SCNN1B, thus increasing the function and activities of the epithelial sodium channel (ENaC) and enhancing Na+ reabsorption and fluid or water retention.

This QES illustrated that the hypermethylation of some genes, including the angiotensin-1-converting enzyme 2 (ACE2) gene at promoters CpG4 and CpG5, directly correlated with hypertension. Available data observed DNA hypermethylation in general to suppress gene transcription, resulting in gene silencing [30]. Overall, mDNA influenced protein-DNA interaction, gene expression, chromatin structure and genome stability. Specifically, the hypermethylation of CpG 4 and CpG5 of the ACE2 promoter may result in renin-angiotensin system (RAS) dysregulation. With the observed dense DNA methylation of ACE2, implying transcription inactivation, and the AGTR1 gene upregulation, there appeared to be an RAS imbalance and subsequent vasoconstriction, resulting in essential HTN.

Although mDNA at CpG inhibits or represses transcription, it is not fully understood if exon methylation of most genes inversely or directly correlates with transcriptional activities, despite the observed inverse correlation between NR3C1 1F exon methylation in major depressive disorders [31]. While several methods have been utilized for epigenomic modulation detection, the current method involves bisulfite sequencing. With this process, the unmethylated cytosine residues were converted to uracil via the application of sodium bisulfite and alkaline treatment, while the methylated cytosine remain unconverted, and thereafter the bisulfite-treated was sequenced to identify the methylated cytosine [31]. Whereas aberrant epigenomic modulations remain a pathway to disease etiology, prognosis, survival and morality as well as subpopulation differences in health outcomes, more investigations with high potentials for causal inference are required in this trajectory for effective intervention mapping and treatment effect homogeneity.

Despite the strength of this study in implicating gene and environment interactions in HTN predisposition, there are some limitations. First, QES is a retrospective study, implying the potentials for information, selection and misclassification biases. Second, as a literature review, implying studying studies prior to scientific statement generation and evidence-based data on HTN causation or association, there is a potential for unmeasured confounding in the studies that constitute this QES. Third, because of the design's sample and sampling technique, patient and bioassay heterogeneity, there is potential for reverse causation in the observation of the DNA hyper- and hypo-methylation of the candidate genes involved in HTN. Specifically, since the individual studies that constitute this QES are non-experimental epidemiologic designs, mainly case-control, cautious optimism should be applied in the causal inference application of these findings. Further, epigenomic modulation is reversible, and the timing of the collection of the specimen is essential in such investigations, implying caution in the application of this QES in intervention mapping or specific risk characterization in HTN prevention and control.

16.3 Summary

In summary, dense DNA methylation of ACE, ACE2, SCNN1B, IFN-γ and CKG correlated with essential HTN, as well as DNA hypomethylation of ACE2, IFN-γ, TLR2, SCNN1A/1B, GCK, ADD1 and AGTR1 in HTN. The observed DNA methylation played a role in hemodynamic imbalance, leading to abnormal cardiac output and increased peripheral resistance, hence essential, primary or idiopathic HTN. Epigenomic investigations reflecting the detection of aberrant modulation involved the assessment of hereditable changes in gene expression that occurred in the absence of underlying DNA sequence as observed in epigenomic mechanistic processes, namely DNA methylation, histone protein modifications, phosphorylation, microRNA and DNA microarray. Unlike DNA or basic inherited structure remaining constant during ontogeny, epigenomic codes or programing undergoes dramatic modification during embryogenesis, reflecting differential patterns in gene expression and related tissue development and cellular function. These epigenomic signatures, although transgenerational, are reversible, implying societal collective effort and responsible action in changing the environment for socially disadvantaged individuals and groups, thus reducing black-white risk differences in HTN incidence and mortality in the United States.

16.4 Questions for Review

1 Characterize the genes involved in essential hypertension in this study.
2 Describe the epigenomic modulations process utilized in this study based on the original articles.
3 Discuss the statistical analysis in these findings and identify the limitations.
4 Describe aberrant epigenomic modulations of the ACE II in essential hypertension based on this finding.
5 What are the advantages and disadvantages of this study on the implications of aberrant epigenomic modulations in essential hypertension?

References

1 Holmes L, Hossain J, Ward D, Opara F. Racial/ethnic variability in hypertension prevalence and risk factors in national health interview survey. *ISRN Hypertens.* 2013;2013:257842. doi: 10.5402/2013/257842.

2 Fountain JH, Lappin SL. *Physiology, Renin Angiotensin System*. (Treasure Island, FL; Petersburg, FL: StatPearls Publishing, 2019). [Updated 2019 May 5].

3 Kanagy NL. α2-Adrenergic receptor signalling in hypertension. *Clin. Sci.* 2005;109:431–437. doi: 10.1042/CS20050101.

4 Jang HS, Shin WJ, Lee JE, Do J.T. CpG and Non-CpG Methylation in Epigenetic Gene Regulation and Brain Function. Genes. 2017;8:148. doi: 10.3390/genes8060148.

5 Chen L, Deng H, Cui H, Fang J, Zuo Z, Deng J, Li Y, Wang X, Zhao L. Inflammatory responses and inflammation-associated diseases in organs. *Oncotarget*. 2017;9:7204–7218. doi: 10.18632/oncotarget.23208.

6 Muñoz-Durango N, Fuentes CA, Castillo AE, González-Gómez LM, Vecchiola A, Fardella CE, Kalergis AM. Role of the renin-angiotensin-aldosterone system beyond blood pressure regulation: Molecular and cellular mechanisms involved in end-organ damage during arterial hypertension. *Int. J. Mol. Sci.* 2016;17:797. doi: 10.3390/ijms17070797.

7 Mengesha HG, Petrucka P, Spence C, Tafesse TB. Effects of angiotensin converting enzyme gene polymorphism on hypertension in Africa: A meta-analysis and systematic review. *PLoS One*. 2019;14:e0211054. doi: 10.1371/journal.pone.0211054.

8 Kiang KMY, Leung GKK. A review on adducin from functional to pathological mechanisms: Future direction in cancer. *BioMed. Res. Int.* 2018;2018:3465929. doi: 10.1155/2018/3465929.

9 National Center for Biotechnology Information KRT13-Keratin 13 (Human), NCBI Gene=3860. Available online: https://pubchem.ncbi.nlm.nih.gov/gene/KRT13/human [Accessed on 2 Oct. 2019].

10 Pollard TD. Actin and actin-binding proteins. *Cold Spring Harb. Perspect. Biol.* 2016;8:a018226. doi: 10.1101/cshperspect.a018226.

11 López-Jaramillo P, Camacho PA., Forero-Naranjo L. The role of environment and epigenetics in hypertension. *Expert Rev. Cardiovasc. Ther.* 2009;11:1455–1457. doi: 10.1586/14779072.2013.846217.

12 Boslaugh SE. *The SAGE Encyclopedia of Pharmacology and Society*. (Saunders Oaks, CA: SAGE Publications, 2016). Centers for Disease Control and Prevention.

13 Fernández-Sanlés A, Sayols-Baixeras S, Curcio S, Subirana I, Marrugat J, Elosua R. DNA methylation and age-independent cardiovascular risk, an epigenome-wide approach. *Arter. Thromb. Vasc. Biol.* 2018;38:645–652. doi: 10.1161/ATVBAHA.117.310340.

14 Schiano C, Vietri MT, Grimaldi V, Picascia A, De Pascale MR, Napoli C. Epigenetic-related therapeutic challenges in cardiovascular disease. *Trends Pharmacol. Sci.* 2015;36:226–235. doi: 10.1016/j.tips.2015.02.005.

15 Agency for Healthcare Research and Quality Multiple Chronic Conditions Chartbook, 2014. Available online: https://www.ahrq.gov/sites/default/files/wysiwyg/professionals/prevention-chronic-care/decision/mcc/mcchartbook.pdf [Accessed on 13 June 2018].

16 Wu SY, Green A. *Projection of Chronic Illness Prevalence and Cost Inflation*. (Santa Monica, CA: RAND Corporation, 2000). Graph illustration in number of people with chronic conditions in millions. Available online: https://www.fightchronicdisease.org/sites/default/files/docs/GrowingCrisisofChronicDiseaseintheUSfactsheet_81009.pdf [Accessed on 12 June 2018].

17 Institute of Medicine Committee on Assessing Interactions Among Social, Behavioral, and Genetic Factors in Health. Genetics and Health. In: Hernandez LM,

Blazer DG, (eds.). *Genes, Behavior, and the Social Environment: Moving Beyond the Nature/Nurture Debate.* (Washington, DC: National Academies Press, 2006, pp. 44–67). Available online: https://www.ncbi.nlm.nih.gov/books/NBK19932/ [Accessed on 18 July 2018].

18 De Geus EJ, Bartels M, Kaprio J, Lightfoot JT, Thomis M. Genetics of regular exercise and sedentary behaviors. *Twin Res. Hum. Genet.* 2014;17:262–271. doi: 10.1017/thg.2014.42.

19 Wise IA, Charchar FJ. Epigenetic modifications in essential hypertension. *Int. J. Mol. Sci.* 2016;17:451. doi: 10.3390/ijms17040451.

20 Bogdarina I, Welham S, King PJ, Burns SP, Clark AJ. Epigenetic modification of the renin-angiotensin system in the fetal programming of hypertension. *Circ. Res.* 2007;100:520–526. doi: 10.1161/01.RES.0000258855.60637.58.

21 Waterland RA, Jirtle RL. Transposable elements: Targets for early nutritional effects on epigenetic gene regulation. *Mol. Cell. Biol.* 2003;23:5293–5300. doi: 10.1128/MCB.23.15.5293–5300.2003.

22 Alkemade FE, Van Vliet P, Henneman P, Van Dijk KW, Hierck BP, Van Munsteren JC, Scheerman JA, Goeman JJ, Havekes LM, de Groot ACG et al. Prenatal exposure to apoE deficiency and postnatal hypercholesterolemia are associated with altered cell-specific lysine methyltransferase and histone methylation patterns in the vasculature. *Am. J. Pathol.* 2010;176:542–548. doi: 10.2353/ajpath.2010.090031.

23 Párrizas M, Brugnara L, Esteban Y, Gonzalez-Franquesa A, Canivell S, Murillo S, Gordillo-Bastidas E, Cusso R, Cadefau JA, Garcia-Roves PM et al. Circulating miR-192 and miR-193b are markers of prediabetes and are modulated by an exercise intervention. *J. Clin. Endocrinol. Metab.* 2015;100:407–415. doi: 10.1210/jc.2014-2574.

24 Silveira AC, Fernandes T, Soci UPR, Gomes JLP, Barretti DL, Mota GGF, Negrão CE, Oliveira EM. Exercise training restores cardiac MicroRNA-1 and MicroRNA-29c to nonpathological levels in obese rats. *Oxidative Med. Cell. Longev.* 2017;2017:1549014. doi: 10.1155/2017/1549014.

25 DerSimonian R, Laird N. Meta-analysis in clinical trials. *Control. Clin. Trials.* 1986;7:177–188. doi: 10.1016/0197–2456(86)90046-2.

26 Ray EC, Rondon-Berrios H, Boyd CR, Kleyman TR. Sodium retention and volume expansion in nephrotic syndrome: Implications for hypertension. *Adv. Chronic Kidney Dis.* 2015;22:179–184. doi: 10.1053/j.ackd.2014.11.006.

27 Stoll S, Wang C, Qiu H. DNA methylation and histone modification in hypertension. *Int. J. Mol. Sci.* 2018;19:1174. doi: 10.3390/ijms19041174.

28 Mao S, Gu T, Zhong F, Fan R, Zhu F, Ren P, Yin F, Zhang L. Hypomethylation of the Toll-like receptor-2 gene increases the risk of essential hypertension. *Mol. Med. Rep.* 2017;16:964–970. doi: 10.3892/mmr.2017.6653.

29 Mao SQ, Sun JH, Gu TL, Zhu FB, Yin FY, Zhang LN. Hypomethylation of interleukin-6 (IL-6) gene increases the risk of essential hypertension: A matched case–control study. *J. Hum. Hypertens.* 2017;31:530–536. doi: 10.1038/jhh.2017.7.

30 Fouse SD, Nagarajan RP, Costello JF. Genome-scale DNA methylation analysis. *Epigenomics.* 2010;2:105–117. doi: 10.2217/epi.09.35.

31 Holmes L, Shutman E, Chinaka C, Deepika K, Pelaez L, Dabney K. Aberrant epigenomic modulation of glucocorticoid receptor gene (NR3C1) in early life stress: Systematic review and quantitative evidence synthesis. *Int. J. Environ. Res. Public Health.* 2019;16:4280. doi: 10.3390/ijerph16214280.

INDEX

Printed in the United States
by Baker & Taylor Publisher Services